Thalassemia Syndromes - New Insights and Transfusion Modalities

Edited by Marwa Zakaria, Tamer Hassan, Laila Sherief and Osaro Erhabor

Published in London, United Kingdom

Thalassemia Syndromes - New Insights and Transfusion Modalities
http://dx.doi.org/10.5772/intechopen.104338
Edited by Marwa Zakaria, Tamer Hassan, Laila Sherief and Osaro Erhabor

Contributors
Yavuz Memis Bilgin, Abdulrahman Abdulbasit Opeyemi, Adesola Precious Oyeyemi, Adeyeye Kamaldeen, Osaro Erhabor, Kolawole A. Fasakin, Josephine O. Akpotuzor, Edward Yaw Afriyie, Godswill Chikwendu Okara, Tosan Erhabor, Donald Ibe Ofili, Teddy Charles Adias, Idris Ateiza Saliu, Evarista Osime, Alhaji Bukar, Oyetunde B. Akinloye, Zakiya Abdul-Mumin, John Ocquaye-Mensah Tetteh, Edwin G. Narter-Olaga, Andrews Yashim-Nuhu, Folashade Aturamu, Ayodeji Olusola Olayan, Adeyinka Babatunde Adedire, Oyeronke Suebat Izobo, Onyeka Paul, Collins Ohwonigho Adjekuko, Elliot Eli Dogbe, Uloma Theodora Ezeh, Atish Bakane, Saksham Singh, Chittala Kiran Sri, Manit Nuinoon, Amrita Panja, Tuphan Kanti Dolai, Sujata Maiti Choudhury, Brahmarshi Das, Simran Patel, Armaan Shah, Raj Wadgaonkar, Ryan Kaiser, Charity Iheanacho, Christiana Okeke, Kenneth Oshiokhayamhe Iyevhobu, Lucky E. Omolumen, Tobechukwu Joseph Okobi, Edidiong Raphael Usoro, A. Airefetalor Ivie, O. Omokpo Victoria, Benedicta A. Ken-Iyevhobu

First published in London, United Kingdom, 2023 by IntechOpen
IntechOpen is the global imprint of INTECHOPEN LIMITED, registered in England and Wales, registration number: 11086078, 5 Princes Gate Court, London, SW7 2QJ, United Kingdom

British Library Cataloguing-in-Publication Data
A catalogue record for this book is available from the British Library

Additional hard and PDF copies can be obtained from orders@intechopen.com

Thalassemia Syndromes - New Insights and Transfusion Modalities
Edited by Marwa Zakaria, Tamer Hassan, Laila Sherief and Osaro Erhabor
p. cm.
Print ISBN 978-1-83768-399-4
Online ISBN 978-1-83768-400-7
eBook (PDF) ISBN 978-1-83768-401-4

For EU product safety concerns:
IN TECH d.o.o., Prolaz Marije Krucifikse Kozulić 3, 51000 Rijeka, Croatia,
info@intechopen.com or visit our website at intechopen.com.

Meet the editors

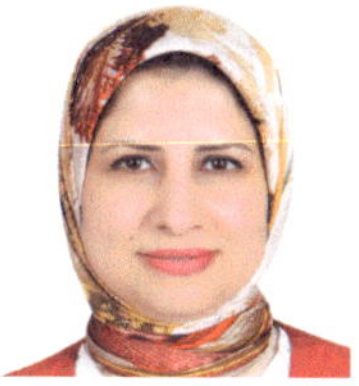

Prof. Marwa Zakaria is an Associate Professor of Pediatrics and Pediatric Hematology and Oncology at Zagazig University, Egypt. She is an active member of the International Society of Pediatric Oncology (SIOP), European Hematology Association (EHA), Histiocytosis Association of America (HAA), and Egyptian Pediatric Hematology Oncology Society (EPHOS). She has participated in several professional trainings and workshops as well as many international and national pediatric and hematology conferences. She received training from the Society for Neuro-Oncology (SNO) and completed a post-graduate training program in pediatric nutrition at the School of Medicine, Boston University, USA. She also completed several preceptorships. She received an award from SIOP in 2018 and EHA-HOPE Cairo scholarships in 2017 and 2018. Prof. Zakaria has been a guest speaker at numerous pediatric oncology and hematology meetings. She has more than fifty publications to her credit, including books and book chapters. She is also a reviewer for several journals, an active member of the Sharkia Thalassemia Association, in Egypt, and a member of the Egyptian National Guidelines Committee (NEGC) for evidence-based clinical practice. Prof. Zakaria has served as co-investigator and sub-investigator in many hematology clinical trials.

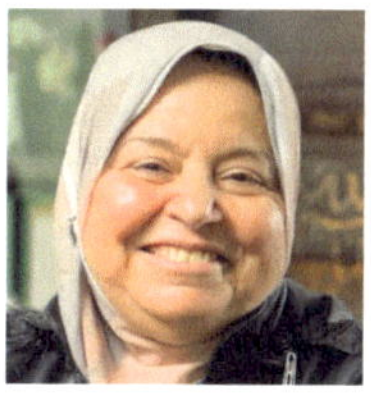

Laila Sherief is a Professor of Pediatrics and Pediatric Hematology and Oncology at the Faculty of Medicine, Zagazig University, Egypt. She has more than fifty publications to her credit and is a peer reviewer for more than thirty-eight international journals. She is also an editorial board member for several other journals. Prof. Sherief maintains memberships in many professional societies, including the International Society of Paediatric Oncology (SIOP), the International Society on Thrombosis and Haemostasis (ISTH), the Egyptian Pediatric Hematology Oncology Society (EPHOS), and Egyptian societies of thalassemia. She is the president of the Sharkia Thalassemia Association, in Egypt, and a member of the Egyptian National Guidelines Committee (NEGC) for evidence-based clinical practice.

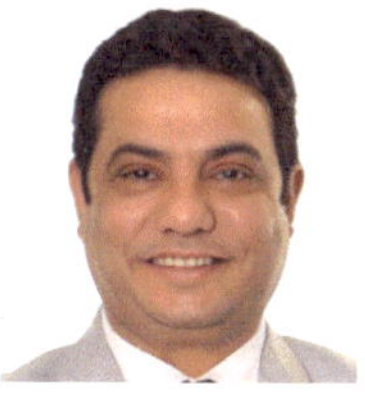

Tamer Hassan is a Professor of Pediatrics and Pediatric Hematology and Oncology, at Zagazig University, Egypt. He is an active member of the International Society of Paediatric Oncology (SIOP), European Hematology Association (EHA), Histiocytosis Association of America (HAA), and Egyptian Pediatric Hematology Oncology Society (EPHOS). He has been a guest speaker at numerous pediatric oncology and hematology meetings. Prof. Hassan has more than fifty publications to his credit. He completed training in pediatric stem cell transplantation at Ulm University, Germany, as well as several preceptorships. He is co-editor of three books and author of six book chapters. He is also a journal reviewer and editor. Prof. Hassan has served as primary investigator in four clinical trials and sub-investigator in ten clinical trials.

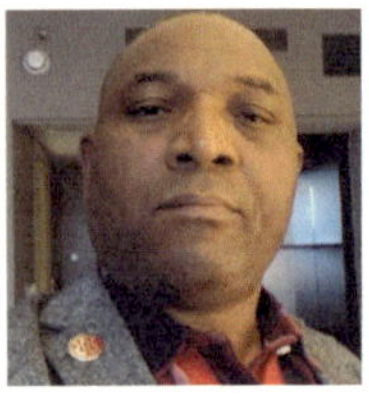

Erhabor Osaro is a Professor of Haematology and Blood Transfusion Science in the Department of Haematology and Blood Transfusion Science, Usmanu Danfodiyo University, Sokoto, Nigeria. He received his Ph.D. in Immuno-Haematology from the Rivers State University of Science and Technology, Nigeria. He is an alumni of the University of Greenwich, UK, and Francis Tuttle College of Technology, USA. He is on the Science Council of the UK register as a chartered scientist and an examiner (registration and specialist portfolio verifier) for the Institute of Biomedical Science (IBMS), UK. He is a fellow of several renowned scientific bodies including the British Blood Transfusion Society (BBTS), the Medical Laboratory Science Council of Nigeria (MLSCN), and the West African Postgraduate College of Medical Laboratory Science (WAPCMLS). He is the chairman of the Blood Transfusion Faculty, WAPCMLS, and a member of the council of the BBTS. He has authored four books and six book chapters. He is the editor-in-chief of the Sokoto Journal of Medical Laboratory Science and an editorial board member and expert reviewer for several international journals. He has received several awards and honors, including the Margaret Kenwright Award from the British Blood Transfusion Society (BBTS). He is the president of Nelon Medical Limited UK. His research interests include infectious diseases, transfusion medicine, laboratory haematology, and laboratory total quality management.

Contents

Preface

Thalassemia syndromes are perhaps some of the least well-defined of the hereditary hemolytic diseases from the standpoint of genetic background, classification, basic biochemical abnormalities, and clinical and hematologic findings. It is hardly necessary to mention the difficulties encountered in fitting in the varied clinical pictures of thalassemia with the simple concept of heterozygosity or homozygosity for the responsible abnormal. The thalassemia group of diseases is caused by a series of multiple interrelated genetic defects, not necessarily closely linked, which in various combinations give rise to a graduated series of hematologic aberrations, starting with the mildest asymptomatic state, in which the diagnosis can often only be inferred, and ending with severe, chronic microcytic hypochromic hemolytic anemia referred to as Cooley's anemia. This book contains four sections: "Beta Thalasemia Overview", "Thalassemia Syndromes", "Treatment Modalities in Beta Thalassemia", "Blood and Blood Components Transfusion Modalities". It reviews some of the many problems related to this complex and interesting group of diseases. More careful genetic, hematologic, and biochemical studies are needed to complete our understanding of this syndrome.

Marwa Zakaria, Laila Sherief and Tamer Hassan
Professor of Pediatric Hematology,
Pediatric Department,
Zagazig University,
Zagazig, Egypt

Osaro Erhabor
Blood Transfusion Faculty,
West African Postgraduate College of Medical Laboratory Science,
Wupa, Nigeria

Professor of Haematology and Blood Transfusion Science,
Department of Haematology and Blood Transfusion Science,
Usmau Danfodiyo University Sokoto,
Sokoto, Nigeria

Section 1

Beta Thalasemia Overview

Chapter 1

Overview of Beta-Thalassemia

Kenneth Oshiokhayamhe Iyevhobu, Lucky E. Omolumen, Tobechukwu Joseph Okobi, Edidiong Raphael Usoro, A. Airefetalor Ivie, Benedicta A. Ken-Iyevhobu and O. Omokpo Victoria

Abstract

Beta-thalassemias are a group of hereditary blood disorders characterized by anomalies in the synthesis of the beta chains of hemoglobin resulting in variable phenotypes ranging from severe anemia to clinically asymptomatic individuals. Three main forms have been described: thalassemia major, thalassemia intermedia, and thalassemia minor. Individuals with thalassemia major usually present within the first 2 years of life with severe anemia, requiring regular red blood cell (RBC) transfusions. Patients with thalassemia intermedia present later in life with moderate anemia and do not require regular transfusions. Thalassemia minor is clinically asymptomatic, but some subjects may have moderate anemia. Beta-thalassemias are caused by point mutations or, more rarely, deletions in the beta-globin gene on chromosome 11, leading to reduced (beta+) or absent (beta0) synthesis of the beta chains of hemoglobin (Hb). Transmission is autosomal recessive; however, dominant mutations have also been reported. Diagnosis of thalassemia is based on hematologic and molecular genetic testing. Laboratory tests that are conventionally performed to diagnose the β-thalassemia and HbE are classified into two groups, based on the purposes, including the screening tests and confirmatory tests.

Keywords: beta, thalassemia, hemoglobin, anemia, globin

1. Introduction

The term thalassemia is deduced from the Greek, namely thalassa (ocean) and haima (blood). Thalassemia is among the most common heritable diseases in the world [1–3]. The thalassemias are conditions caused by dropped expression of one of the two globin chains of the hemoglobin patch, namely α (HBA) and β (HBB). Inherited through an autosomal sheepish pathway, point mutations and elisions on the genes that decode for the globin chains beget dropped hemoglobin (Hb) product, leading to severe anemia [4]. Thalassemia cases depend on lifelong medical care, entering routine blood transfusions and supplemental curatives [5]. Thus, timely opinion and forestallment is essential, especially in regions with high frequency of this complaint [6–8]. Beta-thalassemia characterized by reduced or absent β-globin chain conflation is one of the most common inherited blood diseases in the world and hence a major interference to public health. Beta-thalassemia is a blood complaint that reduces the product of hemoglobin [9]. The protein in red blood cells called hemoglobin, which contains iron, transports oxygen to every cell in the body. Low hemoglobin levels in beta-thalassemia patients cause an oxygen shortage in a number of bodily passageways [10]. A lack of red blood cells in affected people (anemia) can result in pale skin, weakness, weariness, and more severe problems. Beta-thalassemia patients are more likely to get irregular blood clots [11]. Beta-thalassemia runs are a group of heritable blood diseases characterized by reduced or absent beta-globin chain conflation, performing in reduced Hb in red blood cells (RBC), dropped RBC product and anemia. Beta-thalassemia major was first described in the medical literature in 1925 by an American croaker-Thomas Cooley. Beta-thalassemia includes three main forms, namely thalassemia major, perfectly appertained to as "Cooley's Anemia" and "Mediterranean Anemia", thalassemia intermedia, and thalassemia minor also called "beta-thalassemia carrier", "beta-thalassemia particularity", or "heterozygous beta-thalassemia" [10, 11]. Piecemeal from the rare dominant forms, subjects with thalassemia major are homozygotes or emulsion heterozygotes for beta0 or beta genes, subjects with thalassemia intermedia are substantially homozygotes or emulsion heterozygotes, and subjects with thalassemia minor are substantially heterozygotes. Although wide, the major at- threat populations are substantially from Mediterranean, Middle East, and Southeast Asian countries [12, 13]. The thalassemia category of hemoglobin conflation illnesses differs from the others in that there is either little or no-globin chain conflation. The main forms of β-thalassemia are two. The two types of thalassemia are β^{O}-thalassemia, in which no-globin chain is made, and -thalassemia, in which some globin is produced but at a lower level than usual [14]. Microcytosis, often known as thalassemia minor clinically, affects heterozygotes for either type of allele. A more severe phenotype known as β-thalassemia intermedia, which involves anemia, hemolysis, iron loading, and the sporadic need for transfusion, is present in homozygous heterozygotes for two thalassemia alleles or one and one β^0 allele. The most severe form of the condition, known asthalassemia major, is present in people who have two β^0-thalassemia alleles and results in transfusion-dependent anemia, severe transfusional iron overload, reduced life expectancy, and chelation therapy. A severe form of thalassemia with no globin chain product is called β^0-thalassemia. Point mutations in the rendering region (exon) or exon-intron junction of the β-globin gene, which result in an unseasonable stop codon or the production of aberrant β-globin mRNA, are the primary cause. Absence of the β-globin chain product is the result of these anomalies [14]. The frequency of thalassemia is growing mainly in non-indigenous regions, similar as Northern Europe, North America, and Australia, due to increased mobility and migration overflows of populations in recent decades [12, 15–18]. The global burden of hemoglobinopathies necessitates perpetration of public health interventions, similar as webbing programs and antenatal opinion, indeed in non-indigenous countries with high rates of immigration [15]. The genes that render for globin proteins are located on β-and α-globin gene clusters on chromosome 11 and 16, independently [4]. Expression of each globin gene varies throughout the embryonic and fetal development, which is why the Hb patterns of babe and grown-ups differ from each other [19, 20].

2. Epidemiology of beta-thalassemia

Beta-thalassemia is an in actuality normal blood inconvenience round the field. A huge amount of babies are considered with beta-thalassemia consistently.

Beta-thalassemia happens limit of the time in people from Mediterranean nations, North Africa, the Center East, Central Asia, Southeast Asia, India, southern China, and the Far East, notwithstanding nations close by the northern coast of Africa and within side the South America. The most extreme exceptional carrier repeat is situated in Cyprus (14%), Sardinia (10.3%), and Southeast Asia [21]. High-incredible repeat of beta-thalassemia in those districts might be extremely probably to be perceived with the special strain of wilderness fever Plasmodium falciparum [21]. Populace resettlement and intermarriage among unique ethnic congregations have incited thalassemia in virtually all nations of the field, along with northern Europe, wherein thalassemia in the past did now presently do not exist. It has been normal that round 1.5% of the field's general population (80 to 90 million people) are organizations of beta-thalassemia, with cycle 60,000 characteristic individuals transforming into pregnant every year, the especially gigantic a piece of the scene. Without a doubt the yearly cost of interesting people is normal at 1 out of 100,000 worldwide and 1 out of 10,000 within side the European Affiliation [10]. Regardless, there might be a deficiency of explicit records on delivery costs in several people gatherings, for the most part in areas of the field which can be perceived or anticipated to be emphatically impacted [12, 21]. As indicated by the Thalassemia Overall Association, around 200,000 victims stay with thalassemia dominating and are enrolled for standard cure worldwide [21]. The excellent perceived total of beta-thalassemia with phenomenal Hb or number one Hb form with thalassemic homes is HbE/beta-thalassemia, that is typically huge in Southeast Asia, wherein carrier.

2.1 Types and clinical description of beta-thalassemia

The aggregates of homozygous or hereditary heterozygous compound beta-thalassemias incorporate Cooley's frailty and thalassemia intermedia [10]. People with Cooley's frailty ordinarily come to clinical consideration inside the essential 2 years of life and need standard RBC bondings to endure. Those introducing later do not need bonding and get an analysis of thalassemia intermedia [22]. Thalassemia intermedia incorporates patients who present later and do not need customary bonding. Besides inside the uncommon predominant structures, heterozygous beta-thalassemia prompts the clinically quiet transporter state. HbE/beta-thalassemia and HbC/beta-thalassemia display a superb home as far as variety of aggregates and range of seriousness [11].

2.1.1 Beta-thalassemia major (Cooley's anemia)

Beta-thalassemia significant alludes to a serious clinical aggregate that happens when patients are homozygous or compound heterozygous for more extreme beta chain transformations (for example serious B+/B+ changes, B+/B0, B0/B0) [10, 11].

Clinical show of thalassemia major happens somewhere in the range of 6 and 2 years. Youngsters foster dangerous weakness. They do not put on weight and develop at the normal rate (inability to flourish) and may create yellowing of the skin and whites of the eyes (jaundice) and become logically pale. Influenced people might have an amplified spleen, liver, and heart, and their bones might be distorted. Taking care of issues, looseness of the bowels, peevishness, repetitive episodes of fever, and reformist amplification of the midsection brought about by spleen and liver augmentation might happen. The clinical picture of thalassemia major is described by development impediment, paleness, jaundice, helpless musculature, genu valgum, hepatosplenomegaly, leg ulcers, improvement of masses from extramedullary hematopoiesis, and skeletal changes brought on by extension of the bone marrow in some developing nations where patients are untreated or ineffectively bonded due to a lack of resources. Skeletal modifications include frequent craniofacial changes and deformations of the long bones of the legs (bossing of the skull, conspicuous malar greatness, gloom of the extension of the nose, inclination to a mongoloid inclination of the eye, and hypertrophy of the maxillae, which will in general uncover the upper teeth). A few youths with thalassemia significant experience deferred adolescence. Many individuals with thalassemia major have such extreme manifestations that they need incessant blood bondings to recharge their red platelet supply. Over the long haul, a convergence of iron-containing hemoglobin from ongoing blood bondings can prompt a development of iron in the body, bringing about liver, heart, and chemical issues.

On the off chance that a customary bonding program that keeps a base Hb centralization of 9.5 to 10.5 g/dL is started, development and advancement will in general be ordinary up to 10 to 12 years [15]. Bonded patients might foster difficulties identified with iron over-burden. Entanglements of iron over-burden in youngsters incorporate development hindrance and disappointment or postponement of sexual development. Later iron over-burden-related inconveniences incorporate inclusion of the heart (widened myocardiopathy or once in a while arrythmias), liver (fibrosis and cirrhosis), and endocrine organs (diabetes mellitus, hypogonadism, and inadequacy of the parathyroid, thyroid, pituitary, and, less regularly, adrenal organs) [23]. Consistence with iron chelation treatment essentially impacts recurrence and seriousness of the iron over-burden-related complexities [24].

2.1.2 Beta-thalassemia intermedia

Beta-thalassemia intermedia is in the middle of clinical aggregate with heterogeneous hereditary changes that actually consider some beta chain creation (e.g., B+/B0, B+/B+). Some uncommon cases likewise exist in which both beta and alpha transformations exist together [11, 12].

Individuals with thalassemia intermedia present later than thalassemia major, have milder anemia and by definition do not require or only occasionally require transfusion. At the severe end of the clinical spectrum, patients present between the ages of 2 and 6 years and although they are capable of surviving without regular blood transfusion, growth and development are retarded. At the opposite finish of the range are patients who are totally asymptomatic until grown-up existence with just gentle frailty. The signs and side effects of thalassemia intermedia show up in youth or sometime down the road. Influenced people are gentle to direct sickliness and may likewise have slow development and bone anomalies. Hypertrophy of erythroid marrow with the chance of extramedullary erythropoiesis, a compensatory system of bone marrow to beat ongoing iron deficiency, is normal. It leads to common facial and bone deformities, osteoporosis with pathologic breaks in long bones, and the growth of erythropoietic masses that have a significant impact on the spleen, liver, lymph nodes, chest, and spine. The spleen's important role in clearing damaged red blood cells from the circulatory system contributes to its growth. Extramedullary erythropoiesis may result in neurological problems, such as intrathoracic masses and spinal rope pressure with paraplegia. Gallstones may develop in thalassemia intermedia individuals more frequently than in thalassemia major because to ineffective erythropoiesis and fringe hemolysis [25]. Patients with thalassemia intermedia often foster leg ulcers and have an expanded inclination to apoplexy when contrasted with thalassemia major, particularly if splenectomised. Such occasions incorporate profound vein apoplexy, entrance vein apoplexy, stroke, and aspiratory embolism [26].

In spite of the fact that people with thalassemia intermedia are in danger of iron over-burden optional to expanded digestive iron retention, hypogonadism, hypothyroidism, and diabetes are not normal [27]. Ladies might have effective unconstrained pregnancies. Nonetheless, if blood bondings are fundamental during pregnancy, those never or negligibly bonded are in danger of creating hemolytic alloantibodies and erythrocyte autoantibodies. Intrauterine development hindrance, in spite of a customary bonding routine, has been accounted for [28]. Cardiovascular inclusion in thalassemia intermedia results chiefly from a high-yield state and aspiratory hypertension, while systolic left ventricle work is generally protected [29]. Pseudoxantoma elasticum, a diffuse connective tissue issue with vascular indication brought about by degeneration of the versatile lamina of the blood vessel divider and calcium statement, has been portrayed in such patients [30].

2.1.3 Beta-thalassemia minor (Beta-thalassemia carrier/trait)

Beta-thalassemia minor is a gentle clinical aggregate when one typical duplicate of the beta globulin quality is available (e.g., B+/B, B0/B). Transporters of thalassemia minor are normally clinically asymptomatic, however, here, and there have a gentle weakness. At the point when the two guardians are transporters, there is a 25% danger at every pregnancy of having kids with homozygous thalassemia [10, 11].

2.1.4 Dominant beta-thalassemia

Conversely, with the old style latent types of beta-thalassemia, which lead to a diminished creation of ordinary beta-globin chains, some uncommon transformations bring about the union of incredibly unsteady beta-globin variations which hasten in erythroid forerunners causing insufficient erythropoiesis [11]. These transformations are related with a clinically perceptible thalassemia aggregate in the heterozygote and are in this way alluded to as prevailing beta-thalassemias. The presence of hyper-temperamental Hb ought to be suspected in any person with thalassemia intermedia when the two guardians are hematologically ordinary, or in families with an example of autosomal prevailing transmission of the thalassemia intermedia aggregate. Beta-globin quality sequencing sets up the conclusion [6].

Most people who are heterozygous for a beta-thalassemia change have clinicopathological highlights depicted as "thalassemia minor"; for example, the blood count and film are strange yet there are no unusual actual discoveries or indications. Notwithstanding, a few transformations produce clinically obvious anomalies in heterozygotes, mostly splenomegaly, frailty, jaundice, and an expanded occurrence of gallstones. This is alluded to as predominant beta-thalassemia [6]. Predominant beta-thalassemia is uncommon; however, cases are found dissipated all through the world. The clinicopathological highlights are those of thalassemia intermedia. Red cell endurance is not exactly in run of the mill beta-thalassemia attribute and the reticulocyte count is expanded. Patients might require incidental blood bondings. There is extramedullary hematopoiesis, and iron over-burden might happen. The blood film is typically exceptionally unusual with conspicuous basophilic texturing and circling nucleated red cells. The bone marrow shows erythroid hyperplasia and dyserythropoiesis [6].

2.1.5 Beta-thalassemia associated with other Hb anomalies

The participation of HbE and beta-thalassemia achieves thalassemia totals going from a condition unclear from thalassemia major to a delicate sort of thalassemia intermedia. Dependent upon the earnestness of signs, three characterizations may be perceived [31]:

- **Mild HbE/beta-thalassemia:** It is seen in around 15% of all cases in Southeast Asia. This get-together of patients stays aware of Hb levels some place in the scope of 9 and 12 g/dl and by and large does not cultivate clinically basic issues. No treatment is required.

- **Moderately genuine HbE/beta-thalassemia:** The vast majority of HbE/beta-thalassemia cases fall into this class. The Hb levels stay at 6–7 g/dl, and the clinical signs resemble thalassemia intermedia. Bondings are not required aside from if sicknesses support further fragility. Iron over-weight may occur.

- **Severe HbE/beta-thalassemia:** The Hb level can be basically just about as low as 4–5 g/dl. Patients in this social event show signs like thalassemia major and are treated as thalassemia critical patients [10].

Patients with HbC/beta-thalassemia may live freed from signs and be examined during routine tests. Exactly when present, clinical appearances are iron lack and improvement of the spleen. Blood bondings are just every so often required. Microcytosis and hypochromia are found for every circumstance. The blood film shows specific Hb C valuable stones with straight equivalent edges, target cells, and irregularly contracted cells with components of thalassemia like microcytosis [11]. The relationship of acquired ingenuity of fetal Hb (HPFH) with beta-thalassemia mitigates the clinical appearances which change from normal to thalassemia intermedia. Individuals with HbS/beta-thalassemia have a clinical course like that of Hb SS [10].

2.1.6 Beta-thalassemia associated with other features

Rarely, the beta-globin quality group does not contain the beta-thalassemia defect. The sub-atomic damage has been discovered in the quality encoding the record factor TFIIH (beta-thalassemia attribute related with tricothiodystrophy) or in the X-connected record factor GATA-1 (X-connected thrombocytopenia with thalassemia) in cases where the beta-thalassemia characteristic is related with different elements [32–34].

2.2 Signs and symptoms of beta-thalassemia

The majority of people with beta-thalassemia quality do not show any symptoms. Depending on the type of disorientation gained, different people will experience different side effects. Children with beta-thalassemia intermedia or major may not display any symptoms at all, although they usually develop them during the first 2 years of life. Beginning with one person and progressing to the next, the symptoms and severity of beta-thalassemia vary dramatically [10].

The most serious kind of beta-thalassemia is beta-thalassemia major. Children that are born with this type of personality will show signs early on in life, such as

- Pale skin
- Tiredness
- Shortness of breath
- Fussy
- Having a poor appetite
- Having many infections.

Over time more symptoms will appear, including:

- Slowed growth
- A fast heartbeat
- Moodiness
- Belly (abdominal) swelling
- Yellowish skin and eyes (jaundice).

Individuals with beta-thalassemia or intermedia typically have a development of iron within the body, either from the particular illness or from the rehashed blood bondings. Abundance iron will hurt the center, liver, and endocrine framework. While not treatment, the spleen, liver, and heart become broadened. Bones will likewise end up to be meager, weak, and twisted. People with this condition would force continuous blood bondings and will not stick with it with a typical lifespan. Iron develops within the heart and totally different organs from blood bondings. This may cause vast breakdown as right time because the teenagers or middle 20s people with beta-thalassemia might need different real medical problems, including:

Thalassemia minima: this type often causes no symptoms but may have a mild anemia. Many individuals with beta thalassemia minor go through life never knowing they carry an altered gene for the disorder.

Thalassemia intermedia: folks determined to own beta monogenic disorder intermedia have a typically shifted articulation of the difficulty. Creditably extreme weakness is traditional, and influenced folks may need intermittent blood bondings. Each individual case is one among a form. This type will create aspect effects of moderate serious sickliness including:

- Pallor
- Extreme tiredness (fatigue)
- Pale skin
- Jaundice
- Leg ulcers

- Gallstones (cholelithiasis)
- Slow or delayed growth
- Weak bones
- Abnormal enlargement of the liver and spleen
- Moderate to severe skeletal malformations.

Predominant Beta-Thalassemia: Prevailing beta-thalassemia is a very uncommon structure where people who have one changed HBB quality foster specific manifestations related with beta-thalassemia. Influenced people might create gentle to direct sickliness, jaundice, and a strangely broadened spleen (splenomegaly).

2.3 Etiology of beta-thalassemia

Hemoglobin is made of two alpha proteins and two beta proteins. A quality change (transformation) in the alpha proteins causes alpha thalassemia. A quality change in the beta proteins causes beta-thalassemia. Most beta-thalassemia cases are brought about by a transformation in the HBB quality. In incredibly uncommon cases, a deficiency of hereditary material (erasure) that incorporates the HBB quality causes the issue [11]. In beta-thalassemia, the quality change causes an irregularity of hemoglobin proteins. The irregularity causes sickliness in light of the fact that [10]:

- Red platelets separate quicker than ordinary.
- Fewer RBCs are made.
- Less hemoglobin is made.

The awkwardness additionally prompts clinical issues during the bones, bone marrow, and different organs. In excess of 200 changes have been so far announced; the larger part is point transformations in practically significant districts of the beta-globin quality [35]. Erasures of the beta-globin quality are remarkable. The beta-globin quality transformations cause a diminished or missing creation of beta-globin chains. Transformations in the HBB quality reason beta-thalassemia. The HBB quality gives guidelines to making a protein called beta-globin. Beta-globin is a part (subunit) of hemoglobin. Hemoglobin comprises four protein subunits, ordinarily two subunits of beta-globin and two subunits of another protein called alpha-globin [35].

The development of any beta-globin is prevented by a few modifications to the HBB quality. The term beta-zero (β^0) thalassemia refers to a lack of beta-globin. Additional HBB quality alterations allow for the creation of some beta-globin, but in smaller amounts. Beta in addition to (β^+) thalassemia is characterized by a decreased level of beta-globin. Possessing either a β^0 or β^+ thalassemia does not necessarily indicate how bad your condition will be; people with these two types have been found to have thalassemia major and thalassemia intermedia, respectively.

An absence of beta-globin prompts a diminished measure of practical hemoglobin. Without adequate hemoglobin, red platelets do not grow regularly, causing a deficiency of mature red platelets. People with beta-thalassemia have pallor and other related medical problems due to the low quantity of developed red platelets. Beta-thalassemia is the result of damaged or absent components. There are two distinct traits present. There are various varieties of this problem:

Cooley's weakness (beta-thalassemia major). There are two damaged characteristics. The most severe form of this issue is this. Those with this ailment will need further blood bondings. They might not live out a typical lifespan.

Beta-thalassemia minor or thalassemia attribute. Just a single quality is harmed. This causes less extreme pallor. Individuals with this kind have a half shot at passing the quality to their kids. On the off chance that the other parent is not influenced, their kids will likewise have this type of the problem. This sort is additionally isolated into

- **Thalassemia minima:** There are few or no symptoms.
- **Thalassemia intermedia:** This causes moderate to severe anemia.

Many individuals with this problem are given iron substitution unintentionally. This happens when an absence of iron is accepted to cause their pallor. An excessive amount of iron can be hurtful. So, get the right determination.

2.3.1 Genetic modifiers

The modifying qualities are characterized by being hereditary variations that give rise to contrasts in the aggregate of the infection. In homozygous beta-thalassemia, the essential inherited modifiers that affect the clinical severity of the infection contain inherited variations that are ready to reduce the irregularity of the globin chain, creating a milder form of thalassemia [11]. These elements are the presence of quiet or mild beta-thalassemia alleles associated with a high residual yield of beta-globin, the co-inheritance of alpha-thalassemia, and, in addition, hereditary determinants ready for the incessant production of gamma-globin chains of support (HbF) in adult life [36]. Some beta-thalassemia transformations (e.g., deleting and not canceling delta-beta-thalassemia, local 5′ deletions of beta-globin quality) "essentially" increase the performance of gamma-globin quality [10]. Several transformations that extend HbF production are associated with deletional and non-deletional HPFH associated with the beta-globin quality package. Recently, the genome-wide affiliation approach, which specifically focuses on quantitative quality loci (QTL) that cause elevated HbF levels, has inherited components (e.g., changing the severity of homozygous beta-zero thalassemia [37].

The clinical aggregate of homozygous beta-thalassemia may also be altered by the interaction of other planned heritable variations outside the globin groups. These additional heritable modifiers have a profound effect in confounding the aggregate of thalassemia [11]. Some additional heritable modifiers have been recognized in recent years. The appearance of polymorphism (TA) 7 in the uridine diphosphate glucuronosyltransferase quality-reporting site, which in the homozygous state is associated with Gilbert's disease, is a risk factor for the progression of cholelithiasis in patients with thalassemia major and intermedia [38]. Other competing qualities to alter the aggregate of thalassemia are the apolipoprotein E 4 allele and some HLA haplotypes, which appear to be inherited risk factors for left ventricular disappointment in homozygous beta-thalassemia [10, 39, 40]. For qualities related to iron digestion (e.g., C282Y and H63D-HFE quality transformations), less stable information was considered, probably since its effects on iron deposition are obscured by treatment (e.g., B. iron deposits auxiliary to the binding of red blood cells and iron chelation) and for qualities related to bone digestion [41–43]. Recently, a polymorphism in the quality of glutathione transferase M1 has been associated with an increased risk of heart iron overload in thalassemia major [44].

In certain cases, heterozygous beta-thalassemia could trigger the intermediate aggregation of thalassemia instead of the asymptomatic transporter state [10]. Most of these patients have an abundance of practical alpha globin qualities (triple or quadruple alpha quality), which increases the asymmetry in the ratio of the combination of alpha/non-alpha globin chains [36, 45].

2.3.2 Pathophysiology

A general oversupply of unbound alpha globin chains that speed in erythroid precursors in the bone marrow cause their unexpected passing and consequently lead to insufficient erythropoiesis. This is caused by a decreased amount (beta+) or nonexistence (beta0) of beta-globin chains. The concept of the transformation at the beta-globin quality located on chromosome 11 controls the degree of globin chain decline. As opposed to thalassemia intermedia, fringe hemolysis, which exacerbates illness, occurs when insoluble alpha globin attaches rapid layer damage to the fringe erythrocytes. Paleness animates the creation of erythropoietin with resulting concentrated yet inadequate development of the bone marrow (up 25 to multiple times ordinary), which thusly causes the regular recently portrayed bone disfigurements. Delayed and serious paleness and expanded erythropoietic drive additionally result in hepatosplenomegaly and extramedullary erythropoiesis [31].

2.3.3 Hereditary transmission

The beta-thalassemias square measures nonheritable in AN chromosome latent approach. The guardians of AN influenced juvenile square measure commit heterozygotes and convey a solitary duplicate of illness inflicting beta simple protein quality amendment. Mediterranean anemia intermedia square measures non-heritable in an chromosome passive example, which means the 2 duplicates of the HBB quality in each cell have changes. The parents of an individual with an autosomal recessive condition each carry one copy of the mutated gene, but they typically do not show signs and symptoms of the condition [11]. At times, in any case, people with just one HBB quality amendment in each cell foster light paleness. These somewhat influenced people square measure same to own Mediterranean anemia minor. At origination, each offspring of heterozygotes guardians has 25th shot at being influenced, shot at being AN symptomless transporter, and 25th shot at being unaffected and not transporter. The guardians of the proband have 25% hazard of getting to boot influenced youngsters in every gestation [31].

Predominant varieties of beta-thalassemia, connected with transformations that outcome within the creation of deeply unsound transferrin variations and prompting a clinically showing combination of beta-thalassemia in heterozygotes, are talked regarding on top of within the clinical portrayal section. In an exceedingly very little level of families, the HBB quality transformation is nonheritable in AN chromosome predominant approach. In these cases, one duplicate of the changed quality in each cell is up to cause the signs and manifestations of beta Mediterranean anemia [10].

3. Diagnosis beta-thalassemia

Beta-thalassemia is regularly found in individuals who are from Greek, Italian, African, or Asian beginning. The determination is frequently made somewhere in the range of 6 and 12 years of age. Thalassemia major is normally suspected in a newborn child more youthful than 2 years old with extreme microcytic frailty, gentle jaundice, and hepatosplenomegaly. Thalassemia intermedia presents at a later age with comparative yet milder clinical discoveries. Transporters are typically asymptomatic, however, at times might have gentle paleness. People with thalassemias have more modest measured red platelets than unaffected individuals just as low red platelet counts (pallor). Thalassemia major and thalassemia minor would now be able to be analyzed (and recognized from each other) by ordinary clinical and blood testing, yet additionally by atomic and hereditary tests. These tests license exact finding to be made whenever, even before birth (indeed, a long time before the beta chains are even incorporated) [33].

3.1 Hematologic diagnosis

RBC lists show microcytic iron deficiency. Thalassemia major is portrayed by diminished Hb level (50 < 70 fl and mean corpuscolar Hb (MCH) > 12 < 20 pg. Thalassemia intermedia is portrayed by Hb level somewhere in the range of 7 and 10 g/dl, MCV somewhere in the range of 50 and 80 fl and MCH somewhere in the range of 16 and 24 pg. Thalassemia minor is portrayed by diminished MCV and MCH, with expanded Hb A2 level [31].

Complete blood count (CBC): This test really looks at the size, number, and development of various platelets in a set volume of blood.

3.2 Smear of peripheral blood

Affected individuals have RBC morphologic alterations, including nucleated RBC, microcytosis, hypochromia, anisocytosis, and poikilocytosis (spiculated tear-drop and extended cells) (i.e., erythroblasts). After splenectomy, the number of erythroblasts significantly increases and is correlated with the degree of frailty. Compared to influenced people, transporters exhibit less severe RBC morphologic alterations. Usually, erythroblasts are not visible [22].

3.3 HPLC/electrophoresis

The Hb design in beta-thalassemia changes as indicated by beta-thalassemia type. In beta0 thalassemia, homozygotes HbA is absent and HbF constitutes the 92-95% of the total Hb. In beta+ thalassemia homozygotes and beta+/ beta0 genetic compounds HbA levels are between 10 and 30% and HbF between 70-90%. HbA2 is variable in beta-thalassemia homozygotes, and it is upgraded in beta-thalassemia minor [22]. Hb electrophoresis and HPLC likewise identify different hemoglobinopathies (S, C, E, OArab, Lepore) that might cooperate with beta-thalassemia [11].

Hemoglobin electrophoresis with hemoglobin F and A2 quantitation: A lab test that separates the kinds of hemoglobin [10]. Subjective and quantitative Hb investigation distinguishes the sum and kind of Hb present [10].

3.4 Molecular genetic analysis

The pervasiveness of a predetermined number of changes in every populace has incredibly worked with sub-atomic hereditary testing. Generally happening transformations of the beta-globin quality are recognized by PCR-based systems [33, 46]. The most generally utilized techniques are converse dab smudge examination or groundwork explicit enhancement, with a bunch of tests or preliminaries corresponding to the most well-known transformations in the populace from which the influenced individual started. Whenever designated change examination neglects to recognize the transformation, beta-globin quality succession investigation can be utilized to distinguish changes in the beta-globin quality [12].

3.5 Differential diagnosis

Barely any conditions share similitudes with homozygous beta-thalassemia [11]:

- Not really settled sideroblastic anemias are effortlessly separated in view of ring sideroblasts in the bone marrow and dynamically raised serum grouping of erythrocyte protoporphyrin. Most sideroblastic anemias are related with abandons in the heme biosynthetic pathway, particularly delta-aminolevulinic corrosive synthase.

- Congenital dyserythropoietic anemias do not have high HbF and do have other unmistakable components, like multinuclearity of the red platelet forerunners.

- A few obtained conditions related with high HbF (adolescent ongoing myelomonocytic leukemia with ordinary karyotype, aplastic weakness both inherent and procured during the recuperation stage) might be confused with beta-thalassemia, despite the fact that they have exceptionally trademark clinical and hematological provisions [10].

Normal beta-thalassemia transporters are distinguished by examination of RBC files, which shows microcytosis (low MCV) and diminished substance of Hb per red cell (low MCH), and by subjective and quantitative Hb investigation, which shows the increment of HbA2 [11]. These examinations should be possible from a solitary blood test. In a pregnant lady, the child is analyzed utilizing CVS (chorionic villus inspecting) or amniocentesis.

Entanglements in transporter distinguishing proof by hematologic testing are:

- Coinheritance of alpha-thalassemia, which might standardize the RBC records. Nonetheless, in alpha/beta twofold heterozygotes, the HbA2 fixation stays in the beta-thalassemia transporter reach and consequently is indicative. Accordingly, HbA2 assurance ought to consistently be performed for beta-thalassemia transporter ID.

- Coinheritance of delta-thalassemia, which might diminish to ordinary the expanded Hb A2 levels common of the beta-thalassemia transporter state. Twofold heterozygosity for delta-and beta-thalassemia can be recognized from the most well-known alpha-thalassemia transporter state by globin chain blend or globin quality examination [10].

- Silent transformations, i.e., extremely gentle changes related with reliable remaining yield of Hb beta chains and with ordinary RBC files and typical or fringe HbA2. The above detailed gatherings of transporters are alluded to as abnormal transporters.

At the point when the hematologic investigation is unusual, atomic hereditary testing of beta-globin quality is performed to distinguish the infection causing change [46].

3.6 Genetic counseling and prenatal diagnosis

Anticipation of beta-thalassemia depends on transporter distinguishing proof, hereditary advising, and pre-birth analysis [47]. Transporter identification has been recently portrayed. Hereditary guiding gives data to people and in danger couples (e.g., the two transporters) with respect to the method of legacy, the hereditary danger of having influenced kids and the regular history of the sickness including the accessible therapy and treatments being scrutinized. Pre-birth detection for pregnancies with a higher risk of complications is possible by analyzing the DNA of fetal cells obtained by amniocentesis, which is typically done at roughly 15 to 18 weeks of gestation, or by chorionic villi inspection at 11 weeks of development. Before pre-birth testing can be carried out, both alleles that cause the illnesses must be identified. Currently, fetal DNA in maternal plasma and fetal cells in maternal blood are being examined for the presence of the father's transformation [48]. Families with the identified disease-causing mutations may be eligible for preimplantation hereditary conclusion.

3.7 Management of beta-thalassemia

3.7.1 Management of beta-thalassemia major

Babies with thalassemia major are well upon entering the world due to a unique type of hemoglobin present in the hatchling and infant [49]. At last, notwithstanding, this hemoglobin is supplanted by deficient hemoglobin. Manifestations arise late in the main year of life. The youngster creates fair skin, crabbiness, development impediment, expanding of the midsection because of extension of the liver and spleen (hepatosplenomegaly) with jaundice. This is related with serious iron deficiency with burst of the red platelets (hemolytic weakness). The kid with thalassemia major becomes reliant upon blood bondings and, despite the fact that they do help, they make further issues including iron over-burden. Folic corrosive supplementation is frequently given. Right now, the essential medicines are aimed at diminishing manifestations of the sickness. Chosen patients might fit the bill for bone marrow or undifferentiated cell transfers. Quality treatment stays a likely treatment for what is to come. The drawn-out trust is that thalassemia significant will be restored by addition of the ordinary beta-chain quality through quality treatment or by one more methodology of atomic medication [33, 49].

3.7.2 Transfusions

The objectives of bonding treatment are amendment of pallor, concealment of erythropoiesis, and hindrance of gastrointestinal iron retention, which happens in non-bonded patients as an outcome of expanded, albeit insufficient, erythropoiesis.

The choice to begin bonding in patients with affirmed determination of thalassemia ought to be founded on the presence of serious weakness (Hb < 7 g/dl for over about 14 days, barring other contributory causes like contaminations). Nonetheless, additionally in patients with Hb > 7 g/dl, different variables ought to be thought of, including facial changes, helpless development, proof of hard extension and expanding splenomegaly. Whenever the situation allows, the choice to begin ordinary bondings ought not be postponed until after the 2nd-3rd year, because of the danger of fostering various red cell antibodies and resulting trouble in discovering reasonable blood givers. A few diverse transfusional regimens have been proposed throughout the long term, yet the most broadly acknowledged focuses on a pretransfusional Hb level of 9 to 10 g/dl and a post-bonding level of 13 to 14 g/dl. This forestalls development hindrance, organ harm and bone deformations, permitting ordinary action and personal satisfaction [23].

3.7.3 Management of thalassemia intermedia

Treatment of people with thalassemia intermedia is indicative [23, 50]. As hypersplenism might cause demolishing sickliness, hindered development and mechanical unsettling influence from the huge spleen, splenectomy is an applicable part of the administration of thalassemia intermedia. Dangers related with splenectomy incorporate an expanded helplessness to contaminations fundamentally from exemplified microbes (Streptococcus Pneumoniae, Haemophilus Influenzae, and Neisseria Meningitidis) and an increment in thromboembolic occasions [49]. Sepsis after splenectomy can be prevented through vaccination against the aforementioned microbes, anti-infection prophylaxis, and early anti-toxin therapy for fever and agitation. The gallbladder should be examined during splenectomy and removed if necessary to treat or prevent gallstones due to the increased prevalence of cholelithiasis and the risks of cholecystitis in splenectomized patients. Radiation therapy with hydroxycarbamide is used to treat extramedullary erythropoietic masses that are detected by attractive reverberation imaging. Managing a leg ulcer after it has developed is extremely difficult. Zinc supplementation and pentoxifylline, and the utilization of an oxygen chamber have been proposed for ulcer treatment. Hydroxycarbamide additionally has some advantage, either alone or with erythropoietin. As of late encouraging outcomes have been gotten with platelet inferred development factor. Since patients with thalassemia intermedia have a high danger of apoplexy, exacerbated by splenectomy, know about thrombotic inconveniences. Suggested treatment choices incorporate appropriate anticoagulation before careful or other high danger systems, platelet hostile to totaling specialists if there should arise an occurrence of thrombocytosis (platelet count higher than 700,000/mm^3) and low sub-atomic weight heparin in patients with recorded apoplexy [33]. Since people with thalassemia intermedia may foster iron over-burden from expanded gastrointestinal assimilation of iron or from incidental bondings, chelation treatment is begun when the serum ferritin fixation surpasses 300 ng/ml or when iron over-burden is exhibited by immediate or circuitous techniques [51]. Beneficial folic corrosive can be recommended to patients with thalassemia intermedia to keep inadequacy from hyperactive bone marrow.

3.7.4 Improving ineffective erythropoiesis (IE) in thalassemia

Several various therapy modalities are currently being researched throughout the world thanks to recent developments in our understanding of the pathogenic mechanism behind thalassaemia. The investigational drug products that have recently entered the clinical phase are discussed in the section that follows, with an emphasis on their present and potential future relevance for clinical practice. The current standard of care for IE in thalassaemia, which includes blood transfusions and stem cell transplants as well as novel therapeutic approaches based on gene therapies, is not covered in this study and is available elsewhere.

The US Food and Drug Administration (FDA) in 2019 and the European Medicines Agency (EMA) in 2020 have both approved the first treatment for thalassemia, luspatercept, for TDT patients.

Mitapivat is a small-molecule, oral allosteric activator of RBC pyruvate kinase (PK-R), a crucial enzyme to control the synthesis of ATP through glycolysis (**Figure 1**).

3.7.5 Hematopoietic stem cell transplantation for thalassemia

Hemoglobinopathies are treated by allogeneic HSCT; following conditioning to get beyond the immune barrier, allogeneic stem cells are employed as vehicles to rectify the fundamental genetic flaw by re-inserting genes required for healthy hematopoiesis. Allogeneic HSCT is essentially allogeneic stem cell gene therapy in the treatment

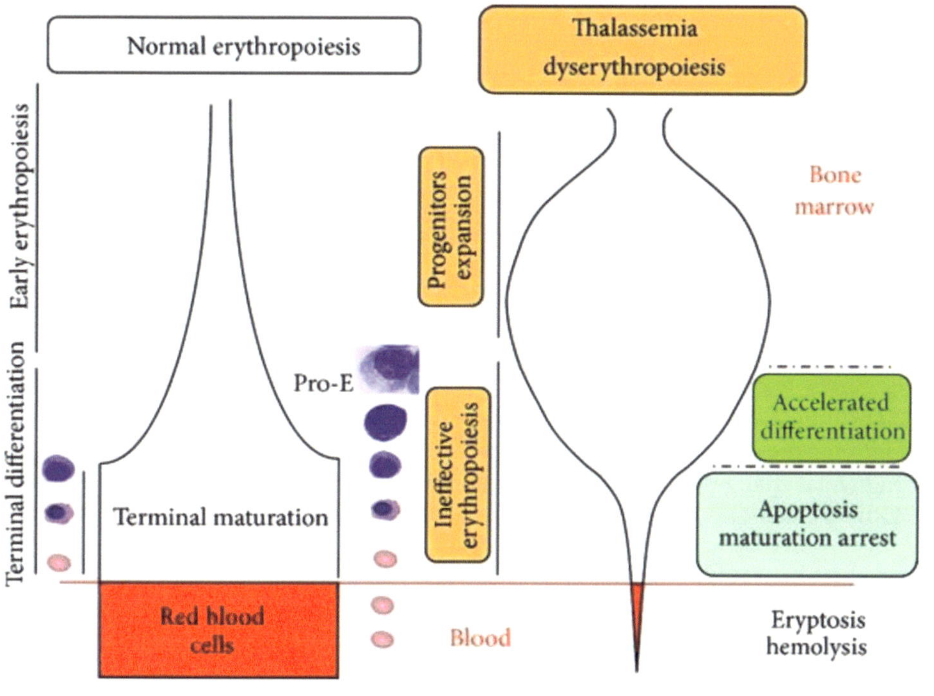

Figure 1.
Distinction between healthy and erythropoiesis that is unsuccessful due to β-thalassemia [52, 53]. Erythropoiesis, which involves a number of proliferative and differentiation phases, is the process that converts hematopoietic stem cells into adult RBCs. The production of cell surface proteins, cell size reduction, progressive hemoglobinization, nuclear condensation, and nuclear extrusion are all temporally regulated processes that occur in conjunction with erythroid differentiation. The growth of extremely early erythroid precursors (proerythroblasts and earlier stages) and subsequent inefficient erythropoiesis are characteristics of β-thalassemia dyserythropoiesis in humans. A proliferating pool of immature erythroblasts is subject to ineffective erythropoiesis, which is characterized by (1) rapid erythroid differentiation, (2) maturation inhibition during the polychromatophilic stage, and (3) death of erythroid precursors [54–56].

of various disorders. Autologous stem cells altered by the insertion of healthy genes may 1 day be used as vectors, but there is currently little sign that this strategy will be available in clinics anytime soon.

Thalassemia treatment with allogeneic hematopoietic stem cell transplantation (HSCT) has been a key component in the growth of HSCT. The allogeneic HSC with successful erythropoiesis is substituted for the thalassemic HSC having deficient erythropoiesis in order to treat thalassemia. This cellular replacement therapy results in the replacement of the entire hematopoietic system rather than just the damaged erythropoietic component. Nonetheless, it is a useful method to achieve a long-lasting, possibly permanent, clinically successful correction of hemolytic anemia, eliminating the need for transfusions and the difficulties that go along with them (i.e., iron overload).

3.8 Risk factors and complications of beta-thalassemia

Family ancestry and heritage are factors that increment the danger of beta-thalassemia. Contingent upon family ancestry, in case an individual's folks or grandparents had beta-thalassemia major or intermedia, there is a 75% (3 out of 4) likelihood of the transformed quality being acquired by a posterity. Regardless of whether a youngster does not have beta-thalassemia major or intermedia, they can in any case be a transporter, potentially bringing about people in the future of their posterity having beta-thalassemia. Another danger factor is lineage. Beta-thalassemia happens regularly in individuals of Italian, Greek, Center Eastern, Southern Asian, and African heritage [57].

Complexities of beta-thalassemia change contingent upon the kind:

- Thalassemia minima is gentle and causes no issues. However, the singular will be a transporter of the issue.

- Thalassemia intermedia can cause issues dependent on the seriousness of the weakness. These issues incorporate postponed development, feeble bones, and augmented spleen.

- Beta-thalassemia significant messes major up and can bring about early passing. Entanglements might incorporate postponed development, bone issues causing facial changes, liver and nerve bladder issues, expanded spleen, augmented kidneys, diabetes, hypothyroidism, and heart issues.

3.9 Prevention of beta-thalassemia

Beta-thalassemia is an innate sickness taking into consideration a safeguard therapy via transporter screening and pre-birth conclusion. It very well may be forestalled in the event that one parent has ordinary qualities, leading to screenings that engage transporters to choose accomplices with typical hemoglobin [58]. This screening technique demonstrated obtuse in populaces of West African family line in light of the markers has high pervasiveness of alpha thalassemia. Nations have programs dispersing data about the regenerative dangers related with transporters of haemoglobinopathies. Thalassemia transporter screening programs have instructive projects in schools, military, and through broad communications just as giving guiding to transporters and transporter couples [12]. Screening has shown diminished rate; by 1995 the commonness in Italy decreased from 1:250 to 1:4000, and a 95%

abatement around there. The reduction in occurrence has helped those influenced with thalassemia, as the interest for blood has diminished, accordingly working on the stock of treatment.

4. Conclusions

Thalassemia is a perplexing condition that needs in-depth approach for lab testing and analysis. High-throughput testing algorithms and procedures are needed for population screening in high-prevalence areas, which increases the difficulty of the diagnosis. Despite this, current best-practice guidelines and protocols are capable of the successful regulation of complicated laboratory procedures, coupled with essential EQA programs. Many novel methods are now being developed that have the potential to improve the accuracy, throughput, and efficacy of laboratory diagnostics of thalassemia and other hemoglobinopathies.

The majority of families cannot afford the estimated US $ 3200 per child per year expense of treating serious thalassemia disease. Thalassemia management is not only distressing for the family but also has a significant socioeconomic impact on the nation, making its prevention and control a top priority. So, the first step toward easing the disease's burden is to prevent the birth of any afflicted fetuses.

Prenatal diagnosis (PND), genetic counseling, carrier screening, and termination of the afflicted fetus are all parts of prevention. This strategy is affordable and reducing the prevalence of thalassemia in many nations with remarkable results. Understanding the range and distribution of thalassemia mutations in a given population is a requirement for an efficient and quick prenatal diagnosis/genetic counseling.

Author details

Kenneth Oshiokhayamhe Iyevhobu[1*], Lucky E. Omolumen[2], Tobechukwu Joseph Okobi[3], Edidiong Raphael Usoro[4], A. Airefetalor Ivie[1], Benedicta A. Ken-Iyevhobu[5] and O. Omokpo Victoria[6]

1 CEPI/ISTH Lassa Fever Epidemiology Study, Irrua Specialist Teaching Hospital (ISTH), Nigeria

2 Faculty of Medical Laboratory Science, Department of Chemical Pathology, Ambrose Alli University, Nigeria

3 Biology Department, Georgetown University, Washington, USA

4 Department of Biomedical Sciences, Augusta University, Augusta, USA

5 Department of Microbiology, Ambrose Alli University, Nigeria

6 Department of Biological Sciences, School of Applied Science, Auchi Polytechnic Auchi, Nigeria

*Address all correspondence to: kennylamai@yahoo.com

References

[1] De Sanctis V, Kattamis C, Canatan D, Soliman AT, Elsedfy H, Karimi M, et al. β-Thalassemia distribution in the old world: An ancient disease seen from a historical standpoint. Mediterranean Journal of Hematology and Infectious Diseases. 2017;**9**:e2017018

[2] Modell B, Darlison M. Global epidemiology of haemoglobin disorders and derived service indicators. Bulletin of the World Health Organization. 2008;**86**:480-487

[3] Williams TN, Weatherall DJ. World distribution, population genetics, and health burden of the hemoglobinopathies. Cold Spring Harbor Perspectives in Medicine. 2012;**2**:a011692

[4] Thein SL. The molecular basis of β-thalassemia. Cold Spring Harbor Perspectives in Medicine. 2013;**3**:a011700

[5] Taher AT, Weatherall DJ, Cappellini MD. Thalassaemia. Lancet. 2018;**391**:155-167

[6] Bain BJ. The alpha, beta, delta and gamma thalassaemias and related conditions. In: Haemoglobinopathy Diagnosis. 2nd ed. Oxford: Wiley-Blackwell; 2006. pp. 63-138

[7] Cao A, Kan YW. The prevention of thalassemia. Cold Spring Harbor Perspectives in Medicine. 2013;**3**:a011775

[8] Angastiniotis M, Eleftheriou A, Galanello R, Harteveld CL, Petrou M, Traeger-Synodinos J, et al. Prevention of Thalassaemias and Other Haemoglobin Disorders: Volume 1: Principles [Internet]. Old J, editor. 2nd ed. Nicosia (Cyprus): Thalassaemia International Federation; 2013. PMID: 24672827

[9] Flint J, Harding RM, Boyce AJ, Clegg JB. The population genetics of the haemoglobinopathies. Baillière's Clinical Haematology. 1998;**11**(1):1-51

[10] Origa R. Beta-Thalassemia. 2000 Sep 28 [updated 2018 Jan 25]. In: Adam MP, Ardinger HH, Pagon RA, Wallace SE, LJH B, Stephens K, Amemiya A, editors. GeneReviews® [Internet]. Seattle; 1993-2020: Seattle (WA): University of Washington; 2020 Available from: http://www.ncbi.nlm.nih.gov/books/NBK1426/CitationonPubMed

[11] Rund D, Rachmilewitz E. Beta-thalassemia. The New England Journal of Medicine. 2005;**353**(11):1135-1146

[12] Akhavan-Niaki H, Derakhshandeh-Peykar P, Banihashemi A, Mostafazadeh A, Asghari B, Ahmadifard MR, et al. A comprehensive molecular characterization of beta thalassemia in a highly heterogeneous population. Blood Cells, Molecules & Diseases. 2011;**47**(1):29-32

[13] Islam MT, Sarkar SK, Sultana N, Begum MN, Bhuyan GS, Talukder S, et al. High resolution melting curve analysis targeting the HBB gene mutational hot-spot offers a reliable screening approach for all common as well as most of the rare beta-globin gene mutations in Bangladesh. BMC Genetics. 2018;**19**(1):1

[14] Thein SL. Genetic modifiers of beta-thalassemia. Haematologica. 2005;**90**(5):649-660

[15] Aguilar Martinez P, Angastiniotis M, Eleftheriou A, Gulbis B, Manú Pereira M, Del Petrova-Benedict R, et al. Haemoglobinopathies in Europe: Health & migration policy perspectives. Orphanet Journal of Rare Diseases. 2014;**9**:97

[16] Angastiniotis M, Vives Corrons JL, Soteriades ES, Eleftheriou A. The impact of migrations on the health services for rare diseases in Europe: The example of haemoglobin disorders. Scientific World Journal. 2013;**2013**:727905

[17] Modell B, Darlison M, Birgens H, Cario H, Faustino P, Giordano PC, et al. Epidemiology of haemoglobin disorders in Europe: An overview. Scandinavian Journal of Clinical and Laboratory Investigation. 2007;**67**:39-70

[18] Piel FB, Tatem AJ, Huang Z, Gupta S, Williams TN, Weatherall DJ. Global migration and the changing distribution of sickle haemoglobin: A quantitative study of temporal trends between 1960 and 2000. The Lancet Global Health. 2014;**2**:e80-e89

[19] Sankaran VG, Orkin SH. The switch from fetal to adult hemoglobin. Cold Spring Harbor Perspectives in Medicine. 2013;**3**:a011643

[20] Wang X, Thein SL. Switching from fetal to adult hemoglobin. Nature Genetics. Apr 2018;**50**(4):478-480. DOI: 10.1038/s41588-018-0094-z. PMID: 29610477; PMCID: PMC6419756

[21] Vichinsky EP. Changing patterns of thalassemia worldwide. Annals of the New York Academy of Sciences. 2005;**2005**(1054):18-24

[22] Cao A, Galanello R. Beta-thalassemia. Genetics in Medicine. 2010;**12**:61-76

[23] Borgna-Pignatti C, Galanello R. Thalassemias and related disorders: Quantitative disorders of hemoglobin synthesis. In: Wintrobe's Clinical Hematology. 11th ed. Vol. 42. Philadelphia: Lippincott Williams & Wilkins; 2004. pp. 1319-1365

[24] Borgna-Pignatti C, Cappellini MD, De Stefano P, Del Vecchio GC, Forni GL, Gamberini MR, et al. Survival and complications in thalassemia. Annals of the New York Academy of Sciences. 2005;**1054**:40-47

[25] Galanello R, Piras S, Barella S, Leoni GB, Cipollina MD, Perseu L, et al. Cholelithiasis and Gilbert's syndrome in homozygous betathalassemia. British Journal of Haematology. 2001;**115**:926-928

[26] Taher AT, Otrock ZK, Uthman I, Cappellini MD. Thalassemia and hypercoagulability. Blood Reviews. 2008;**22**:283-292

[27] De Sanctis V, Tangerini A, Testa MR, Lauriola AL, Gamberini MR, Cavallini AR, et al. Final height and endocrine function in thalassemia intermedia. Journal of Pediatric Endocrinology & Metabolism. 1998;**11**:965-971

[28] Nassar AH, Naja M, Cesaretti C, Eprassi B, Cappellini MD, Taher A. Pregnancy outcome in patients with beta-thalassemia intermedia at two tertiary care centers, in Beirut and Milan. Haematologica. 2008;**93**:1586-1587

[29] Aessopos A, Farmakis D, Deftereos S, Tsironi M, Tassiopoulos S, Moyssakis I, et al. Thalassemia heart disease: A comparative evaluation of thalassemia major and thalassemia intermedia. Chest. 2005;**127**:1523-1530

[30] Aessopos A, Farmakis D, Loukopoulos D. Elastic tissue abnormalities resembling pseudoxanthoma elasticum in beta thalassemia and the sickling syndromes. Blood. 2002;**99**:30-35

[31] Galanello R, Origa R. Beta-thalassemia. Orphanet Journal of Rare Diseases. 2010;**5**:11. DOI: 10.1186/1750-1172-5-11

[32] Freson K, Matthijs G, Thys C, Marien P, Hoylaerts MF, Vermylen J, et al. Different substitutions at residue D218 of the X-linked transcription factor GATA1 lead to altered clinical severity of macrothrombocytopenia and anemia and are associated with variable skewed X inactivation. Human Molecular Genetics. 2002;**11**:147-152

[33] Jarjour RA, Murad H, Moasses F, Al-Achkar W. Molecular update of β-thalassemia mutations in the Syrian population: Identification of rare β-thalassemia mutations. Hemoglobin. 2014;**38**(4):272-276

[34] Viprakasit V, Gibbons RJ, Broughton BC, Tolmie JL, Brown D, Lunt P, et al. Mutations in the general transcription factor TFIIH result in beta- thalassemia in individuals with trichothiodystrophy. Human Molecular Genetics. 2001;**10**:2797-2802

[35] Giardine B, van Baal S, Kaimakis P, Riemer C, Miller W, Samara M, et al. HbVar database of human hemoglobin variants and thalassemia mutations: 2007 update. Human Mutation. 2007;**28**:206

[36] Galanello R, Cao A. Relationship between genotype and phenotype. Thalassemia intermedia. Annals of the New York Academy of Sciences. 1998;**850**:325-333

[37] Uda M, Galanello R, Sanna S, Lettre G, Sankaran VG, Chen W, et al. Genome-wide association study shows BCL11A associated with peristent fetal hemoglobin and amelioration of the phenotype of beta-thalassemia. Proceedings of the National Academy of Sciences of the United States of America. 2008;**105**:1620-1625

[38] Origa R, Galanello R, Perseu L, Tavazzi D, Domenica Cappellini M, Terenzani L, et al. Cholelithiasis in thalassemia major. European Journal of Haematology. 2009;**82**:22-25

[39] Economou-Petersen E, Aessopos A, Kladi A, Flevari P, Karabatsos F, Fragodimitri C, et al. Apolipoprotein E epsilon4 allele as a genetic risk factor for left ventricular failure in homozygous betathalassemia. Blood. 1998;**92**:3455-3459

[40] Kremastinos DT, Flevari P, Spyropoulou M, Vrettou H, Tsiapras D, Stavropoulos-Giokas CG. Association of heart failure in homozygous beta-thalassemia with the major histocompatibility complex. Circulation. 1999;**100**:2074-2078

[41] Dresner Pollack R, Rachmilewitz E, Blumenfeld A, Idelson M, Goldfarb AW. Bone mineral metabolism in adults with β-thalassemia major and intermedia. British Journal of Haematology. 2000;**111**:902-907

[42] Longo F, Zecchina G, Sbaiz L, Fischer R, Piga A, Camaschella C. The influence of hemochromatosis mutations on iron overload of thalassemia major. Haematologica. 1999;**84**:799-803

[43] Perrotta S, Cappellini MD, Bertoldo F, Servedio V, Iolascon G, D'Agruma L, et al. Osteoporosis in β-thalassemia major patients: Analysis of the genetic background. British Journal of Haematology. 2000;**111**:461-466

[44] Origa R, Satta S, Matta G, Galanello R. Glutathione S-transferase gene polymorphism and cardiac iron overload in thalassemia major. British Journal of Haematology. 2008;**142**:143-145

[45] Sollaino MC, Paglietti ME, Perseu L, Giagu N, Loi D, Galanello R. Association of alpha globin gene quadruplication and heterozygous beta thalassemia in

patients with thalassemia intermedia. Haematologica. 2009;**94**:1445-1448

[46] Vrettou C, Traeger-Synodinos J, Tzetis M, Malamis G, Kanavakis E. Rapid screening of multiple betaglobin gene mutations by real-time PCR on the LightCycler: Application to carrier screening and prenatal diagnosis of thalassemia syndromes. Clinical Chemistry. 2003;**49**:769-776

[47] Cao A, Galanello R, Rosatelli MC. Prenatal diagnosis and screening of the haemoglobinopathies. Baillière's Clinical Haematology. 1998;**11**:215-238

[48] Mavrou A, Kouvidi E, Antsaklis A, Souka A, Kitsiou Tzeli S, Kolialexi A. Identification of nucleated red blood cells in maternal circulation: A second step in screening for fetal aneuploidies and pregnancy complications. Prenatal Diagnosis. 2007;**27**:150-153

[49] Wonke B. Clinical management of beta-thalassemia major. Seminars in Hematology. 2001;**38**(4):350-359

[50] Borgna-Pignatti C. Modern treatment of thalassaemia intermedia. British Journal of Haematology. 2007;**138**:291-304

[51] Origa R, Galanello R, Ganz T, Giagu N, Maccioni L, Faa G, et al. Liver iron concentrations and urinary hepcidin in beta-thalassemia. Haematologica. 2007;**92**:583-588

[52] Centis F, Tabellini L, Lucarelli G. The importance of erythroid expansion in determining the extent of apoptosis in erythroid precursors in patients with β-thalassemia major. Blood. 2000;**96**(10):3624-3629

[53] Yuan J, Angelucci E, Lucarelli G. Accelerated programmed cell death (apoptosis) in erythroid precursors of patients with severe β-thalassemia (Cooley's anemia). Blood. 1993;**82**(2):374-377

[54] de Franceschi L, Bertoldi M, de Falco L. Oxidative stress modulates heme synthesis and induces peroxiredoxin-2 as a novel cytoprotective response in β-thalassemic erythropoiesis. Haematologica. 2011;**96**(11):1595-1604

[55] Leecharoenkiat A, Wannatung T, Lithanatudom P. Increased oxidative metabolism is associated with erythroid precursor expansion in β0-thalassaemia/ Hb E disease. Blood Cells, Molecules and Diseases. 2011;**47**(3):143-157

[56] Mathias LA, Fisher TC, Zeng L. Ineffective erythropoiesis in β-thalassemia major is due to apoptosis at the polychromatophilic normoblast stage. Experimental Hematology. 2000;**28**(12):1343-1353

[57] Mayo Clinic. Risk factors. 2017. Available from: http://www.mayoclinic.org/diseases-conditions/thalassemia/symptoms-causes/dxc-20261829). Retrieved 14 Oct 2020

[58] Cousens NE, Gaff CL, Metcalfe SA, Delatycki MB. Carrier screening for Betathalassaemia: A review of international practice. European Journal of Human Genetics. 2010;**18**(10):1077-1083

Chapter 2

Effects of Beta-Thalassemia on COVID-19 Outcomes

Simran Patel, Armaan Shah, Ryan Kaiser and Raj Wadgaonkar

Abstract

Beta-thalassemia is a hemoglobinopathy caused by mutations in the beta-globin chain. This disrupts hemoglobin production and can potentially result in severe anemia. There has been a rise in COVID-19 cases over the last 2 years, with a predominant effect on the respiratory and vascular systems of the body. Since beta-thalassemia is the most common inherited single-gene disorder in the world, investigating the impact of COVID-19 on these patients is important. Some theories suggest that patients with beta-thalassemia will be more susceptible to COVID-19 and have worse outcomes due to their underlying comorbid conditions. However, majority of the literature found that beta-thalassemia is protective against COVID-19. This could be because SARS-CoV-2 proteins can attack the beta chain of normal hemoglobin, resulting in impaired oxygen transfer and increased ferritinemia. Thus, in hemoglobinopathies with beta-chain defects and low hepcidin levels, susceptibility to COVID-19 infection is potentially decreased. Higher levels of Hemoglobin F in thalassemia patients may also be protective against viral infections. Surprisingly, most studies and case reports focus on patients with beta-thalassemia major. There is yet much to learn about the outcomes of patients with thalassemia minor and other hemoglobinopathies.

Keywords: thalassemia, beta-thalassemia, COVID-19, SARSCoV-2, coronavirus

1. Introduction

Thalassemias are a group of autosomal recessive blood disorders caused by variations in alpha or beta globin genes that disrupt hemoglobin production and lead to ineffective erythropoiesis and hemolysis [1]. Given that hemoglobin serves as the oxygen-carrying component of red blood cells (RBCs), inadequate production can cause severe anemia and other life-threatening complications requiring frequent blood transfusions to maintain hemoglobin levels. Individuals affected by these disorders can start presenting with symptoms early in childhood and last for their entire lifetime.

Hemoglobin is made up of two chains: alpha-globin and beta-globin chains. Alpha thalassemia is generally caused by alpha-globin gene deletion that results in either reduced or absent alpha-globin production. Since the alpha-globin gene has four alleles, disease severity is dependent on the number of deleted alleles. One deletion can be clinically silent, whereas four deletions can be incompatible with life and lead

IntechOpen

to hydrops fetalis [1]. Beta thalassemia is generally caused by beta-globin gene point mutations that are classified based on the zygosity of the gene mutation. A heterozygous mutation will result in one defective and one normal gene allowing for some production of the beta-globin chains. This is the mildest form of beta-thalassemia. A homozygous mutation will result in two defective genes causing a total absence of beta-globin chains. This mutation can lead to moderate to severe symptoms. Since the alpha and beta-globin chains are insoluble alone, they can precipitate and lead to damage to RBC membranes and intravascular hemolysis [1].

The impact of severe acute respiratory syndrome coronavirus 2 (SARS-CoV-2) has reached the entire globe over the last 2 years and resulted in millions of deaths. It primarily targets the respiratory and vascular systems of the body. Since beta-thalassemia is the most common inherited single-gene disorder in the world and can affect the oxygen-carrying capacity of the body, investigating the impact of COVID-19 on these patients is important given the limited research data currently available [2].

2. Classifications of beta-thalassemia

The disease burden of beta-thalassemia depends on the zygosity of the beta-globin chain gene mutation. There are three main types of beta-thalassemia: beta-thalassemia major, beta-thalassemia intermedia, and beta-thalassemia minor [3].

2.1 Beta-thalassemia major

Individuals who are homozygous for the beta-globin chain mutation are classified as having beta-thalassemia major and completely lack beta chains. The manifestations of beta-thalassemia major are much more severe than beta-thalassemia minor and can result in jaundice, growth retardation, hepatosplenomegaly, endocrine abnormalities, and severe anemia. Symptoms begin at the age of 6 months when fetal hemoglobin is completely replaced by defective globin chains that accumulate and damage RBC membranes. Patients at this stage may present with failure to thrive and require lifelong blood transfusion and iron chelation therapy [3]. The classic clinical picture of beta-thalassemia major is primarily seen in underdeveloped countries where long-term transfusion facilities are not widely available. Patients who are inadequately treated for beta-thalassemia major commonly present with brown pigmentation of the skin, poor musculature, genu valgum, development of masses from extramedullary hematopoiesis, and skeletal changes in the long bones of the legs and craniofacial structures due to expansion of the bone marrow. Individuals not receiving regular transfusion therapy may die from high-out cardiac failure. Adequate maintenance of a minimum hemoglobin level between 9.0 and 10.5 g/dl ineffective erythropoiesis can be inhibited and regular growth and development can occur up to 10–12 years [3]. However, the complications of iron overload from repeated transfusions may manifest in children with growth retardation and failure of sexual maturation and in adults with liver fibrosis and cirrhosis, endocrine dysfunction resulting in diabetes mellitus and parathyroid insufficiency, and cardiac disease including dilated cardiomyopathy and arrhythmias. Hence, adequate iron chelation therapy is necessary as well. In the early 2000s, 50% of beta-thalassemia major patients died before the age of 35 due to all these complications. With the advent of new developments of noninvasive methods to measure organ iron levels and chelation therapy, the prognosis of beta thalassemia major has greatly improved [1–3].

2.2 Beta-thalassemia intermedia

Patients with beta-thalassemia intermedia can present much later in life than those with beta-thalassemia major. They have milder anemia symptoms and may still require transfusions but much less frequent, if at all. They can remain asymptomatic until adulthood, during which they may develop clinical features such as pallor, jaundice, cholelithiasis, hepatosplenomegaly, extramedullary masses of hyperplastic erythroid marrow, osteopenia, osteoporosis, and thrombotic complications. Patients can present with cardiac manifestations as well, including high-cardiac output and pulmonary hypertension with preserved systolic function [3]. Pseudoxanthoma elasticum, a disease caused by the accumulation of calcium deposits in elastic fibers in the skin, eyes, and blood vessels, is also common among beta-thalassemia intermedia patients [3]. Although the rate of iron loading is slower in these patients, similar complications can still occur if proper iron chelation therapy is not administered [1–3].

2.3 Beta-thalassemia minor

Heterozygotes of the beta-globin chain mutation are classified as having beta-thalassemia minor in which beta chains are being produced to a lesser degree than normal. Patients are generally asymptomatic or have mild anemia symptoms [1–3].

3. Epidemiology of beta-thalassemia

Beta-thalassemia is most prevalent in the Mediterranean and Middle East populations but is also common in regions of Southeast Asia. It has been less prevalent in regions of Northern Europe and North America. It is reported that 80–90 million people are carriers of this disease, making up about 1.5% of the global population [4]. According to a report published by the World Health Organization in 2008, more than 40,000 infants are born with beta-thalassemia annually, the majority of whom are transfusion-dependent. Roughly 205,000 newborns with beta-thalassemia are born in Southeast Asia, 10,000 in the Eastern Mediterranean region, 1000 in Europe, and 350 in North, Central, and South America. Thailand alone has close to 4000 new cases of beta-thalassemia annually. Only a few European countries have reported incidences of beta-thalassemia major, including Belgium which reported 1 in 25,000 neonates being born with beta-thalassemia, and 1 in 113,000 neonates in France between 2005 and 2008. In the United States, an incidence of 1 in 55,000 newborns was reported in California [4]. The high prevalence of beta-thalassemia in certain regions can be explained by multiple factors. There is a higher carrier rate and a cultural preference for consanguineous marriages in the Middle East. Increases in rates of migration from areas with a higher prevalence of beta-thalassemia to non-endemic areas have led to a higher prevalence of the disease in some European and Northern American regions. Also, with the improvement of health resources and access to blood transfusion centers, and adequate iron chelation therapy, survival rates have increased significantly, adding to the prevalence of beta-thalassemia [3, 4].

Comprehensive prevention programs have been put in place in endemic areas of beta-thalassemia, with a focus on public education, genetic counseling, population screening, and prenatal diagnostic testing. The Greek National Registry for Hemoglobinopathies reported a lower incidence of beta-thalassemia compared to what was expected based on the prevalence of carriers in the population [4]. Similar trends have been noted in Iran and Iraq as well, suggesting that thalassemia these programs have been effective in reducing the prevalence of the disease in some regions.

4. Beta-globin gene mutations causing beta-thalassemia

The beta-globin chain is encoded by a structural gene on chromosome 11 that is clustered with five other beta-like genes including ε(HBE), Gγ (HBG2), Aγ (HBG1), δ (HBD), and β (HBB) [5]. These genes are arranged on the chromosome based on the order of their developmental expression and are dependent on local promotor sequences and upstream control regions which bind to various erythroid-specific transcription factors (e.g. GATA-1, GATA-2, NF-E2, KLF1) and co-factors (e.g. FOG, p300). The controlled gene expression leads to the production of specific hemoglobin tetramers including embryonic (Hb Gower-1 (ζ2ε2), Hb Gower-2 (α2ε2), and Hb Portland (ζ2β2)), fetal (α2γ2), and adult (HbA, α2β2 and HbA2, α2δ2). Each is produced at a distinct stage of development, allowing for the process of hemoglobin switching to occur between the embryonic, fetal, and adult stages of life [5].

Fetal hemoglobin (HbF) is the primary hemoglobin from birth till about 6 months of age. Since it is made up of two alpha and two gamma chains and no beta chains, the manifestations of beta-thalassemia are not seen until after 6 months. When HbF levels drop and make up less than 5% of the total hemoglobin content of the body, it is replaced with adult hemoglobin (HbA), which is made up of two alpha and two beta chains. Since beta chain production is disrupted in beta-thalassemia, symptoms begin during this time. Hydroxyurea is an agent that upregulates gamma-globin gene production leading to increased HbF production. Though this therapy is widely used in sickle cell disease, its efficiency in beta-thalassemia is still being investigated [5–7].

There have been more than 300 beta-thalassemia alleles reported in the literature. However, only about 40 account for more than 90% of beta-thalassemia worldwide likely because only a few mutations are common in endemic regions. Downregulation of the beta-globin chain can be caused by a variety of molecular changes such as point mutations, small deletions limited to the beta-globin genes, or even extensive deletions of this region. However, most mutations are non-deletional. They may be single-base substitutions and small insertions or deletions of only a few bases within the gene. These mutations can lead to downregulation of the beta-globin gene throughout all stages of gene expression including transcription of the gene from DNA into mRNA to translation of the mRNA into a functional protein [5, 6]. Very rarely do larger deletions in the beta-globin gene result in beta-thalassemia. There are 18 deletions specifically on the beta-globin gene that have been found to cause beta-thalassemia. They range from 25 base pairs to about 6000 base pairs [5].

5. Pathophysiology of beta-thalassemia

Hemoglobin A is a tetrameter made up of two heterodimers each consisting of one alpha and one beta globin chain, attached to a heme moiety in the center. A balanced production these chains is crucial and tightly regulated. Once the globin chains combine, they are highly soluble in RBCs. However, if left unbound, these globin chains are highly insoluble and can accumulate in the blood. In beta-thalassemia, excess alpha-globin chains begin aggregating as soon as they accumulate in erythroid precursors and precipitate adjacent to the RBC membrane in early marrow erythroid precursors. This disrupts proper membrane assembly and can accelerate apoptosis [8–11].

5.1 Effects of beta-thalassemia on red blood cells

In normal physiology, hemoglobin in RBCs is oxidized to methemoglobin and subsequently reduced back to native hemoglobin. However, in patients with beta-thalassemia, the unpaired alpha chains attached to a heme moiety are more susceptible to oxidation and proteolysis, leading to the formation of hemichromes. These hemichromes can generate reactive oxygen species that in turn oxidize adjacent RBC membrane proteins and lipids. This can cause damage to the membrane by affecting the globin chains that bind to the membrane and directly altering cytoskeletal and integral membrane proteins [8–11].

Normal RBC precursors undergo cytoskeletal and membrane assembly via spectrin, band 4.1, band 3, and several other proteins. The asymmetry of the phospholipid bilayer that naturally exists between the inner and outer leaflets of the membrane is disrupted with oxidative damage and results in a disorderly and discontinuous pattern of membrane protein incorporation, especially in the regions with alpha chain aggregates [12]. There is also a lack of membrane stability caused by an oxidative injury that hinders the ability and inability to handle sheer stress [13]. All these changes are responsible for the abnormal maturation of RBCs in beta-thalassemia. Although the use of proteases may be used to treat membrane damage caused by an accumulation of globin chains by directly attacking and partially destroying the chains, they do not aid in their elimination from the body [14].

Beta-thalassemia can also affect the hydration of RBCs and result in their dehydration. This may be due to excessive activation of the potassium-chloride cotransport system, which is responsible for controlling potassium chloride loss in the body. Excessive activation results in the loss of these ions, leading to the loss of water as well. The resultant dehydration can cause a high mean cell hemoglobin concentration and a dense appearance on peripheral blood smears [13]. The flexible nature of RBCs allows for them to travel through the capillary circulation and the reticuloendothelial system lined by phagocytic cells lie within the spleen, liver, and lungs. The dehydration of RBCs caused by beta-thalassemia can affect this essential property and cause a delay in RBC passage and increased engulfment by macrophages [13, 15].

5.2 Causes of anemia in beta-thalassemia

Ineffective erythropoiesis refers to a decrease in the production of RBCs due to the destruction of maturing erythroblasts from either apoptosis or hemolysis. In patients with thalassemia, ineffective erythropoiesis leads to the expansion of the erythroid progenitor cell population and acceleration of differentiation, and mature arrest at the polychromatophilic erythroblast stage [16].

Some causes of ineffective erythropoiesis include apoptosis of erythroid precursors. Studies have shown that a possible mechanism for this apoptosis in beta-thalassemia patients involves the sequestration of heat shock proteins by free alpha-globin chains contained within the cytoplasm of precursor RBCs. These heat shock proteins are generally expressed in response to stress and play an important role in the stabilization of the cell [17]. The caspase and cytochrome proteins, which regulate apoptosis, were also found to be abnormally phosphorylated in the bone marrow erythroblasts of some beta-thalassemia patients [18]. Apoptosis of cells can result in the movement of phosphatidylserine from the inner to the outer leaflet of RBC membranes, which serves as a signal for the removal of the cell by macrophages in the reticuloendothelial system [19].

Adverse consequences of ineffective erythropoiesis can arise at peripheral locations and result in extramedullary hematopoiesis, which is the production of RBCs outside of the bone marrow. This process is driven by a rise in erythropoietin levels and can manifest with the expansion of bone marrow cavities that can distort long bone, head, and facial bones that are not common sites of erythropoiesis. Ineffective erythropoiesis can also result in increased iron absorption, which is accompanied by its own set of complications.

Hemolysis can also lead to anemia in beta-thalassemia patients and can shorten the lifespan of the RBC by a third. This hemolysis is caused by the aggregation and oxidation of RBC membranes, resulting in mechanical property changes such as increased rigidity and dehydration that inhibit their smooth passage within the reticuloendothelial system and allow more time for macrophages to phagocytose the cells. Studies show that patients who have undergone splenectomies are more likely to be observed with unstable and deformed RBCs [20–22].

6. COVID-19

In late 2019, the first cases of mysterious pneumonia of unspecified origin were seen in Wuhan, the capital of Hubei province, China. Later, it would be confirmed that these cases were caused by the coronavirus disease 2019 (COVID-19). This pathogen belongs to the enveloped RNA beta coronavirus family. Due to its similarities with the original severe acute respiratory syndrome coronavirus (SARS-CoV-2) and Middle East Respiratory Syndrome (MERS) viruses, it was named SARS-CoV-2. Over the past 2–3 years, a staggering number of studies have explored the epidemiology and clinical presentation of COVID-19. However, there remains much to be learned regarding how the virus impacts the respiratory system both in the short and long term and how it affects those with chronic conditions such as hemoglobinopathies. Taking a macroscopic view, data classifies the presentation of the disease as mild, severe, or critical [23, 24]. A common symptom that is independently associated with in-hospital mortality is the severity of hypoxemia; this symptom has been described as a potentially important predictor of whether a patient requires intensive care.

6.1 Pathophysiology of hypoxemia in COVID-19

Arterial hypoxemia, an early sequela of COVID-19 infection, is caused mainly due to a V/Q mismatch. Continued blood flow to non-ventilated alveoli increased the P(A-a) O2 gradient. Infection also causes interstitial edema, particularly in structures with elastic properties responsible for withstanding stress and strain. This edema can lead to the appearance of ground-glass opacities and consolidation on chest X-ray or computerized tomographic imaging. Additionally, the edema causes loss of surfactant and increased superimposed pressure on lung parenchyma, eventually leading to alveolar collapse. While this occurs, a moderate amount of cardiac output continues to perfuse these collapsed areas, causing intrapulmonary shunting. The body's response to this is increased effort of breathing and use of accessory muscles, causing a rise in tidal volume, and subsequently, negative inspiratory intrathoracic pressure. Inflammation also causes increased lung permeability, which when combined with the increase in negative intrathoracic pressure, leads to progressive edema, alveolar flooding, and effusions. Over time, this causes a severe decline in the quality of oxygenation and increases shunt fraction which is difficult to correct by increasing FiO2 [25].

While useful, clinicians should take caution when using oxygen saturation measured by pulse oximetry (SpO2) to detect hypoxemia. Tachypnea and hyperpnea due to infection, as described above, cause respiratory alkalosis and subsequent drop in PaCO2. This leads to a left shift in the oxyhemoglobin dissociation curve. Increased affinity of hemoglobin for oxygen during these periods can result in a paradoxical finding of preserved SpO2 during states of low PaO2 [25–27]. Another theory for the left-ward shift of the oxy-hemoglobin curve in COVID-19 was put forth by Rapozzi et al. Their hypothesis states that serum heme levels increase in COVID-19 infection, along with harmful iron ions ($Fe3+$) which cause inflammation and cell death. However, the interaction of the virus and abnormal heme groups remains to be studied. The apparently increased oxygen affinity of hemoglobin leads to lower tissue perfusion and extremity ischemia in patients with normal hemoglobin structure. However, for patients with thalassemias or sickle cell disease that may be on HbF treatment, the changes in the oxy-hemoglobin curve may shed light on if having hemoglobinopathies is protective or not against infection [26].

Further exploration of how COVID-19 affects erythrocytes and hemoglobin was done by the group. They propose that viral protein ORF8 and a surface glycoprotein of COVID-19 damaged the 1-beta chain of deoxyhemoglobin via docking with porphyrin and lead to the release of iron-free porphyrins. This interaction is intriguing. If it can be proven in vitro settings, this apparent interaction could explain cases where having beta-thalassemia has been shown to be protective against COVID- 19 infections. An absence of a beta-hemoglobin chain would leave the virus unable to negatively affect the oxygen binding capacity of existing hemoglobin chains, especially in patients that have increased HbF due to hydroxyurea therapies [26].

6.2 COVID-19 and beta-thalassemia

Multiple studies have been conducted to study the relationship between beta-thalassemia and COVID-19 infection. These studies have been piloted by groups mainly from countries where thalassemias have a higher prevalence, such as the Mediterranean and Middle Eastern nations. Researchers from these nations posit two hypotheses regarding the susceptibility of beta-thalassemia patients to COVID-19. One theory states that patients with beta-thalassemia may be more susceptible to COVID-19 infection and have worse outcomes due to chronic conditions such as heart disease, liver disease, iron overload, adrenal insufficiency, diabetes, and splenectomy. Being in a prolonged state of oxidative stress can lead to immunosuppression and thus worsen the body's innate ability to combat infection. A latent effect of beta-thalassemia is the need for ongoing medical treatment and attention that these patients need. Frequent visits to hospitals or medical centers for blood transfusion and complication management increase these patients' exposure to COVID-19. A second theory, however, proposes a different possibility. It suggests that patients who are heterozygous for beta-thalassemia may have immunity against COVID-19 infection. This is in part because beta-thalassemia patients have a higher concentration of HbF, which possesses a unique tetramer structure. The exact protective potential of HbF in COVID-19 infection remains to be studied [27].

Figure 1 is a hypothetical representation of the interaction between the SARS-CoV-2 virus and the erythrocytes infected [28]. The internalization process is the virus is dependent on TMPRSS2, a serine protease, and angiotensin-converting enzyme type 2 (ACE-2), which allow entry of the virus into the cell. Once in the cell, the infection would activate metabolic processes that would result in oxidative stress. This negatively affects erythrocytes and would cause their destruction. The release of Fe^{2+} from damaged erythrocytes would further propel the metabolic reactions leading to oxidative stress. Remnants of alpha and beta hemoglobin chains would also be released into the intercellular space [28].

6.2.1 Review of published studies

A study from Iran describes 43 patients with beta-thalassemia from the ages of 9–67 years who contracted COVID-19. These patients were both transfusion-dependent and transfusion-independent. Results showed that transfusion-independent patients had a higher mortality rate (27.3%) than patients who were receiving regular transfusions (4.71%). Patients in the transfusion-independent category were found to be in a persistent chronic anemic state with hypercoagulability. Additionally, micro thrombosis made these patients more likely to develop pulmonary artery hypertension and heart failure. However, overall, the study found that the prevalence of COVID-19 infections in the beta-thalassemia population was lower than in the general population. Another report from the same group describes that in 48 patients with beta-thalassemia from ages 9–67, 8 (16.7%) died from COVID-19. Compared to the general population, while patients with beta-thalassemia had a lower prevalence of COVID-19 infection, those that did contract the disease had higher mortality [29, 30].

An Italian group studied individuals with thalassemia who contracted COVID-19 and had 15 days of follow-up from symptom onset of positive SARS-CoV2 positivity. They collected data on 11 patients, mainly centered in northern Italy. Patients ranged from ages 31–61 years with a majority being female. Ten patients were transfusion-dependent, and one was not. Eight of these patients were splenectomized and all patients had thalassemia-associated comorbidities. Six of the patients were hospitalized with mild-moderate upper respiratory symptoms but did not require mechanical

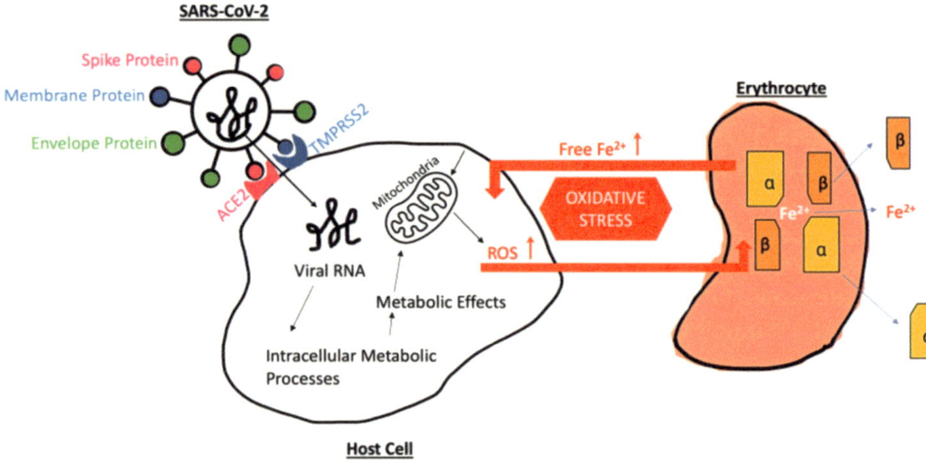

Figure 1.
SARS-CoV-2 entry into host cell and resultant erythrocyte damage.

ventilation. Three patients were asymptomatic. One patient developed severe symptoms of high fever, agranulocytosis, and lymphopenia. This patient also required intensive ventilation support with continuous positive airway pressure. Of the six hospitalized patients, the clinical course ranged from 10 to 29 days. Splenectomy was not found to affect the clinical course of any of the patients. One surprising finding was the apparent lack of severe acute respiratory syndrome in the patients, as well as a lack of signs of cytokine storm or death given the mean age and comorbidities of the patient population. From their preliminary data, the research team concluded that thalassemia did not increase the severity of COVID-19 disease progression [31].

A French study showed that most of the cases of COVID-19 and thalassemia had a favorable outcome in France. The study proposed that this was most likely due to the rarity of the most severe hemochromatosis-related complications such as diabetes, heart failure, cirrhosis, or iron overload in transfusion-dependent patients. However, the study also reported that patients with signs of iron overload detectable via MRI had an increased risk of thromboembolism events, particularly renal or hematological side effects [32].

Most recently, a systematic review meta-analysis of three papers from France in July 2022 described the susceptibility of beta-thalassemia carriers and COVID-19 susceptibility. Based on their findings and after conducting statistical analysis the study found that beta-thalassemia patients were less susceptible to COVID-19 but had higher mortality if infected when compared to the general population. Those that had an ICU course that did not result in death tended to have a shorter ICU stay when compared to patients with no hemoglobinopathies. While the sample size of this systematic review was small, it shows interesting evidence to further showcase the potential protective effects of beta-thalassemia in COVID-19 infections [33].

6.2.2 Review of case reports

A multitude of case reports showcasing the outcomes of COVID-19 infection in patients with hemoglobinopathies has been published. From Indonesia, four beta-thalassemia pediatric patients developed mild COVID-19 infection with one developing thrombosis supported by elevated D-dimer [34]. In Italy, a 59-year-old woman who was transfusion-dependent developed a mild COVID-19 infection [35]. In Pakistan, two patients developed a mild infection as well, with one of the patients having a prior splenectomy [36]. Most case reports describe the infection progression in pediatric patients, while also reporting benign infection courses for all patients.

6.2.3 Summary of findings

Almost universally, the presented studies highlight the relatively young population of patients with COVID-19 and thalassemia had a favorable outcome probably due to the rarity of the most severe hemochromatosis complications. Specific risks related to both thalassemia-related co-morbidities and long-term treatments should be considered. No clear-cut separation between the direct effect of thalassemia on hemoglobin structure and the effect of systemic comorbidities on COVID-19 outcomes has been established.

SARS-CoV-2 proteins can attack the beta chain of hemoglobin, resulting in impaired oxygen transfer and increased ferritinemia. Thus, in hemoglobinopathies with beta chain defects and low hepcidin levels, susceptibility to COVID-19 infection might decrease. Higher levels of HbF in thalassemia patients may be protective against viral infections; the anti-parasitic effect of HbF has been well-documented in areas where malaria is endemic. Studies have attributed lower COVID-19-related mortality in tropical countries where there is a higher prevalence of thalassemias/sickle cell disease due to the increased use of hydroxyurea which induces HbF production. This theory supports the pursuit of clinical studies analyzing the role of HbF-inducing therapies as treatment for COVID-19. Hydroxyurea is a medication used in patients with thalassemia intermedia. Its anti-inflammatory function, antiviral effect, and induction of HbF levels might suggest the benefit of hydroxyurea against the severe forms of COVID-19 [37, 38].

Splenectomy is a common therapeutic intervention in thalassemias, but it might increase the risk of coagulopathy and cytokine storms. However, there is no evidence that splenectomy increases the risk of severe COVID-19 in asplenic/hyposplenic patients [39]. High ferritin levels might be a negative prognostic factor in patients with COVID-19, and iron chelation might be beneficial against COVID-19 [40]. Patients with hemoglobinopathies, including those with thalassemias, are at increased risk of developing severe complications of COVID-19. Lifestyle and nutrition controls are important in controlling their infection, and vitamin D supplementation is beneficial against viral and bacterial infections. Two trace elements, zinc, and selenium are involved in the immune system's integrity and are necessary for beta-thalassemia patients during the COVID-19 pandemic.

6.2.4 Socio-economic factors affecting patients with beta-thalassemia

Most infants born with beta-thalassemia are in Southeast Asia and the Middle East. Nations in these geographical locations are still developing standardized and accessible healthcare for their citizens. While patient education and screening measures have been taken and some countries, such as Iran and Greece, have reported a lower incidence of thalassemias, there remains a stark asymmetry in access to proper healthcare in developing nations when compared to nations of the European Union and North America. As a result, it is possible that many patients who suffer from hemoglobinopathies may not have access to or be educated about when to seek healthcare. This results in lower data from clinical sources for studies such as those listed above. Additionally, due to the small sample size of the studies listed above, the power of each outcome is low. While some of the results reported are seen as significant after statistical analysis, it is not possible to generalize these findings without further inquiry. The potential protective nature of thalassemias in COVID-19 infection may not be relevant if patients who do contract the disease have higher mortality when compared to the general population [41].

6.3 Vaccines for patients with beta-thalassemia

While exact SARS-CoV-2 vaccination rates among patients with thalassemias are difficult to ascertain, vaccination is imperative in this community. The efficiency of the humoral response to the new vaccines against SARS-CoV-2 is currently a topic of great scientific relevance. The importance of vaccination in vulnerable patients is highlighted by the increased mortality rates in patients with hemoglobinopathies that contract COVID-19. A recent study by Anastasia et al. describes the humoral immune system response to the Comirnaty vaccine in beta-thalassemia major patients. In the study, beta thalassemia major patients were boosted with BNT162b2, an mRNA vaccine, produced by Pfizer-Biontech. Sixty-seven patients met the inclusion criteria.

Blood samples were collected from participants after receiving two doses of the vaccine. Antibody titers were measured against the receptor binding domain (RBD) in the S1 subunit of the Spike protein by using a quantitative Elecsys anti-SARS-CoV-2 ROCHE automated system. The study observed that 73.3% of splenectomized transfusion-dependent thalassemia patients showed anti-S ab titers in the second quartile, while non-splenectomized transfusion-dependent thalassemia patients had anti-S ab titers below 800 BAU/mL.

One month after administration of the second vaccine dose, there were no notable side effects in the patients. The production of immunoglobulin levels was robust in asplenic patients, arising several issues concerning the unusual humoral immune response in this vulnerable population. The group suggests that after splenectomy, memory B cells are deficient in patients. The role of humoral immunity then falls on perilymphatic tissue and bone marrow. The group suggests that this paradoxical increase in antibody titers in splenectomized patients may be due to unknown interactions between a novel mRNA vaccine and pathways in the immune system yet to be elucidated [42].

7. Conclusion

In conclusion, the current literature supports the conclusion that beta-thalassemia is protective against COVID-19. Surprisingly, most studies and case reports focus on patients with beta-thalassemia major. There is yet much to learn about the outcomes of patients with thalassemia minor and other hemoglobinopathies. The relative protective factors of beta-thalassemia major may not be present in other manifestations of the disease. Due to the limited patient population and lack of resources in nations where thalassemia is more common, it is possible a widescale study is not feasible. A lack of evidence-based medicine for such patients is glaring in the age of modern medicine. Leaders and researchers in hematology should focus efforts on expanding the current data available by controlled testing using in vitro samples. A keen understanding of the interactions between COVID-19 and abnormal hemoglobin chains is needed to better treat this vulnerable patient population.

Conflict of interest

The authors declare no conflict of interest.

Author details

Simran Patel, Armaan Shah, Ryan Kaiser and Raj Wadgaonkar*
SUNY Downstate Health Sciences University, Brooklyn, USA

*Address all correspondence to: raj.wadgaonkar@downstate.edu

References

[1] Bajwa H, Basit H. Thalassemia. In: StatPearls. Treasure Island (FL): StatPearls Publishing; 2022

[2] Sotiriou S, Samara AA, Vamvakopoulou D, et al. Susceptibility of beta-thalassemia heterozygotes to COVID-19. Journal of Clinical Medicine. 2021;**10**(16):3645. DOI: 10.3390/jcm10163645

[3] Kattamis A, Forni GL, Aydinok Y, Viprakasit V. Changing patterns in the epidemiology of beta-thalassemia. European Journal of Haematology. 2020;**105**(6):692-703. DOI: 10.1111/ejh.13512

[4] Origa R. beta-Thalassemia. Genetics in Medicine. 2017;**19**(6):609-619. DOI: 10.1038/gim.2016.173

[5] Thein SL. Molecular basis of β thalassemia and potential therapeutic targets. Blood Cells, Molecules & Diseases. 2018;**70**:54-65. DOI: 10.1016/j.bcmd.2017.06.001

[6] Needs T, Gonzalez-Mosquera LF, Lynch DT. Beta Thalassemia. In: StatPearls. Treasure Island (FL): StatPearls Publishing; 2022

[7] Yasara N, Premawardhena A, Mettananda S. A comprehensive review of hydroxyurea for β-haemoglobinopathies: The role revisited during COVID-19 pandemic. Orphanet Journal of Rare Diseases. 2021;**16**(1):114. DOI: 10.1186/s13023-021-01757-w

[8] Advani R, Sorenson S, Shinar E, Lande W, Rachmilewitz E, Schrier SL. Characterization and comparison of the red blood cell membrane damage in severe human alpha- and beta-thalassemia. Blood. 1992;**79**(4):1058-1063

[9] Scott MD, Rouyer-Fessard P, Lubin BH, Beuzard Y. Entrapment of purified alpha-hemoglobin chains in normal erythrocytes. A model for beta thalassemia. The Journal of Biological Chemistry. 1990;**265**(29):17953-17959

[10] Scott MD, Rouyer-Fessard P, Ba MS, Lubin BH, Beuzard Y. Alpha- and beta-haemoglobin chain induced changes in normal erythrocyte deformability: Comparison to beta thalassaemia intermedia and Hb H disease. British Journal of Haematology. 1992;**80**(4):519-526. DOI: 10.1111/j.1365-2141.1992.tb04567

[11] Scott MD, van den Berg JJ, Repka T, et al. Effect of excess alpha-hemoglobin chains on cellular and membrane oxidation in model beta-thalassemic erythrocytes. The Journal of Clinical Investigation. 1993;**91**(4):1706-1712. DOI: 10.1172/JCI116380

[12] Aljurf M, Ma L, Angelucci E, et al. Abnormal assembly of membrane proteins in erythroid progenitors of patients with beta-thalassemia major. Blood. 1996;**87**(5):2049-2056

[13] Schrier SL, Rachmilewitz E, Mohandas N. Cellular and membrane properties of alpha and beta thalassemic erythrocytes are different: Implication for differences in clinical manifestations. Blood. 1989;**74**(6):2194-2202

[14] Sancar GB, Cedeno MM, Rieder RF. Rapid destruction of newly synthesized excess beta-globin chains in HbH disease. Blood. 1981;**57**(5):967-971

[15] Dondorp AM, Chotivanich KT, Fucharoen S, et al. Red cell deformability,

splenic function and anaemia in thalassaemia. British Journal of Haematology. 1999;**105**(2):505-508. DOI: 10.1111/j.1365-2141.1999.01367.x

[16] Arlet JB, Dussiot M, Moura IC, Hermine O, Courtois G. Novel players in β-thalassemia dyserythropoiesis and new therapeutic strategies. Current Opinion in Hematology. 2016;**23**(3):181-188. DOI: 10.1097/MOH.0000000000000231

[17] Arlet JB, Ribeil JA, Guillem F, et al. HSP70 sequestration by free α-globin promotes ineffective erythropoiesis in β-thalassaemia. Nature. 2014;**514**(7521):242-246. DOI: 10.1038/nature13614

[18] Pootrakul P, Sirankapracha P, Hemsorach S, et al. A correlation of erythrokinetics, ineffective erythropoiesis, and erythroid precursor apoptosis in Thai patients with thalassemia. Blood. 2000;**96**(7):2606-2612

[19] Wiener E, Wanachiwanawin W, Kotipan K, Fucharoen S, Wasi P, Wickramasinghe SN. Erythroblast- and erythrocyte-bound antibodies in alpha and beta thalassaemia syndromes. Transfusion Medicine. 1991;**1**(4):229-238. DOI: 10.1111/j.1365-3148.1991.tb00038.x

[20] Galili U, Korkesh A, Kahane I, Rachmilewitz EA. Demonstration of a natural antigalactosyl IgG antibody on thalassemic red blood cells. Blood. 1983;**61**(6):1258-1264

[21] Yuan J, Kannan R, Shinar E, Rachmilewitz EA, Low PS. Isolation, characterization, and immunoprecipitation studies of immune complexes from membranes of beta-thalassemic erythrocytes. Blood. 1992;**79**(11):3007-3013

[22] Wanachiwanawin W, Siripanyaphinyo U, Fucharoen S, et al. Activation of monocytes for the immune clearance of red cells in beta zero-thalassaemia/HbE. British Journal of Haematology. 1993;**85**(4):773-777. DOI: 10.1111/j.1365-2141.1993.tb03222.x

[23] Wu Z, McGoogan JM. Characteristics of and important lessons from the coronavirus disease 2019 (COVID-19) outbreak in China: Summary of a report of 72 314 cases from the Chinese Center for Disease Control and Prevention. Journal of the American Medical Association. 2020;**323**(13):1239-1242. DOI: 10.1001/jama.2020.2648

[24] Omer SB, Malani P, Del Rio C. The COVID-19 pandemic in the US: A clinical update. Journal of the American Medical Association. 2020;**323**(18):1767-1768. DOI: 10.1001/jama.2020.5788

[25] Gattinoni L, Chiumello D, Caironi P, et al. COVID-19 pneumonia: Different respiratory treatments for different phenotypes? Intensive Care Medicine. 2020;**46**(6):1099-1102. DOI: 10.1007/s00134-020-06033-2

[26] Rapozzi V, Juarranz A, Habib A, Ihan A, Strgar R. Is haem the real target of COVID-19?. Photodiagnosis and Photodynamic Therapy. 2021;**35**:102381. DOI: 10.1016/j.pdpdt.2021.102381

[27] Karimi M, Haghpanah S, Azarkeivan A, et al. Prevalence and mortality in β-thalassaemias due to outbreak of novel coronavirus disease (COVID-19): The nationwide Iranian experience. British Journal of Haematology. 2020;**190**(3):e137-e140. DOI: 10.1111/bjh.16911

[28] Mendonça MM, da Cruz KR, Pinheiro DDS, et al. Dysregulation in erythrocyte dynamics caused by SARS-CoV-2 infection: Possible role in

shuffling the homeostatic puzzle during COVID-19. Hematology, Transfusion and Cell Therapy. 2022;**44**(2):235-245. DOI: 10.1016/j.htct.2022.01.005

[29] de Sanctis V, Canatan D, Corrons JLV, et al. Preliminary data on COVID-19 in patients with hemoglobinopathies: A multicentre ICET-A study. Mediterranean Journal of Hematology and Infectious Diseases. 2020;**12**(1):e2020046. DOI: 10.4084/MJHID.2020.046

[30] Karimi M, Haghpanah S, Azarkeivan A, Matin S, Safaei A, De Sanctis V. Coronavirus disease 2019 (COVID-19) severity in patients with thalassemias: A nationwide iranian experience. Mediterranean Journal of Hematology and Infectious Diseases. 2021;**13**(1):e2021008. DOI: 10.4084/MJHID.2021.008

[31] Motta I, Migone De Amicis M, Pinto VM, et al. SARS-CoV-2 infection in beta thalassemia: Preliminary data from the Italian experience. American Journal of Hematology. 2020;**95**(8):E198-E199. DOI: 10.1002/ajh.25840

[32] Telfer P, De la Fuente J, Sohal M, et al. Real-time national survey of COVID-19 in hemoglobinopathy and rare inherited anemia patients. Haematologica. 2020;**105**(11):2651-2654. DOI: 10.3324/haematol.2020.259440

[33] Edouard L, Emmanuel D, Carsten B. Beta-Thalassemia minor and SARS-CoV-2, prevalence, severity, morbidity and mortality: A systematic review study, medRxiv doi: 10.1101/2022.07.25.22278009

[34] Marhaeni W, Wijaya AB, Khairiyadi, Munawaroh, Hendriyono. Coagulation abnormalities due to COVID-19 in a child with thalassemia. Indian Journal of Pediatrics. 2021;**88**(4):396-397. DOI: 10.1007/s12098-020-03600-9

[35] Okar L, Ali M, Parengal J, Yassin MA. COVID-19 and thalassemia beta major in splenectomized patient: Clinical case progression and literature review. Clinical Case Reports. 2020;**8**(12):2918-2922. DOI: 10.1002/ccr3.3345

[36] Torti L, Maffei L, Sorrentino F, De Fabritiis P, Miceli R, Abruzzese E. Impact of SARS CoV-2 in hemoglobinopathies with immune disfunction and epidemiology. A protective mechanism from beta chain hemoglobin defects? Mediterranean Journal of Hematology and Infectious Diseases. 2020;**12**(1):e2020052. DOI: 10.4084/MJHID.2020.052

[37] Yadav U, Pal R. Challenging times for children with transfusion-dependent thalassemia amid the COVID-19 pandemic. Indian Pediatrics. 2020;**57**(5):478. DOI: 10.1007/s13312-020-1831-9

[38] Lee CK, Leung JNS, Cheng P, Lung DC, To KKW, Tsang DNC. Absence of SARS-CoV-2 viraemia in a blood donor with COVID-19 post-donation. Transfusion Medicine. 2021;**31**(3):223-224. DOI: 10.1111/tme.12724

[39] d'Arqom AG, Putri M, Savitri Y, Rahul Alfaidin AM. Vitamin and mineral supplementation for β-thalassemia during COVID-19 pandemic. Future Science OA. 2020;**6**(9):FSO628. DOI: 10.2144/fsoa-2020-0110

[40] Cavezzi A, Troiani E, Corrao S. COVID-19: Hemoglobin, iron, and hypoxia beyond inflammation. A narrative review. Clinics and Practice. 2020;**10**(2):1271. DOI: 10.4081/cp.2020.1271

[41] Khanna AK, Prabhakaran A, Patel P, Ganjiwale JD, Nimbalkar SM. Social, psychological and financial burden on caregivers of children with chronic illness: A cross-sectional study. Indian

Journal of Pediatrics. 2015;**82**(11):1006-1011. DOI: 10.1007/s12098-015-1762-y

[42] Anastasi E, Marziali M, Preziosi A, et al. Humoral immune response to Comirnaty (BNT162b2) SARS-Cov2 mRNA vaccine in Thalassemia major patients. Microbes and Infection. 2022;**24**(6-7):104976. DOI: 10.1016/j.micinf.2022.104976

Section 2

Thalassemia Syndromes

Chapter 3

Newborn Screening and Thalassaemia Syndrome

Charity Iheanacho and Christiana Okeke

Abstract

Haemoglobin variants or haemoglobin disorders are a group of clinical disorders characterised by impairment of synthesis of normal adult haemoglobin, due to genetically determined abnormality in the formation of the globin moiety of the molecule. These disorders fall into two broad groups, that is qualitative (haemoglobinopathies) and quantitative (thalassaemias). In the anthropoids, the most common congenital single-gene disorder is the alteration of the globin genes which account for about 270 million carriers globally. These globin gene alterations cause low/no globin expression (thalassaemia) or abnormal globin protein production (haemoglobinopathy). The clinical manifestation of haemoglobin disorder is the culminated measure of one's genetic and molecular makeup. Summarily, the study, diagnosis and management of thalassaemia are models of biological principles of human disease. Newborn screening, however, is a system that aims at improving management and/or eradication of genetic disorders from the neonatal stage of life. This chapter will be dealing with the definition and steps involved in newborn screening for thalassaemia.

Keywords: thalassaemia, newborn screening, confirmatory diagnosis, haemoglobin disorders, next-generation sequencing (NGS)

1. Introduction

The haemoglobin (Hb) is a tetramallic, metalloprotein consisting of two alpha α and/or α-like alleles (α or ζ) and two β and/or β-like alleles (ε, γ, δ or β) globin chains with a chemical formula ($C_{2952}H_{4664}O_{832}N_{812}S_8Fe_4$) [1, 2]. Each polypeptide globin chain is folded around a haem molecule (**Figure 1**). The major function of Hb is a gaseous transfer between the tissue and the lungs. The globin chains are encrypted by their various genes sited on chromosome 11 and chromosome 16 and they all have more than one allele [4]. These alleles codes for the various globin chains at various stages of human life from the embryonic to adult life in varying concentrations (**Tables 1** and **2**). Many of these alleles undergo point mutations during DNA sequencing resulting in single amino acid substitution in the globin portion, leading to the production of haemoglobin derivatives (variants) [6]. Haemoglobin variants or haemoglobin disorders are a group of clinical disorders characterised by impairment of synthesis of normal adult haemoglobin, due to genetically determined abnormality in the formation of the globin moiety of the molecule. These disorders fall into two broad groups, that is, qualitative (haemoglobinopathies) and quantitative

IntechOpen

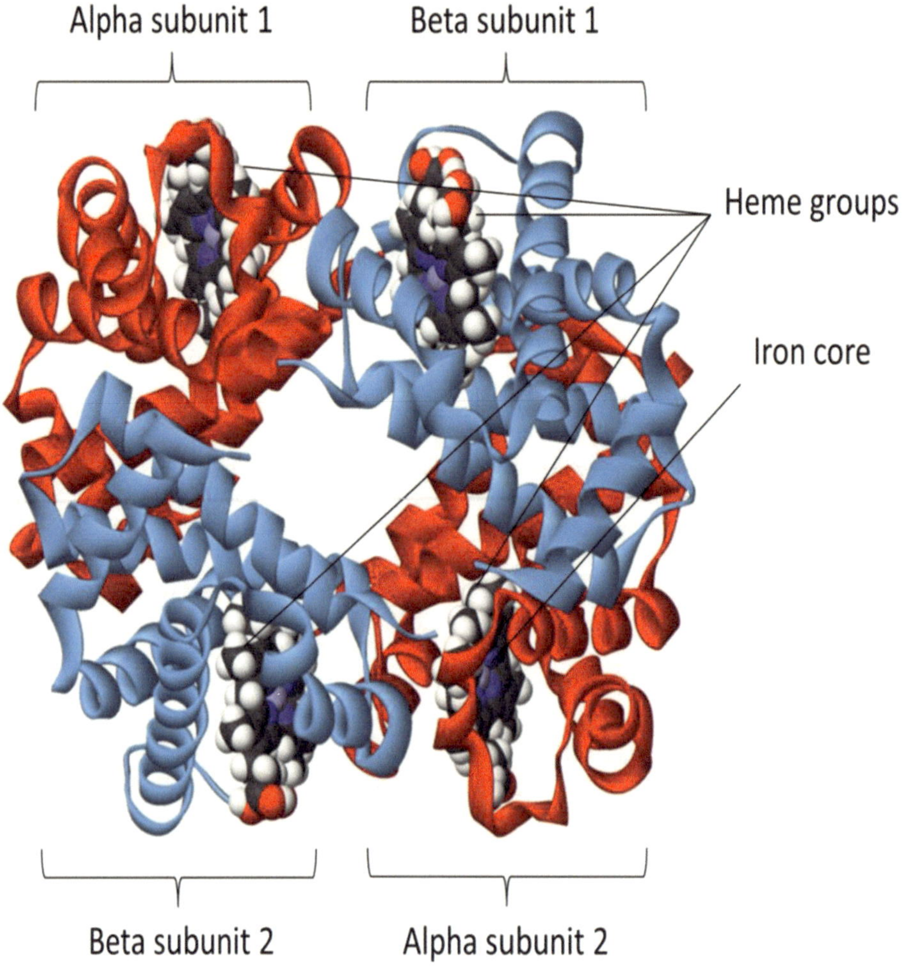

Figure 1.
Haemoglobin structure. A molecule of haemoglobin is made up of four subunits; two alpha-like subunits and two beta-like subunits. Each subunit contains a haem group with a ferrous core to which an oxygen molecule can reversibly bind. Image adapted from [3].

(thalassaemias) [7]. In the anthropoids, the most common congenital single-gene disorder is the alteration of the globin genes which account for about 270 million carriers globally and 0.4 million of such births annually [8]. These globin gene alterations cause low/no globin expression (thalassaemia) or abnormal globin protein production (haemoglobinopathy). The clinical manifestation of haemoglobin disorder is the culminated measure of one's genetic and molecular makeup. Summarily, the study, diagnosis and management of thalassaemia is a model of biological principles of human disease. Newborn screening however is a system that aims at improving management and/or eradication of genetic disorders from the neonatal stage of life.

1.1 The haemoglobin nature and structure

The anatomy and genetic structure of the human haemoglobin are demonstrated in the tables and figures below.

Haemoglobin specie	Globin chains present	Period when normally present
A	$\alpha_2\beta_2$ (alpha$_2$ & beta$_2$)	Major haemoglobin in adult life
A_2	$\alpha_2\delta_2$ (alpha$_2$ & delta$_2$)	Minor haemoglobin in adult life; even more minor in foetal and neonatal life
F	$\alpha_2\gamma_2$ (alpha$_2$ & gamma$_2$)	Minor haemoglobin in adult life; major haemoglobin in foetal life with a declining percentage through the neonatal period
Gower 1	$\zeta_2\varepsilon_2$ (zeta$_2$ & epsilon$_2$)	Significant haemoglobin during early intrauterine life
Gower 2	$\alpha_2\varepsilon_2$ (alpha$_2$ & epsilon$_2$)	Significant haemoglobin during early intrauterine life
Portland I or Portland II	$\zeta_2\gamma_2$ or $\zeta_2\beta_2$ (zeta$_2$ & gamma$_2$ or beta$_2$)	Significant haemoglobin during early intrauterine life

Modified from: [5].

Table 1.
Haemoglobins normally present during adult, foetal and embryonic periods of life.

Haemoglobin	Structure	Levels at birth	Levels in adult	Comments
A	$\alpha_2\beta_2$	20–25%	97%	Reaches adult levels by one year of age.
A_2	$\alpha_2\delta_2$	0.5%	2.5%	Elevated in β thalassaemia trait
F	$\alpha_2\gamma_2$	75–80%	<1%	Reaches adult levels by one year of age
HbH	β_4	15–20% in HbH disease	NA	HbH produces Heinz bodies in the erythrocytes and haemolysis
Hb Bart	γ_4	100% in hydrops feotalis, 15–25% in HbH disease	NA	Increased in carriers of α thalassaemia trait at birth

Courtesy: [3].

Table 2.
Normal and variant haemoglobin at birth and in older children.

1.2 What is newborn screening?

Newborn screening is an entire system of identification, treatment, management and possibly eradication of genetic disorders from the neonatal stage of life. Newborn screening starts from the recruiting stage through the diagnosis of the infant and management. It is generally applied for the early recognition of infants affected by disorders that benefit from early treatment to avoid irreversible health problems [9]. It is supreme for early diagnosis and enrolment of affected children into a comprehensive health care programme. This has created diagnostic and treatment opportunities for several children with genetic or metabolic diseases across the globe with a resultant healthier life. However; in many countries, the screening programmes have not started or have been limited to a few disease conditions [10]. These delays are tied to financial incapabilities of the citizens and lack of government-established organisation for screening. However, the physician's suspicion and or awareness is heightened by accurate identification of risk factors of haemoglobin disorders and family history [11]. The ultimate benefit of newborn screening programmes is the improved health status in patients diagnosed early and treated optimally. However, issues such as false positives and false negatives results might occur but the use of novel and molecular technologies for confirmation has over that [12]. Each part of the newborn screening system is important and needs evaluation for any weaknesses. Newborn screening for genetic disorders can be undertaken from two dimensions:

1. Random selection from all neonates aged 0–9 months of life to ensure full development of every haemoglobin gene and mutational characteristics.

2. Collation of family history during antenatal visits or recruiting of all willing pregnant women whose family histories are suggestive of a haemoglobin disorder or the "don't know" subjects.

The family history method might be cost-effective but will likely miss out on the few misinformed questionnaires, so for a start, a random newborn screening of a population site should be of best interest for subsequent studies, government policies and data storage.

1.2.1 Algorithm for newborn screening

1. Create awareness through seminars and meetings for parents/guardians and plead or persuade them to cooperate for the success of the programme.

2. Formulate centres/medical outlets that will be equipped with personnel for recruiting, counselling, sampling and testing.

3. Alternatively, incorporate NBS into an already existing programme such as child immunization and include personnel for haemoglobin disorders screening as in no. 2 above.

4. All prospective thalassaemia syndromes from a well-structured questionnaire are issued a consent form to the parents/guardians.

5. Every consented subject should be sampled for screening via dry blood sampling (DBS) in six to eight spots.

6. Communicating positive screening results to a clinician and/or parents and tracking outcomes of confirmatory testing are of primary concern for the final outcome.

7. Follow-up or regular data review processes for newborn screening ensure total inclusion of all infants with thalassaemia syndrome for management and treatment

DOI: http://dx.doi.org/10.5772/intechopen.109302

8. For the collection of whole blood samples for confirmation, ethylenediaminetetraacetic acid (EDTA) is the typical anti-coagulant used. Heparin may interfere with DNA amplification by polymerase chain reaction (PCR). DBS collected from a finger prick; preferably the last finger or the heel is commonly used. To maintain the integrity of haemoglobin molecules, the medium of transportation and storage of DBS must be dry and cool, possibly by means of dry ice.

1.3 The thalassaemias

Thalassaemia is a group of heterogenous genetic disorders of haemoglobin synthesis. These disorders arise from a decrease in production rate of one or more globin chain [13]. The thalassaemias are named α, β, δβ- and γδβ-thalassaemias depending on the globin chain that is produced in a reduced amount. In the occasion where one of the globin chain is not synthesised at all, the condition is known as thalassaemia Null (°), that is, α^0 or β^0 thalassaemias. This condition usually occurs amongst the populace with structural Hb abnormalities, therefore the inheritance of one thalassaemia gene from one parent and the second gene with a structural Hb variant from the next parent is a common finding in such places [14]. Other minor haemoglobins in adults include HbF (foetal haemoglobin, $\alpha_2\gamma_2$) and HbA2 ($\alpha_2\delta_2$) [15].

The α-Thalassaemias: These groups of thalassaemias result from the deletion of one or more alpha-globin genes and are subgrouped in order of the number of the α-globin gene deletions. Hence, one gene deletion is α^+-thalassaemia, α^0-thalassaemia is two gene deletion from the same chromosome, Hb-H syndrome is a three-gene deletion while hydrops feotalis with the Hb-Barts is a four-gene deletion. The haemoglobin being a tetrametric protein of 4 globin gene $\alpha_2\beta_2$, it has been observed that deletion of only one α gene will not result in a significant haematological abnormality and is therefore referred to as a "silent carrier" state. On the other hand, deletions of two α-genes can occur in two ways i.e. from the same chromosome (in cis) or of the opposite chromosome (in trans). The two α gene deletion is the homozygous state or homozygous α^+-thalassaemia and has similar clinical presentations as mild hyperchromasia and microcytic anaemia but the cis-genotype is common amongst Asians while the trans-form is common in Black African origins [16].

The Hb-H disease is usually associated with haemolysis due to the excessive accumulation of β-globin subunits that self-bond to form soluble β-chain tetramers which are the Hb-H. Because of the relatively unstable nature of the Hb-H, it does not precipitate as the erythrocytes age leading to the formation of inclusion bodies which distorts the red cells' life span [17].

Hydrop's foetalis with Hb-Barts is usually detected at the third trimester or within the early post-natal period. Haemoglobin Barts is not an effective oxygen transporter because it has a very high affinity for oxygen. It is a tetramer of 4γ globin subunits so the foetus or infant will lack Hb F&A, resulting in hypoxia and extreme organ swelling and subsequent deaths [17].

The β-Thalassaemias: The Hb variant resulting from the point-mutation of the β-globin gene is known as the β-thalassaemias. This variant has two main sub-types, that is, the β^0-thalassaemia in which there is complete absence of normal β-globin subunits. And the second is β^+-thalassaemia which has remarkably reduced synthesis of normal β-globin. It was noted that some forms of β-thalassaemia might be due to an unequal crossing over of bridges of the δ & β-globin genes leading to a fusion of δβ-globin gene (thalassaemia), εγδβ-thalassaemia and hereditary persistence of foetal haemoglobin (HPFH) syndromes [18]. It has been reported that β-thalassaemia has over 200 molecular different subtypes but in spite of their heterogeneity; they still possess similar clinical manifestations since they all lack HbA with excess accumulation of α-subunits [19].

1.4 Newborn screening methods for thalassaemias

In the recent past, most newborn screening programmes uses high-performance liquid chromatography (HPLC) as the primary screening method to make a presumptive screening of possible haemoglobinopathy [20]. However, for low-income nations, a simple alkaline or acid globin chain electrophoresis with $_{DL}$-dithiothreitol ($_{DL}$-DTT) and urea in Tris EDTA-borate buffer can suffice for the detection of abnormal haemoglobins [21]. Also, manual HbF quantification and inclusion body detection can serve as a good NBS source for low-income states. All suspected abnormal Hbs or neonates can then be subjected to fully automated, high throughput HPLC for identification, and quantitation of Hb F, HbA_2 and Hb Bart's, enabling thalassaemic screening and classification in the newborn period [20]. According to literatures, an understanding of the specific HPLC retention times will aid the probable identification of thalassaemic disorders such as a Hb S/Hb A ratio >2.0 is highly suggestive of Hb S/β+ thalassaemia rather than Hb AS trait. Secondary or primary screening with HPLC can thus help to streamline the subsequent tests needed for the identification/confirmation of a thalassaemia syndrome in most cases [22].

Globin chain electrophoresis: This is used in the separation of α- and β-globin chains by adding 6 M urea and 2-mercaptoethanol to the buffer. When electrophoresis is applied at alkaline or acid pH, these chains migrate differently revealing the characteristic patterns of migration of abnormal α- and β-chains. This method provides a means of identifying abnormal haemoglobin variants that cannot be identified by routine electrophoretic methods. It is especially helpful when variants other than S and C are present and which have identical migration on both cellulose acetate and citrate agar systems [23].

Determination of distribution of HbF in red cells: This is employed to distinguish hereditary persistence of foetal haemoglobin (HPFH) from β thalassaemias. The acid elution test of Betke-Kleihauer is used to evaluate the distribution of HbF, where fresh thin-blood film fixed with ethanol is examined microscopically. The principle is that HbA on fixing readily wash off from red cells by acid solution while HbF resists acid-elution and remains within the cells. Cells containing more HbF appear dark after staining, while those with no HbF appear unstained and empty or ghost-like [24].

Tests for inclusion bodies: Inclusion bodies that can be detected in thalassaemias include HbH and α chain inclusion and they can be detected as follows:

a. HbH inclusions: These are detected when peripheral blood is incubated with methyl violet in splenectomised patients. They are also precipitated in mature or nucleated red cells as multiple, small, ragged inclusions due to the redox action of dyes such as brilliant cresyl blue. HbH inclusions are usually seen in Hb Bart's hydrops foetalis syndrome, HbH disease, and α-thalassaemia carrier states [23].

b. α chain inclusions: In homozygous β-thalassaemia, α chain inclusions are seen only in nucleated red cells in bone marrow, or in peripheral blood after splenectomy. α chain inclusions appear as single, ragged structures closely attached to the nucleus when peripheral blood or bone marrow sample is incubated with methyl violet, and the prepared films observed under microscope [23].

High-performance liquid chromatography: This is used as a screening test for thalassemias and for the detection, identification and quantification of haemoglobin variants. It is also used for the quantitation of HbA2 and HbF. HPLC is well suited for neonatal screening since it can detect small amounts of haemoglobin and needs small amount of blood. Haemoglobins A, F, S, C, E/A2, D_{Punjab}, $O\text{-}_{Arab}$ and $D_{Philadelphia}$ can be separated and identified with HPLC. In this technique, blood sample is introduced into a column packed with silica gel. Different haemoglobins get adsorbed onto the resin. Elution of different haemoglobins is achieved by changing the pH and ionic strength of the buffer. Haemoglobin fractions are detected as they pass through a detector and are recorded by a computer [25].

1.5 Confirmatory diagnostic testing for the thalassaemias

Demographic information and an EDTA/DBS blood sample from one or both parents are required with that of the newborn to help guide the sequence of confirmatory diagnostic tests for specific thalassaemias. Methods of gene-typing for thalassemia based on PCR techniques are as follows: dot-blot analysis, reverse dot-blot analysis, the amplification refractory mutation system, denaturing gradient gel electrophoresis, mutagenically separated polymerase chain reaction, gap-PCR, restriction endonuclease analysis, real-time polymerase chain reaction, Sanger sequencing, pyrosequencing, multiplex ligation-dependent probe amplification and gene array [26–29] Gap-PCR is used to test for common α-thalassaemia deletions or duplications, as well as all forms of HPFH and Hb Lepore deletions. will identify point mutations in the γ-, α- and β-globin genes are usually captured in direct DNA sequencing but mutations within the alleles as well as large deletions are often missed out. Large β-globin locus deletions account for only a very small number of β-thalassaemia mutations but are the most difficult to detect because gap-PCR relies on knowledge of the deletion breakpoints. Multiplex ligation-dependent amplification (MLPA) becomes a handy method to determine the presence of an unidentified α- or β-globin gene deletion, by assessing DNA ploidy quantity changes [30]. Long-range sequencing using comparative genomic hybridisation (CGH) or microarray-based comparative genomic hybridisation (matrix CGH) method to identify deletion breakpoints and DNA copy numbers with high resolution is employed for beta thalassaemia confirmation [31]. This is a molecular cytogenetic method for analysing "copy number variation" which is related to the number of complete sets of chromosomes in a cell and hence the number of possible alleles for autosomal and pseudo-autosomal genes [32]. These novel methods are summarised in **Table 3**.

The method employed for the detection of unknown mutations is the restriction fragment length polymorphism (RFLP) analysis. This method is based on the fact that each restriction enzyme targets different nucleotide sequences in a DNA strand hence different enzyme cuts at different sites. The distance between the cleavage sites of a certain restriction endonucleotide differs between individuals. Hence, the length of the DNA fragments produced by a restriction endonuclease will certainly differ from organisms and species [33]. The variations that affect restriction sites and produce different fragmentation sizes after digestion are known as restriction fragment length polymorphisms (RFLPs). This polymorphism serves as 'markers' for genetic disorders, especially thalassemias. If the linkage is not close then the crossing

Disorder and mutation type	Diagnostic method
α^0-Thalassaemia	Gap-PCR, MLPA
α^+-Thalassaemia: deletion nondeletion	Gap-PCR, MLPA ASO, RE, DGGE, Sanger sequencing
β-Thalassaemia: deletion non-deletion	Gap-PCR, MLPA ASO, RDB, ARMS, RE-PCR, Sanger sequencing
δβ-Thalassaemia	Gap-PCR, MLPA
HPFH deletion	Gap-PCR, MLPA ASO, ARMS, RE-PCR, Sanger sequencing

The main diagnostic approaches commonly used for the diagnosis or confirmation of thalassaemias [28].

Table 3.
The novel methods of DNA diagnosis for thalassaemia.

over of chromosomal material between homologous chromosomes during meiosis may 'separate' the polymorphic site from the abnormal gene; this will lead to a false negative result in the foetus [23].

2. Next-generation sequencing (NGS)

Recently, however, the introduction of technologies such as dosage mutation tests to detect large deletion or duplication mutations and multiple gene panel tests by massively parallel sequencing (next-generation sequencing; NGS) facilitates a more precise molecular diagnosis of thalassaemias and a better understanding of the genomic mechanisms of the disease [34].

In next generation sequencing (NGS), the diagnosis of thalassaemias is based on massively parallel sequencing of clonally amplified DNA molecules, alongside sufficient computational power and appropriate software for efficient data analysis [35]. The procedure can be applied to a whole genome or exome, and to specific targeted regions of the genome. The most critical step in NGS manipulation is the design of the probe-set to be applied for DNA capture which requires a high level of homology between the genes in the alpha and beta clusters. Another critical point for NGS is that it is useful for the detection of single nucleotide substitutions and insertions or small deletions, but it is less accurate for other types of genomic variation.

3. Conclusion

Newborn screening is a system of identification, treatment, management, and possibly eradication of genetic disorders from the neonatal stage of life. The procedure begins at the recruiting site or stage through the diagnosis of the infant and management. It is generally applied for the early recognition of infants affected by disorders that benefit from early treatment to avoid irreversible health problems. It is supreme for early diagnosis and enrolment of affected children into a comprehensive health care programme thus; thousands of children with genetic and/or metabolic diseases have had an opportunity for a healthy life with early diagnosis and

DOI: http://dx.doi.org/10.5772/intechopen.109302

treatment. Thalassaemia syndrome has a high financial and national health burden, national policies and intervention are needed for its success. Each nation should adopt newborn screening and diagnostic/confirmatory methods for thalassaemia syndromes within their financial or economical capacity, maintaining standards. Communication, documentation and follow-up is the key to the success of newborn screening for thalassaemia syndromes.

Author details

Charity Iheanacho[1*] and Christiana Okeke[2]

1 Haematology Department, Jos University Teaching Hospital, Jos, Plateau State, Nigeria

2 44 Nigerian Army Reference Hospital, Kaduna, Kaduna State, Nigeria

*Address all correspondence to: udoanacho@gmail.com

References

[1] Pandya PP, Wapner R, Oepkes D, Sebire N. Fetal Medicine E-Book: Basic Science and Clinical Practice. Amsterdam, Netherlands: Elsevier Health Sciences; 2019

[2] Kreitzberg P, Lucke K, Pennington J, Serang O. Selection on $ X_1+ X_1+\ cdots X_m $ via Cartesian product tree. arXiv preprint arXiv:2008.07023. 2020

[3] Centers for Disease Control and Prevention. Hemoglobinopathies: Current Practices for Screening, Confirmation and Follow-up. Silver Spring, Maryland, U.S: Association of Public Health Laboratories; 2015

[4] Weatherall DJ. The challenge of haemoglobinopathies in resource-poor countries. British Journal of Haematology. 2011;**154**(6):736-744

[5] Esan AJ. Hematological differences in newborn and aging: A review study. Hematology Transfusion International Journal. 2016;**3**(3):178-190

[6] Buseri FI, Okonkwo CN. Abnormal hemoglobin genotypes and ABO and rhesus blood groups associated with HIV infection among HIV-exposed infants in north Western Nigeria. Pathology and Laboratory Medicine International. 2014;**6**:15-20

[7] Shiva Raj KC, Basnet S, Gyawali P. Prevalence of hemoglobinopathies and hemoglobin variants. Nepal Medical College Journal. 2017;**19**(3):121-126

[8] Modell B, Darlison M. Global epidemiology of haemoglobin disorders and derived service indicators. Bulletin of the World Health Organization. 2008;**86**(6):480-487

[9] Giordano P. Newborn screening for haemoglobinopathies. In: Prevention of Thalassaemias and Other Haemoglobin Disorders: Volume 1: Principles. 2nd ed. Strovolos, Cyprus: Thalassaemia International Federation; 2013

[10] Nnodu OE, Sopekan A, Nnebe-Agumadu U, Ohiaeri C, Adeniran A, Shedul G, et al. Implementing newborn screening for sickle cell disease as part of immunisation programmes in Nigeria: A feasibility study. The Lancet Haematology. 2020;**7**(7):e534-e540

[11] Shorter D, Hong T, Aosborn D. Screening programmes for developmental dysplasia of the hip in newborn infants. Evidence-Based Child Health. 2013;**8**(1):11-54

[12] Wilcken B. Newborn screening: How are we travelling, and where should we be going? Journal of Inherited Metabolic Disease. 2011;**34**(3):569-574

[13] Bain BJ. Haemoglobin and the Genetics of Haemoglobin Synthesis. 2nd ed. New Jersey, USA: Blackwell Publishing Ltd.; 2006. pp. 1-23

[14] Thom CS, Dickson CF, Gell DA, Weiss MJ. Hemoglobin variants: Biochemical properties and clinical correlates. Cold Spring Harbor Perspectives in Medicine. 2013;**3**(3):a011858

[15] Langlois S, Ford JC, Chitayat D, Désilets VA, Farrell SA, Geraghty M, et al. Carrier screening for thalassemia and hemoglobinopathies in Canada. Journal of Obstetrics and Gynaecology Canada. 2008;**30**(10):950-959

[16] Forget BG, Bunn HF. Classification of the disorders of hemoglobin. Cold Spring Harbor Perspectives in Medicine. 2013;**3**(2):a011684

[17] Higgs DR, Engel JD, Stamatoyannopoulos G. Thalassaemia. Lancet. 2012;**379**:373-383

[18] Thein SL. The molecular basis of β-thalassemia. Cold Spring Harbor Perspectives in Medicine. 2013;**3**(5):a011700

[19] Nienhuis AW, Nathan DG. Pathophysiology and clinical manifestations of the β-thalassemias. Cold Spring Harbor Perspectives in Medicine. 2012;**2**(12):a011726

[20] Hoppe CC. Prenatal and newborn screening for hemoglobinopathies. International Journal of Laboratory Hematology. 2013;**35**(3):297-305

[21] Dacie JV, Lewis SM. Practical Haematology. 10th ed. Edinburgh, London: Churchill Livingstone; 2006. pp. 398-440

[22] Fucharoen S, Winichagoon P. Thalassemia in South East Asia: Problems and strategy for prevention and control. The Southeast Asian Journal of Tropical Medicine and Public Health. 1992;**23**(4):647-655

[23] Adams TL, Latham GJ, Eisses MJ, Bender MA, Haberkern CM. Essentials of hematology. In: A Practice of Anesthesia for Infants and Children. Amsterdam, Netherlands: Elsevier; 2019. pp. 217-239

[24] Amann C, Geipel A, Müller A, Heep A, Ritgen J, Stressig R, et al. Fetal anemia of unknown cause—A diagnostic challenge. Ultraschall in der Medizin - European Journal of Ultrasound. 2011;**32**(S02):E134-E140

[25] Lo L, Singer ST. Thalassemia: Current approach to an old disease. Pediatric Clinics. 2002;**49**(6):1165-1191

[26] Old J, Henderson S. Molecular diagnostics for haemoglobinopathies. Expert Opinion on Medical Diagnostics. 2010;**4**(3):225-240

[27] Harteveld CL, Kleanthous M, Traeger-Synodinos J. Prenatal diagnosis of hemoglobin disorders: Present and future strategies. Clinical Biochemistry. 2009;**42**(18):1767-1779

[28] Fabry M, Old JM. Laboratory methods for diagnosis and evaluation of hemoglobin disorders. In: Disorders of Hemoglobin: Genetics, Pathophysiology, and Clinical Management. New York: Cambridge University Press; 2009. pp. 658-686

[29] Old J, Harteveld CL, Traeger-Synodinos J, Petrou M, Angastiniotis M, Galanello R. Molecular diagnosis. In: Prevention of Thalassaemias and Other Haemoglobin Disorders: Volume 2: Laboratory Protocols. 2nd ed. Strovolos Cyprus: Thalassaemia International Federation; 2012

[30] Harteveld CL, Voskamp A, Phylipsen M, Akkermans N, den Dunnen JT, White SJ, et al. Nine unknown rearrangements in 16p13. 3 and 11p15. 4 causing α-and β-thalassaemia characterised by high resolution multiplex ligation-dependent probe amplification. Journal of Medical Genetics. 2005;**42**(12):922-931

[31] Phylipsen M, Chaibunruang A, Vogelaar IP, Balak JR, Schaap RA, Ariyurek Y, et al. Fine-tiling array CGH to improve diagnostics for α-and β-thalassaemia rearrangements. Human Mutation. 2012;**33**(1):272-280

[32] Kallioniemi A, Kallioniemi OP, Sudar D, Rutovitz D, Gray JW, Waldman F, et al. Comparative genomic hybridization for molecular cytogenetic analysis of solid tumors. Science. 1992;**258**(5083):818-821

[33] Cheriyedath S. Restriction Fragment Length Polymorphism (RFLP) Technique. 2018

[34] Shang X, Xu X. Update in the genetics of thalassaemia: What clinicians need to know. Best Practice & Research. Clinical Obstetrics & Gynaecology. 2017;**1**(39):3-15

[35] Lohmann K, Klein C. Next generation sequencing and the future of genetic diagnosis. Neurotherapeutics. 2014;**11**(4):699-707

Chapter 4

The Key Genetic Determinants Behind the Phenotypic Heterogeneity of HbE/β-thalassemia Patients and the Probable Management Strategy

Amrita Panja, Brahmarshi Das, Tuphan Kanti Dolai and Sujata Maiti Choudhury

Abstract

HbE/β-thalassemia is the most common severe form of thalassemia which is very prominent in South East Asian countries. It is responsible for nearly one-half of all the severe types of β-thalassemia all over the world. It is also known to represent a wide range of phenotypic diversity which varies from asymptomatic to transfusion-dependent severe phenotype. The most important predictive factor is mutations within the beta-globin gene (*HBB*). Apart from the primary genetic modifiers, there are certain other determinants regulating the phenotypic heterogeneity including, co-inheritance of alpha thalassemia mutations and other secondary modifiers including *Xmn*1 polymorphism, *HBS1L-MYB*, *GATA-1, BCL11A* polymorphism, and presence of HPFH mutations. Although the degree of severity is also determined by other tertiary genetic modifiers like increase in serum erythropoietin due to anemia, previous infection with malaria, environmental factors, splenectomy, etc. This review aimed to reveal the potential genetic predictors of HbE/β-thalassemia patients and the probable management strategy. This also enhances the generation of "personalized medicine" for better patient care. The instability of clinical phenotype and remarkable variation indicate careful monitoring of treatment for each patient and the therapeutic approaches should be monitored over time.

Keywords: HbE/β-thalassemia, genotype, phenotype, genetic modifiers, management strategy

1. Introduction

Thalassemia is a group of congenital anemias which are characterized by deficient synthesis of one or more globin chain of normal hemoglobin molecules. It is primarily caused due to defective synthesis of globin chain production [1]. It is the most prevalent recessive monogenic disorder and it occurs in about 4.4/10,000 live births all over the world [2]. In European Union, annually 1/10,000 people are symptomatic whereas the global incidence rate is 1/100,000 [3]. It has been found that every year approximately 300,000 and 400,000 babies are born with hemoglobin disorders and most of them are reported from low-income countries [4]. India is now known to possess the largest number of thalassemia major children (150,000) [5]. It has been estimated that approximately 10,000–15,000 new cases are added every year in this country. Moreover, there are 42 million β-thalassemia carriers reported with an average prevalence rate of 3–4% [6].

Hemoglobinopathies are broadly classified into two main groups: thalassemia syndrome and structural hemoglobin variants (abnormal hemoglobins). According to the quantitative reduction in the production of globin chain, thalassemia can be categorised into: 1) thalassemia major (the absence of globin synthesis); 2) thalassemia intermedia (reduced synthesis of globin chain); 3) thalassemia minor (silent type) [7]. The main types of thalassemia include α, β, and δβ thalassemias whereas the clinically important hemoglobin variants include HbS, HbC, HbE, and HbD. So far, >800 different types of mutations and structural variants in the Human beta globin (HBB) gene have been well characterized using the existing genomic protocol. Out of which more than 350 different mutations are known to be associated with β-thalassemia [8, 9]. In the case of α-thalassemia, most of the mutations are deletion type, whereas a wide spectrum of β-thalassemia mutations involved one or a limited number of nucleotides situated within the β-globin gene or its immediate flanking region. Beta-thalassemia has over 200 different point mutations that cause several types of clinical variability due to varying levels of arrangements of compound heterozygous alleles [7, 10]. The structural hemoglobin variants result from the substitution of one or more amino acids in the globin chains of the hemoglobin molecule. The prevalence rate of thalassemia is widely variable depending on the ethnicity of a particular geographical domain. All over the world, HbE/beta-thalassemia represents nearly 50% of all the cases affected from severe beta-thalassemia [11]. It is one of the commonest forms of hemoglobinopathies in many Asian countries including India, Bangladesh, Laos, Indonesia, and Sri Lanka [12]. Moreover, in Southern China, thousands of people are suffering from HbE/beta thalassemia where its gene frequency is about 4% [13]. In certain parts of the world, the number has increased up to 70% like in Thailand and Cambodia [14]. HbE and HbE/β-thalassemia are prominently found in the north-eastern parts of India [15, 16]. The incidence of HbE and beta thalassemia carrier rate is 4.4% and 3.9% correspondingly in this country [17].

HbE/β-thalassemia is formed due to differential interaction between β-thalassemia mutant allele and HbE allele. In many cases, there is interface between α-thalassemia allele with HbE which results in a complex series of phenotypes, although the clinical severity is comparatively milder [18]. It is not always possible to predict the appropriate phenotype from the genotype and it needs adequate genetic counseling. The objective of the present study is to describe the wide range of clinical spectrum of HbE/β-thalassemia and the probable primary and secondary genetic modifiers which influence the variable phenotype. At the same time, the probable management strategy and future therapeutic approach of thalassemia have been focussed.

2. Pathophysiology

HbE is a hemoglobin variant which appears mildly unstable and shows increased sensitivity to oxidants. The blood oxygen dissociation curves of patients with homozygous HbE appear to be normal or very slightly right-shifted. HbE is synthesized at a mildly reduced rate and globin chain imbalance. It is formed due to substitution mutation at codon 26 of the β-globin gene (GAG>AAG) which leads to the substitute of lysine for glutamic acid. This mutation activates the cryptic splice site toward the 3′ end of exon 1, which causes abnormal messenger RNA processing [19]. Therefore, the normally spliced β^E messenger RNA is declined as the normal donor site must complete with the newly formed spliced site (**Figure 1**).

In the case of HbE patients, hemoglobin constitutes about 25–30% of the total hemoglobin and the level widely varies between 3 and 11 g/dl. The HbE patients with β + thalassemia mutations are characterized by low levels of HbA% and elevated HbE%. The blood smear reveals hypochromic, microcytic red cells with considerable morphologically altered blood cells with increased numbers of target cells. HbE (EE) homozygous red blood cells are not very flexible while moving through the blood vessels. These blood cells have a smaller outside surface area to carry oxygen. EE red blood cells have a reduced capacity to hold oxygen. The lifespan of these RBCs is also shorter than that of the normal. They appear mildly anemic and their hematological findings are very similar to that of heterozygous β-thalassemia [20].

3. The interactions of hemoglobin E with different forms of thalassemia

The interaction of HbE with other types of hemoglobinopathies can be complex and puzzling. Due to a lack of proper diagnosis and genetic counseling, the chance of different types of hemoglobinopathies can be enhanced [21]. HbE alone cannot lead to any significant clinical complications, although the co-association with α and β-thalassemia leads to a diverse range of clinical syndromes of varying severity.

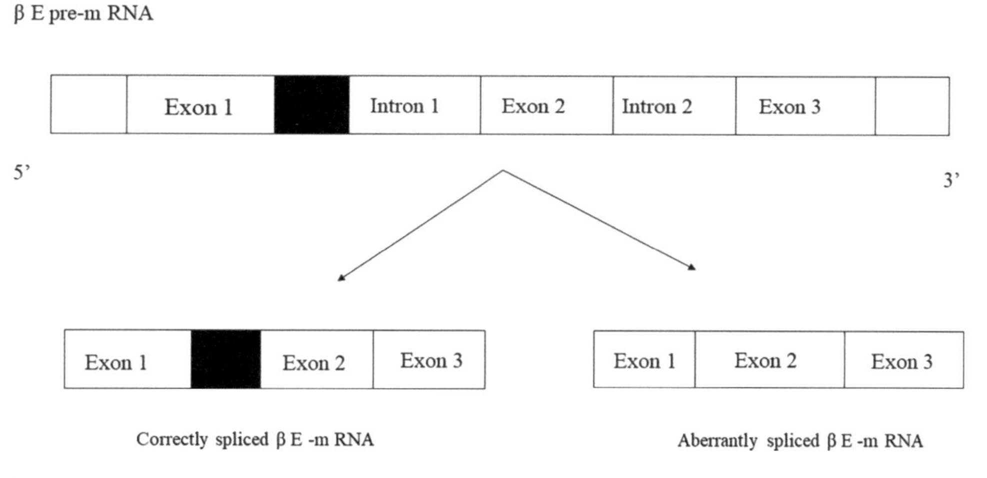

Figure 1.
Simplified schematic representation of abnormal splicing of β^E-globin mRNA. The black box denotes 16 nucleotides at the 3′-end of exon-1 deleted by abnormal splicing mechanism.

Phenotype	Genotype	Anaemia
Asymptomatic		
HbE heterozygote	β^N/β^E	No
HbE heterozygote and α^+-thalassemia heterozygote	β^N/β^E and $\alpha\alpha/\alpha^+$-thal	No
HbE heterozygote and α^0-thalassemia heterozygote	β^N/β^E and $\alpha\alpha/\alpha^0$-thala	No
HbE homozygote	β^E/β^E	No
HbE homozygote and α-thalassemia heterozygote	β^E/β^E and $\alpha\alpha/\ \alpha^+$-thal	No
HbE/HbC	β^E/β^C	No
Symptomatic		
HbE homozygote and Hb CS homozygote	β^E/β^E and Hb CS/ Hb CS	Mild
HbE/β^0-thalassemia	β^0/β^E	Moderate to severe
HbE/β^+-thalassemia	$\beta^E/\ \beta^+$	Mild

N: normal; CS: constant spring; thal: thalassaemia.

Table 1.
Common HbE syndrome and their respective genotype.

In Thailand and different South East Asian countries, the association between HbE and α-thalassemia (−α/αα) causes a various range of phenotypic diversity. Clinical parameters exhibit that level of HbE is almost similar in the case of HbE heterozygous and compound heterozygous for α^+ − thalassemia (−α/αα), whereas the co-association of α^0-thalassemia (−α/−−) have mild thalassemia like syndrome with HbE ranges between 19 and 21%. In certain extreme cases where HbE is associated with HbH disease (−−/−α) which is characterized by 13–15% of HbE and it is called HbAE Bart's Disease [22]. On other hand, the compound heterozygote condition for HbE and β-thalassemia leads to the formation of HbE/β-thalassemia which exhibits a remarkably heterogenous range of phenotypic variability. The phenotypic variability may be influenced by the inheritance of α^0 and α^+ mutant alleles [23]. Heterogenous types of HbE syndromes are also observed due to interaction with other hemoglobinopathies. The symptomatic and asymptomatic forms of HbE syndrome are summarized in **Table 1**. The blood smears of different types of HbE-thalassemia and its co-association with other types of hemoglobinopathies have been depicted in **Figure 2**.

4. Phenotypic heterogeneity of HbE/β-thalassemia

The clinical heterogeneity of HbE/β-thalassemia is not well understood. The condition may present as mild, asymptomatic anemia or life-threatening disorder that may lead to lethality from anemia in the first years of life. The phenotype of HbE/β-thalassemia seems to be unstable. Scanty reports have been found on the clinical heterogeneity of these patients. At one end of the spectrum, there are patients whose clinical severity is alike to that of β-thalassemia major; whereas at another end there are patients who can lead a normal life without the need for regular blood transfusions.

At the time of birth, infants with severe HbE/β-thalassemia patients are asymptomatic as the HbF level becomes high. As the production of HbF becomes low with increasing age and is replaced by HbE, gradually anemia and splenomegaly develop during the first decade of life [18]. Moreover, deficient blood transfusion can lead to

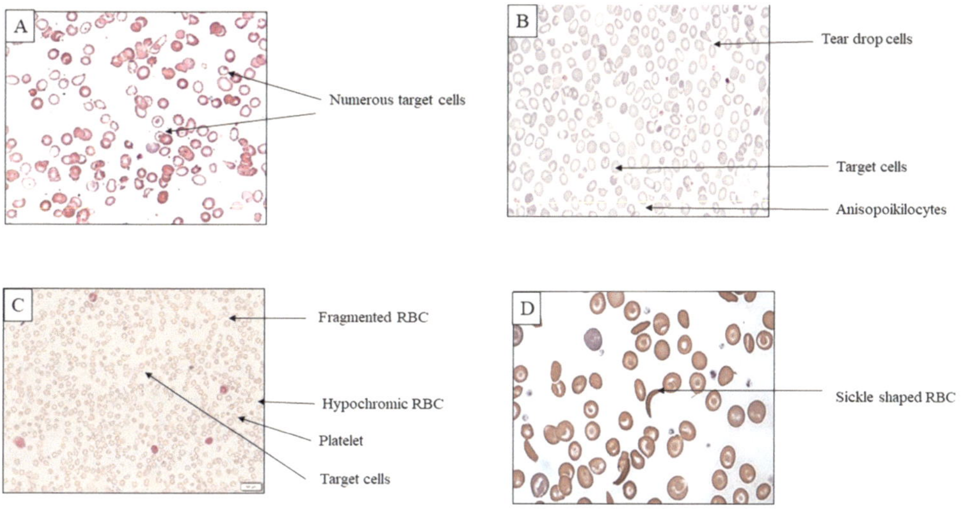

Figure 2.
The peripheral blood film in the (A) homozygous state for hemoglobin E shows large numbers of target cells, (B) HbH disease indicating tear drop cells and anisopoikilocytes, (C) HbE/β-thalassemia contains numerous fragmented RBC, hypochromic RBC, and target cells, (D) HbSE disease having sickle-shaped RBC in blood smear.

anemia, jaundice, hepatomegaly, and growth retardation. Sometimes chronic leg ulcer is also associated with delayed sexual development. Decreased oxygen delivery leads to ineffective erythropoiesis which is like β-thalassemia major. Patients with milder forms of HbE/β-thalassemia tend to grow normally and are generally active. Usually, there is a delayed pubertal growth pattern and under-developed secondary sexual characteristics. Although it is still not distinct whether they further develop complications in the near future. Gradual iron absorption may develop endocrine complications like diabetes. The clinical symptoms of HbE/β-thalassemia has been depicted in **Figure 3**.

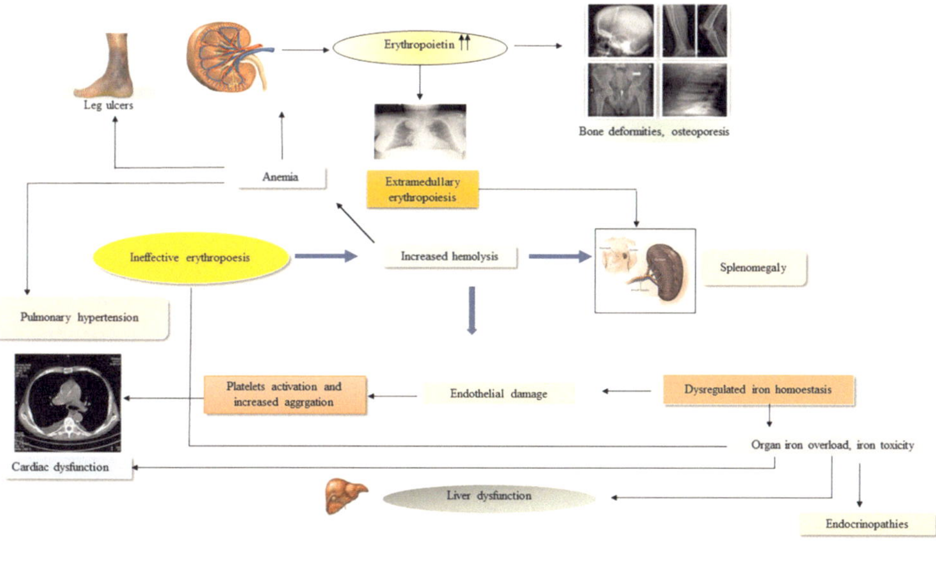

Figure 3.
Clinical heterogeneity of HbE/β-thalassemia patients.

4.1 Asymptomatic forms

HbE trait: Individuals with the HbE trait are clinically normal with minimal changes in blood count and erythrocyte indices. Haemoglobin electrophoresis reveals the presence of HbE is approximately 28.5 ± 1.5%. Likewise, the hemolysate in compound heterozygotes for HbE and $\alpha + -$thalassemia contains 25–30%. Due to the coinheritance of α^0-thalassemia, HbE levels are reduced up to 19–21% and in the case of HbAE Bart's disease syndrome, there is a markedly reduction in HbE (13–15%). On the other hand, the interaction of β-thalassemia can cause the elevation of HbE (>39%). Iron deficiency also causes lower amounts of HbE and MCV, MCH in the case of HbE trait [24].

Homozygous HbE: The clinical symptoms of HbE homozygous appear as normal individuals except few clinical conditions like jaundice and hepatosplenomegaly; although the reticulocyte count and hemoglobin level appear as normal (>10 g/dl). The hematological profile reveals nearly 85–95% of HbE and about 20–80% target cells with reduced osmotic fragility. In these patients, HbE/A2 level is high (10–90%) with lower HbA and HbF levels [25]. The interaction of HbE with different types of hemoglobinopathies has been depicted in **Figure 4** where chromatograms of high performance liquid chromatography have been described.

4.2 Symptomatic forms

The co-inheritance of the HbE and β^0-thalassemia trait can lead to transfusion-dependent form of thalassemia major. Likewise, the co-association between HbE homozygote and Hb CS causes mild anemic condition. In contrast, the association between HbE and β^0 mutant allele can cause moderate to severe thalassemia. The coinheritance of HbE homozygotes with HbH disease (α^o-Thal/$\alpha + -$thal and β^E/β^E)

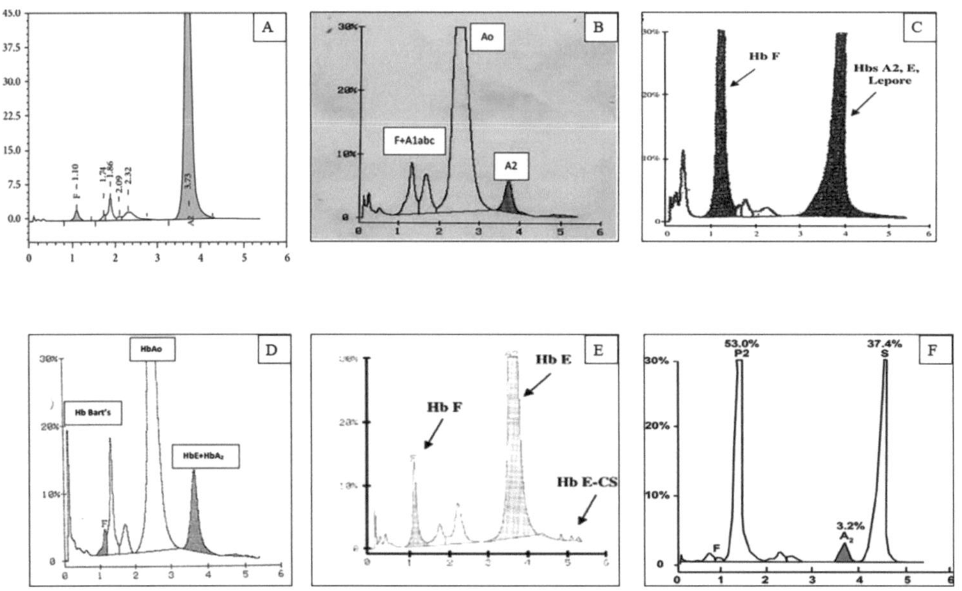

Figure 4.
Chromatograms of HPLC showing interactions of HbE with different hemoglobinopathies (A) HbE homozygous, (B) HbE/β-thalassemia, (C) Hb Lapore, (D) HbAE Bart, (E) HbE-CS, (F) HbSE.

Types of HbE	Clinical symptoms
HbEE	• Hematological findings are similar to that of beta-thalassemia carrier • Hypochromic microcytic red cells with target cells • Reduced mean corpuscular volume (MCV) and mean corpuscular hemoglobin (MCH) • Normal mean corpuscular hemoglobin concentration (MCHC) • Asymptomatic • Enlarged spleen
HbEE and heterozygous alpha-thalassemia	• Phenotype same as that of heterozygous alpha-thalassemia disease • Mild hypochromic anemia • A little elevated HbF levels
HbH (EF Bart disease)	• Moderate anemia and elevated levels of HbF and Bart
HbE beta^0-thalassemia	• The most severe form of HbE syndrome • More severe phenotype than HbE beta$^+$-thalassemia • Haemoglobin level is lower than in HbE disease • Phenotype is similar to that of transfusion-dependent beta-thalassemia major including ineffective erythropoiesis, chronic hemolytic anemia, and iron overload
HbE beta$^+$-thalassemia	Clinical severity is less in comparison to HbE beta^0-thalassemia
HbAE Bart	Small amounts of Hb Bart are present, but hemolytic crises rare
HbEF Bart	HbH is not present, possibly because beta-E chains do not form tetramers; relatively mild form of thalassemia
HbE Constant Spring	Co-inheritance of Hb Constant Spring ameliorates the disease phenotype
HbE Lepore	Mild phenotype
HbE delta-beta-thalassemia	Mild phenotype
HbSE	• Mild anemia with microcytic red cells • Sickling disorder, clinical phenotype like sickle beta$^+$-thalassemia • Vaso-occlusive episodes rare
HbE trait (HbAE)	• Asymptomatic • Minimal morphological abnormalities of red blood cells including reduced MCV, reduced MCH, mild or no anemia • Peripheral smear is characterized by hypochromia, microcytosis, target cells, and irregularly contracted cells

Table 2.
Different types of HbE thalassemia and their clinical symptoms.

and HbH-CS (α^o-Thal/Hb CS and β^E/β^E) lead to form moderate to severe anemia. Severe anemia may also form due to the presence of HbE/β-thalassemia along with HbH disease (α^o-Thal/α^+-thal & β^o/β^E) or HbH-CS disease (α^o-Thal/Hb CS and β^o/β^E) [26].

The different forms of symptomatic and asymptomatic forms of HbE disease have been enlisted in **Table 2**.

5. Genotype-phenotype interaction

The exact reason behind the phenotypic heterogeneity of HbE/β-thalassaemia is not properly understood. For a proper understanding of the clinical severity there is a need for a standardized, robust classification of disease severity; although a lack of suitable clinical severity scoring may impair deciphering of the proper clinical spectrum of HbE/β-thalassemia. According to the phenotypic heterogeneity, patients have been classified into "severe," "moderate," and "mild." There are considerable number of patients who are transfusion-independent while others are regular transfusion-dependent [27–29]. According to the severity of the disease, patients are classified into five groups. Group 1 included those patients who need minimal transfusion requirements as well as normal growth and sexual maturity. Group 2 comprised patients with similar types of quality of life to that of Group 1 except for transfusion history as these patients usually experience longer history of transfusion. Group 3 includes patients who have undergone splenectomy and have an advantageous response to splenectomy. Group 4 comprises patients who are transfusion-dependent and their secondary sexual characteristics and growth rate are not satisfactory. Likewise, Group 5 includes patients who are unable to maintain their regular lifestyle without transfusion [29].

6. Genetic modifiers of HbE/β-thalassemia

The wide range of clinical phenotypes of HbE/β-thalassemia is believed to be regulated through several genetic as well as environmental factors. There is an emerging understanding of the interaction between genetic and environmental factors which triggers the clinical progression and severity.

According to some previous findings, alterations in the *HBB* gene play a crucial role in modulating phenotypic features of HbE/β-thalassemia. Although *HBB* mutations are not only responsible for modulating phenotypic alterations by changing the patterns of gene expression. Currently, genome-wide association study (GWAS) has shown the linked genetic loci to predict phenotype diversity. The genetic modifiers can be classified into the following three groups: the first one is the primary genetic factors including the β-globin gene mutations which are responsible for the manifestation of β-thalassemia; the second one includes loci involved in globin chain synthesis; and the third one is the tertiary factors which are not involved directly in globin chain synthesis but might modulate the disease severity [30].

6.1 Primary modifier

The primary modifier is one of the most important factors responsible for regulating the phenotype variability in β-thalassemia disorder. Such type of defects occurs in the β-globin gene itself [31]. The mutant allele can reduce the synthesis of the β-globin chain or lead to the complete absence of the β^0-globin chain. The patients who inherit a mild β-thalassemia allele with HbE might exhibit minor disease, whereas patients who co-inherit severe β + or β0-thalassemia alleles might exhibit the severe form of the disease [32]. In addition, the severity of β-mutation is an important parameter for determining the clinical diversity of HbE/β-thalassemia. Most of the mutations in the *HBB* gene are point mutation, deletion, or insertion type and situated in the promoter, exon, intron, or at the junction between the intron-exon boundary, and polyadenylation site. Defects in single base substitution in the coding sequence of β-polypeptides will lead to premature stop codon whereas small insertion or deletion may lead to alteration in the reading form of mRNA. Likewise, β + allele defects are generally caused due to single base substitution which causes alteration of mRNA reading frame. The list of mutations responsible for mild and silent types of thalassemia is enlisted in **Table 3**.

Location of mutation	Mild β+	Silent
Transcriptional mutants in the proximal CACC box	−90 (C-T) −88 (C-T) −87 (C-A) −87 (C-T) −87 (C-A) −86 (C-T) −86 (C-G)	−101 (C-T) −92 (C-T)
TATA box	−31 (A-G) −30 (T-A) −29 (A-G)	
5′ UTR	+22 (G-A) +10 (−T) +33 (C-G)	+1 (A-C)
Alternative splicing	CD 19 (A-C), Malay CD 24 (T-A)	CD 27 (G-T), Hb Knossos
Consensus splicing	IVS 1-6 (T-C)	
Intron		IVS 2-844 (C-G)
3′ UTR		+6 (C-G)
Poly-A site	AACAAA AATGAA	
Mild β°-frameshift	CD 6 (−AA) CD 8 (−AA)	

Table 3.
List of HBB *gene mutations responsible for mild β + and silent type thalassemia.*

In the Indian population, five mutations are the most frequently found β-globin gene including IVS 1-5 (G → C), IVS 1-1 (G → T), Codon 41/42 (− TCTT), Codon 8/9 (+G), and 619 bp deletion which account for over 90% of all the mutations associated with β-thalassemia [33, 34], whereas in Malaysian population, IVS1-5(G > C), IVS1-1 (G > T) mutations and Chinese population, CD41/42 (-TCTT), CD71/72(+A), CD 17 (A-T) and − 28 (A-G) mutations are most commonly found. Among the non-sense mutations CD43(G > T), CD35(C > A), CD15(A > G) mutations lead in formation of nonfunctional mRNA, whereas CD8/9(+G), CD15(−T) are frame shift mutations. Certain mutations cause alterations in RNA processing including splice junction changes [CD27/28 + C, CD14/15 + G, CD 95 + A, CD41(-C), CD26 (G > T), IVS1-1 (G > T)]. There are certain deletion mutations including 619 bp del, 3.5 kb del, 45 kb del, and 105 bp del. [35]. Mutation at nucleotide −28 in the ATA box of the β globin gene, was reported earlier among the HbE/β-thalassemia patients [36]. The interaction of two β + globin alleles which is IVS1-5(G > C) and − 28(A > G) resulting in the mild phenotype The beta-thalassemia alleles in "*trans*"-condition to HbE do not seem to have a significant role in regulating phenotypic variation of HbE/β-thalassemia and there must be some other modifying factors. The position of different *HBB* mutations is schematically represented in **Figure 5.** The co-inheritance of β^0-allele with HbE gives rise to widely variable clinical phenotype. Therefore, β-globin gene mutations alone cannot determine the clinical severity.

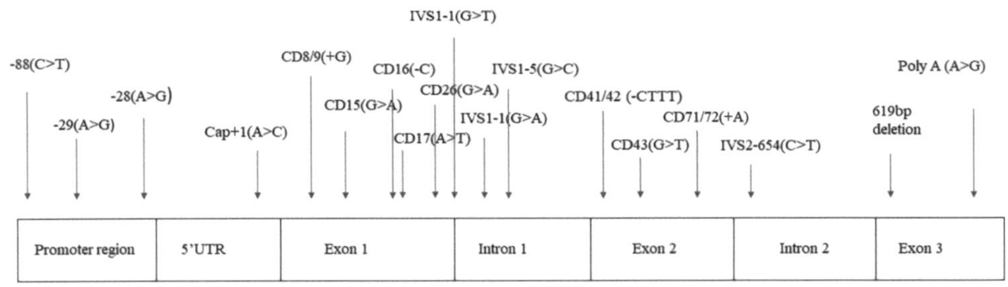

Figure 5.
The position of different HBB *gene mutations within the promoter, 5′ UTR, Exon 1, Intron 1, Exon 2, Intron 2, and Exon 3 region which act as the primary genetic modifiers in HbE/β-thalassemia.*

6.2 Other modifying factors

6.2.1 α-thalassemia

HbE/β-thalassemia patients who co-inherit determinants for α-thalassemia may have some unmatched α-globin chains leading to more balanced globin chain synthesis and resulting in a milder phenotype. According to some previous studies, HbE/β-thalassemia patients with α^+-thalassemia allele demonstrate higher state of hemoglobin in comparison to those who do not have α-thalassemia [37, 38]. One of the studies done on Thai HbE patients revealed that the mean age of clinical presentation was more than those patients who did not possess α-thalassemia mutations [39]. Another study done on Indian HbE/β-thalassemia patients presented that coinheritance of the triplicated α-globin gene led to the formation of mild phenotype and their transfusion requirement was also minimal [40]. Therefore, the coinheritance of the alpha thalassemia gene appears as a major genetic factor regulating the clinical phenotype.

6.2.2 Determining factors for regulating increased HbF level

Xmn1 polymorphism: The presence of G to T substitution at −158 position 5′ to Gγ gene (*Xmn*1 polymorphism) is known to be associated with increased HbF production. Earlier investigations showed that patients with the *Xmn*1 (+/+) genotype were identified only in mildly affected patients; in contrast, patients having the *Xmn*1 (−/−) genotype exhibited severe phenotypes including early age of onset and more transfusion dependency [41, 42]. Overall homozygosity for *Xmn*1 appeared as a crucial genetic determinants for HbE/β-thalassemia; although some conflicting data were presented.

Additional genetic factors: Recently, genome-wide association studies elucidate the role of several additional genetic factors in regulating clinical variability. Numerous single nucleotide polymorphisms (SNPs) in the *BCL11A* gene on chromosome 2p16.1 are known to increase the F-cell number [43]. An extensive genetic association study revealed the presence of quantitative trait loci (QTL) on chromosomes 6q23, 8q, and Xp22 may facilitate the amount of HbF production [44]. Apart from these loci, there are certain other protein molecules including erythropoietin, β-protein 1, *EKLF, GATA-1,* and *NF-E2* which have significant role in regulating the HbF level. The strongest correlation was observed in SNPs in the β-globin gene cluster (chr.11p15), rs2071348 of the *HBBP*1 and intergenic region between the *HBS1L* and *MYB* genes (chr.6q23) which had important significant role in modulating the clinical heterogeneity.

α-hemoglobin stabilizing protein (AHSP) gene: The alpha hemoglobin stabilizing protein (AHSP) is an erythroid-specific protein which has a potential role as a molecular chaperone for binding with the free α-chains of hemoglobin molecule. AHSP participated in the hemoglobin synthesis and reduced the cytotoxic effect of excessive α-globin chain accumulation [45]. Since these proteins are essential for conformational change in many essential proteins required for erythropoiesis, it might have a certain important role in Hb E/β-thalassaemia.

6.2.3 Bilirubin metabolism

The phenotype of HbE disease is also altered by the presence of chronic hyperbilirubinemia, and gallstone formation. The increased level of bilirubin is associated with the polymorphism of the promoter of the UDP-glucuronosyltransferase-1 (UGT1) gene [46]. The UGT1 gene polymorphism is also important in the genesis of gall stone. Investigators found significantly higher bilirubin levels in HbE/β-thalassemia patients [47].

6.2.4 Coinheritance of other hematologic disorders

Coinheritance of other hematologic aberrations may play important role in phenotypic alterations within the patients with HbE/β-thalassemia. The deficiency of pyrimidine 5 nucleotidase 1 (P5N-I) is found to be resulting in hemolytic anemia while co-associated with homozygous HbE [48]. Therefore, the inhibition of P5N-I activity may lead to severe hemolysis related to HbE.

6.2.5 Variation in iron overload

Poor growth and delayed sexual maturation are the common complications found in a majority of HbE/β-thalassemia and it may be resulted in chronic anemia, iron overload, or a combination of these. Many patients with a transfusion history have substantial iron overload and end-organ damage. Some of the previous studies reported that mutations within the *SLC40A1*, hepcidin, and hemojuvelin might play a crucial role in iron overload [49–51]. Although the complete profile of iron overload among the HbE/β-thalassemia patients is not completely understood.

7. Environmental influences on the phenotype of HbE/beta-thalassemia

There are scanty reports available on the environmental influence of HbE/beta-thalassemia. In tropical regions and developing countries, there is a higher incidence of malaria. It is one of the major health issues in many Asian countries and mostly the transmission occurs through *P. falciparum* and *P. vivax*. A population-based study among the HbE/β-thalassemia revealed the level of malarial antibody is significantly high, especially among splenectomized patients rather than those with the intact spleen. Overall, the quantity of malarial antibodies was quite higher in HbE/β-thalassemia patients rather than control population [52]. Studies reported that the growth of malarial parasites was inhibited in HbE cells [53]. Children with HbE/β-thalassemia are more prone to *P. vivax* due to the production of an increased amount of young red cell population. *P. vivax* has high potentiality for invasion within the young red blood cell [54]. Although, the biological pathways linking HbE thalassemia and malarial infection are not completely still understood and yet not investigated so much. Further research is required to elucidate whether there is a positive selection for HbE due to protection against malarial infection. The finding is very important for the treatment purpose of malaria, especially in developing countries like India and other South-East Asian countries where HbE/β-thalassemia is very common. Patients with HbE/β-thalassemia should be provided with prophylaxis against common forms of malaria.

7.1 Treatment strategy

The time of diagnosis, physical examination, and clinical history may give proper information for providing potentially effective treatment strategies. The proper history of appetite, weight gain, energy level, irritability, different major and minor infections, and daily functioning details may help in defining the proper clinical status of a child with thalassemia. Moreover, the genotype of the patients, the presence of α-thalassemia, and polymorphism associated with increased HbF production should also be investigated intermittently. Among the pathological features, Hb concentration, and platelet count should be determined in each visit. Serum EPO level, ferritin, or transferrin saturation should also be considered in the regular interval [55]. In the case of HbE/β-thalassemia patients, there is a significant decrease in the oxygen affinity of hemoglobin in comparison to other types of β-thalassemia diseases which indicates that HbE thalassemia might adapt better to anemia; therefore, proper treatment guidelines should be followed which depends on the clinical severity score of the patient.

7.2 Transfusions

Patients with severe forms of HbE need lifelong RBC transfusions, iron chelation therapy, and management of complications. In contrast, patients with milder forms of disease severity only require occasional blood transfusions. The pre-transfusion hemoglobin concentration of 9–10 g/dl is recommended as this is required for preventing ineffective erythropoiesis. The hemoglobin threshold for determining the increased frequency of disease complications was 7–8 g/dl [56]. The optimal quantity of hemoglobin should be maintained with accessibility to iron chelation therapy. Some patients may need regular transfusion as it is essential to identify phenotypic heterogeneity between "mild" and "severe" within a narrow range of stable stage hemoglobin values [27, 28]. Generally, transfusion-dependent patients should be monitored carefully especially their quality of life, spleen size, signs, and symptoms of anemia. Sometimes, many HbE/β-thalassemia children suffer from different complications due to unnecessary administration of regular transfusion therapy for several years.

7.3 Splenectomy

One of the treatment strategies for transfusion-dependent thalassemia patients is splenectomy which is believed to ameliorate red blood cell transfusion. Although not all patients respond equally to splenectomy. Moreover, splenectomy might facilitate many unfavorable consequences like postoperative infections and thromboembolic events [57]. In recent years, the use of splenectomy is characteristically reduced due to an adequate amount of blood transfusion. When the annual blood transfusion volume exceeds 225–250 ml/kg, splenectomy is prescribed among patients with increased demand for transfusion, hypersplenism, or splenomegaly due to severe hemolysis [58]. Splenectomy might have some benefits in HbE/β-thalassemia patients. Although it is not clear that morbidity and mortality due to infection after splenectomy are higher in all groups of patients.

7.4 Iron chelation therapy

Regular transfusion-dependent patients require iron chelation therapy. Even in the absence of transfusions, chelation therapy may be required in some patients with HbE thalassemia because of excess intestinal iron absorption. In the case of regular blood transfusion, each RBC contains 200 mg of iron which leads to nearly 0.3–0.6 mg/kg per day iron accumulation. Iron chelators are classified into three classes: Deferasirox (DFX), Deferiprone (DFP), and Deferoxamine (DFO) [59]. DFX (Exjade) is recommended as an iron chelator after 2005 for transfusion overloaded [60, 61]. It is found to be effective both in the case of offspring and grownups. Generally, 20–30 mg/kg daily dose is recommended; although in certain cases, the dose is recommended to enhance up to 40 mg/kg daily. DFP is generally absorbed by the gastrointestinal tract and the half-life period of DFP is 1.5–4 hours in plasma. The dose is recommended as 75 mg/kg daily. This dose might be elevated to 100 mg/kg daily [62]. It has efficiency for improving cardiac function by removing iron from cardiac muscle [63]. Deferoxamine (DFO) enters the parenchymal cells of the liver where it chelates the iron as the iron chelator DFO in plasma and bile. The dose and duration of administration differ from patient to patient and depend on how much amount of iron is accumulated after transfusion [64]. Chelation therapy is generally initiated after 20–25 RBC units are transfused between 2 and 4 years of age [65].

Patients should be prescribed iron chelation treatment according to proper guidelines. Quantitative assessment of iron is now recommended among patients before starting chelation therapy [37]. In patients who fail to respond sufficiently to a single iron-chelating drug, the dose can be augmented for betterment [66, 67]. The low molecular weight orally absorbed DFP and DFX quickly access intracellular iron in cytosol and organelles whereas larger DFO molecule contacts with these intracellular iron pools relatively slowly; although it interacts more effectively with lysosomal ferritin iron [68].

7.5 Bone marrow transplantation (BMT)

The bone marrow transplantation is regarded as the main conclusive treatment approach for thalassemia patients [69]. The most effective transplantation was completed in the 1980s. The thalassemia-free survival rate is 70% in very young individuals after satisfactory BMT whereas the rejection rate is 23%, and the mortality rate is 7% [70]. In this therapy, hematopoietic stem cells (HSC) from the bone marrow of healthy individuals are collected and transmitted to thalassemia patients [71]. Although BMT has a few disadvantages like human leukocyte antigen-matched compatible donor is required for the successful attempt. Graft versus host disease (GVHD) is the most clinically important problem associated with bone marrow transplantation which may lead to lethality [72]. In low socioeconomic developing countries, treatment through BMT is still not accessible for all patients and the accessible treatment includes chelation therapy and transfusion of packed red cells.

7.6 Gene therapy

Gene transfer therapy helps in introducing genetic materials into the cells. If the altered gene leads to forming the necessary protein being defective, gene transfer therapy can bring about a normal copy of the gene to regain the proper function of the targeted protein. In gene therapy initially, a hematopoietic stem and progenitor cells (HSPCs) of patients are harvested from the peripheral blood, bone marrow, and umbilical cord blood. Through a lentiviral vector, normal β or γ-gene is transferred into the genome of host cells. Hemoglobin genome is transferred into pluripotent hematopoietic cells and is also performed carefully in humans [73]. The cells that contain expected genes are again implanted into patients where they multiply and proliferate in the bone marrow.

Induced pluripotent stem cells (iPSCs) are also used in future gene therapies. Recently, iPSCs are used as in vitro models to reveal the pathophysiological mechanisms of human diseases. In this technique, somatic cells are first isolated from the patients and then remodeled into a pluripotent form [74]. Induced pluripotent stem cells (iPSCs) are susceptible to acchieve alterations in the gene. Then after, these cells are distinguished into hematopoietic stem and progenitor cells and then transferred back into the individuals.

Gene editing is another approach to future gene therapy. According to this method, human DNA can be cut at specific nucleases, like CRISPR/Cas9 and zinc-finger nucleases [75]. They can either enhance the production of HbF, by reorienting the mutations seen in the hereditary persistence of fetal hemoglobin or act specifically on the erythroid enhancer region that regulates the switch from the γ-globin gene to β-globin gene. Recently, gene editing was done by treating with CRISPR/Cas9 gene-editing method in a thalassemia patient with β0/IVS-1-110 genotype. By editing *BCL11A* gene (chromosome 2) the HbF level was elevated and the patient was transfusion-independent at 12-months follow-up [76].

8. Induction of fetal hemoglobin production

Various drugs are used to induce the production of HbF including Hydroxyurea (HU). It is used for the treatment of sickle cell anemia as well as thalassemia. HU enhances the production of gamma-globin gene and improves the hematological profile of thalassemia patients. It increases the expression of fetal hemoglobin by regulating the expression of GATA-2 (fetal hemoglobin regulating gene) which is related to the cell cycle and apoptosis. It may also facilitate the propagation of progenitor cells and enhance the quantity of erythropoietin [77]. At the same time, 5-azacytidine and butyrate analogs have also been used most frequently to elevate the HbF level [78, 79].

Several HbF inducers inhibit the histone deacetylase (HDAC) activity [80] and can stimulate the HbF level without disturbing the growth and proliferation of other cells. The combined use of HbF inducers may improve the result. Presently, different oligonucleotide (ODN)-based approaches might help design specific treatment strategies for different types of β-thalassemia [81].

9. Molecular therapy for HbE/β-thalassemia

The severity of β-thalassemia, as well as HbE/β-thalassemia, can be reduced by regulating the amount of free α-globin chain synthesis by the coinheritance of α-thalassemia which may reduce the disease severity. The upregulation of AHSP protein or synthesis of such type of similar agent can limit the formation of α inclusion bodies and ineffective erythropoiesis [45].

Moreover, there are some additional prognostic indicators including *Xmn*1 polymorphism, co-existence of Alpha globin gene mutations, and age of onset [82]. Ethnicity and environment are also significant parameters for the analysis of genotype and phenotype correlation. Genetic modifiers that enhance the secondary complications resulting from severe anemia or excessive iron overload due to frequent transfusion are also considered for determining the disease's severity and progression [83]. Therapeutic antisense m RNA is used for correcting aberrent RNA splicing. The use of morpholino oligonucleotides has the ability for high level correction of transcribed mutant β-globin m RNA. These oligonucleotides have been shown to correct the aberrant splice site in a HeLa cell line bearing β^E/IVS1–6 mutations. The repaired β^E-mRNA was stable and translated into mature β^E globin polypeptide [84]. Another approach for molecular therapy of HbE/β -thalassemia in the Ubiquitin-dependent α-chain proteolysis. The excess α-globin chains in β -thalassemia and HbE/β -thalassemia erythrocytes are degraded by ATP and ubiquitin-dependent mechanisms. The cytosolic α-chain precipitation and subsequent cellular damage and haemolysis may be reduced due to efficient proteolysis. Previous experiments demonstrated that radiolabelled α-chains in hemolysates obtained from β-thalassaemia patients were degraded in increased level due to hydrolysis through Ubiquitin aldehyde [85]. *Role of antioxidants in cellular damage* several studies have demonstrated that reactive oxygen species (ROS) play a crucial role in the pathophysiology of thalassemia. Thalassemia patients have very high level of malonyldialdehyde, a biproduct of lipid peroxidation. Transfusion-dependent HbE/β-thalassemia patients have very high level of serum iron and correlates positively with levels of malonyldialdehyde [86]. Treatment with Vitamin C and E is well known to improve the oxidative profile of thalassemia patients [87].

The phenotype heterogeneity of HbE/β-thalassemia causes difficulty in the proper management and classification of the disease. Although some of the genetic factors have been recognized as possible modifiers, the wide range of phenotypic alterations cannot be well understood and it requires thorough investigation from early childhood before substantial medical intervention [88, 89]. With the advancement of molecular technologies, the association studies between genetic polymorphism and thalassemia may help explore potential clinical applications by providing possible risk markers and therapeutic targets. The development of personalized medicine is the main objective and genetic counseling should be included in providing patient care programs in the proper management of HbE/β thalassemia patients in the future.

Acknowledgements

We thank our colleagues for their assistance and constant support provided by them.

Author contributions

Conceptualization, Supervision and Editing: TKD and SMC.
Conceptualization, Original Draft writing formatting and Editing: AP.
Writing and formatting: BD.

Conflict of interest

The authors declare that they have no competing interests.

Appendix A: Mutations in the human beta globin gene cluster-responsible for β0 or β+ type of thalassemias

Mutation position in *HBB* gene	Name of the mutations	HGVS nomenclature	Phenotype
(A) G-gamma, A-gamma, ψβ, δ and Locus control region (hypersensitive sites) of HBB gene	Turkish G gamma (Agamma delta beta)	NG_000007.3:g.45410_81665del36256	β0
	HPFH-6	NG_000007.3:g.45595_124872del79278	β0
	German G gamma (Agamma delta beta)	NG_000007.3:g.(45922_46319)_(98640_99640)del	β0
	Malay-2 Ggamma (Agamma delta beta)	NG_000007.3:g.(47376_47553)_(89149_90149)del	β0
	Italian (Agamma-delta-beta)	NG_000007.3:g.(48103_48100)_(103161_103158) del55059	β0
	Algerian HPFH deletion	U01317.1:g.[(48747_72606)del23860;(72609_72611)delA]	HPFH
	French West-Indies HPFH deletion	U01317.1: g.48762_72489del23728insCAGCAGGAAAGTGTGAGAAG	HPFH
	Chinese Ggamma (A gamma deltabeta)	NG_000007.3:g.48795_127698del78904	β0
	Black Ggamma (Agammadeltabeta)	NG_000007.3:g.49040_84889del35850	β0
	Indian Ggamma Agamma(deltabeta)	NG_000007.3:g.50509_83170del32662	β0
	Japanese (deltabeta)	NG_000007.3:g.51483_165148del113666	β0
	French HPFH deletion	U01317.1:g.[53013_72746del19734;53009_53010insC].	HPFH
	HPFH-3; Indian	NG_000007.3:g.53390_103157del49768	HPFH
	HPFH-2; Ghanaian	NG_000007.3:g.54867_139178del84312	HPFH
	HPFH-1; Black	NG_000007.3:g.59478_144395del84918	HPFH
	Spanish (deltabeta)0-Thal	NG_000007.3:g.60375_153285del92911	(δβ)0
	Black (deltabeta)0-Thal	NG_000007.3:g.(60530_60730)_(72351_72551)del11822	β0
	-125 bp deletion	U01317:g.61953_62077del125	β0
	Kabylian deletion-insertion	U01317.1:g.62009_64049del2040insATAAG	β0
	NG_000007.3:g.(63154-63209)-(70570-70625) del7417	NG_000007.3:g.(63154_63209)_(70570_70625)del7417	(δβ)0

Mutation position in *HBB* gene	Name of the mutations	HGVS nomenclature	Phenotype
	Sicilian (deltabeta)0-Thal	NG_000007.3:g.64336_77738del13403	β0
	Thai (deltabeta)0-Thal	NG_000007.3:g.64384_76993del12610	β0
	~45 kb deletion; the Filipino deletion	NG_000007.3:g.66258_184734del118477	β0
II. 5'-UTR: CAP site	CAP +1 (A->C)	HBB:c.-50A>C	β+
	5'UTR; +10 (-T)	HBB:c.-41delT	β+(Silent)
	5'UTR; +22 (G->A)	HBB:c.-29G>A	β+
	5'UTR; +33 (C->G)	HBB:c.-18C>G	β+ (silent)
	5'UTR; +43 to +40 (-AAAC)	HBB:c.-11_-8delAAAC	β+
(B) Codon ***I. Exon -1***	Initiation codon ATG->GTG	HBB:c.1A>G	β0
	Initiation codon T>A	HBB:c.2T>A	β (0 or + unclear)
	Initiation codon ATG->ACG beta0	HBB:c.2T>C	β0
	Initiation codon ATG->AGG	HBB:c.2T>G	β0
	Initiation codon ATG->ATA	HBB:c.3G>A	β0
	Initiation codon ATG->ATT	HBB:c.3G>T	β0
	Initiation codon ATG->ATC	HBB:c.3G>C	β0
	Codon 1 (-G); GTG(Val)->-TG	HBB:c.4delG	β0
	Codons 2/3/4 (-9 bp; +31 bp)	HBB: c.7_15delinsCCTGAGGTGAAGTCTGCCTGAGGAGAAGTCT	β0
	Codon 5 (-CT); CCT(Pro)->C–	HBB:c.17_18delCT	β0
	Codon 5/6 (-TG)	HBB:c.18_19delTG	β (0 or + unclear)
	HBB:c.20_45del26	HBB:c.20_45del	β0
	Codon 6 (-A); GAG(Glu)->G-G	HBB:c.20delA	β0

DOI: http://dx.doi.org/10.5772/intechopen.109999

Mutation position in *HBB* gene	Name of the mutations	HGVS nomenclature	Phenotype
	HBB:c.8delA	HBB:c.8delA	β0
	Codon 8 (-AA); AAG(Lys)->–G	HBB:c.25_26delAA	β0
	Codons 8/9 (+AGAA)	HBB:c.23_26dup	β0
	Codons 7/8 (+G); GAG AAG(Glu;Lys)->GAG G AAG	HBB:c.24_25insG	β0
	Codons 8/9 (+G); AAG TCT(Lys;Ser)->AAG G TCT	HBB:c.27_28insG	β0
	Codons 9/10 (+T); TCT GCC(Ser;Ala)->TCT T GCC	HBB:c.30_31insT	β0
	Codon 10 (C->A); GCC(Ala)->GCA(Ala)	HBB:c.33C>A	β+
	Codon 11 (-T); GTT(Val)->GT	HBB:c.36delT	β0
	Codons 14/15 (+G); CTG TGG(Leu;Trp)->CTG G TGG	HBB:c.45_46insG	β0
	Codon 15 (-T); TGG(Trp)->-GG	HBB:c.46delT	β0
	Codon 15 (G->A); TGG(Trp)->TAG(stop codon) beta0	HBB:c.47G>A	β0
	Codon 15 (G->A); TGG(Trp)->TGA(stop codon)	HBB:c.48G>A	β0
	Codon 16 (-C); GGC(Gly)->GG	HBB:c.51delC	β0
	Codon 17 (A->T); AAG(Lys)->TAG(stop codon)	HBB:c.52A>T	β0
	Codon 22 (G->T); GAA(Glu)->TAA(stop codon)	HBB:c.67G>T	β0
	Codons 22/23/24 (GAA GTT GGT; Glu Val Gly); deletion of -AAGTTGG	HBB:c.68_74delAAGTTGG	β0
	Codon 24 (T->A); GGT(Gly)->GGA(Gly)	HBB:c.75T>A	β+

Mutation position in *HBB* gene	Name of the mutations	HGVS nomenclature	Phenotype
	44 bp deletion	HBB:c.76_92+27del	β0
	Codon 24; GGT(Gly); (-G; +CAC)	HBB:c.74delinsCAC	β0
	Codons 25/26 (+T); GGT GAG(Gly-Glu)->GGT T GAG(Gly-Term)	HBB:c.78_79insT	β0
	Codon 26 (+T); GAG(Glu)->GTAG	HBB:c.79_80insT	β0
	Codon 26 (G->T); GAG(Glu)->TAG(stop codon)	HBB:c.79G>T	β0
	Codons 27/28 (+C); GCC CTG(Ala Ser)->GCC C CTG	HBB:c.84_85insC	β0
	Codon 28 (-C); CTG(Leu)->-TG	HBB:c.85delC	β0
	Codons 28/29 (-G); CTG GGC(Leu Gly)->CTG -GC	HBB:c.89delG	β0
	25 bp deletion	HBB:c.93-22_95del	β0
II. Exon-2	Codons 36/37 (-T); CCT TGG(Pro-Trp)->CCT -GG	HBB:c.112delT	β0
	Codon 37 (TGG>TAG)	HBB:c.113G>A	β0
	Codon 37 (G->A); TGG(Trp)->TGA(stop codon)	HBB:c.114G>A	β0
	Codons 37/38/39 (-7 nts)	HBB:c.114_120delGACCCAG	β0
	Codons 38/39 (-C); ACC CAG(Thr Gln)->ACC -AG	HBB:c.118delC	β0
	Codon 39 (C->T); CAG(Gln)->TAG(stop codon)	HBB:c.118C>T	β0
	Codon 39 (-A)	HBB:c.119delA	β0
	Codon 40 (-G); AGG(Arg)->AG	HBB:c.123delG	β0
	Codons 40/41 (+T); AGG TTC(Arg-Phe)->AGG T TTC	HBB:c.123_124insT	β0

Mutation position in *HBB* gene	Name of the mutations	HGVS nomenclature	Phenotype
	Codons 41/42 (-TTCT); TTCTTT(Phe-Phe)->- - - -TT	HBB:c.126_129delCTTT	β0
	Codon 41 (-C); TTC(Phe)->TT	HBB:c.126delC	β0
	Codons 42/43 (+G); TTT GAG(Phe Glu)->TTT G GAG	HBB:c.129_130insG	β0
	Codon 43 (G->T); GAG(Glu)->TAG (stop codon)	HBB:c.130G>T	β0
	Codon 44 (-C); TCC(Ser)->TC	HBB:c.135delC	β0
	Codon 45 (-T); TTT(Phe)->-TT	HBB:c.138delT	β0
	Codon 46/47 (+G); GGG GAT(Gly; Asp))->GGG G GAT	HBB:c.142_142dup	β0
	Codon 47 (+A); GAT(Asp)->GAA(Glu) T	HBB:c.143_144insA	β0
	Codons 47/48 (+ATCT); GAT CTG(Asp Leu)->GAT CTATCTG	HBB:c.146_147insATCT	β0
	Codon 51 (-C); CCT(Pro)->-CT	HBB:c.155delC	β0
	Codon 52 (-A)	HBB:c.158delA	β0
	53/54 (+G); GCT GTT(Ala-Val)->GCT G GTT	HBB:c.162_163insG	β0
	Codon 54 (-T); GTT(Val)->GT	HBB:c.165delT	β0
	Codons 54/55 (+A); GTT ATG(Val Met)->GTT A ATG	HBB:c.165_166insA	β0
	HBB:c.166_178del13	HBB:c.166_178delATGGGCAACCCTA	β0
	Codons 56/57/58/59/60 (GGC AAC CCT AAG GTG); duplication of 14 bp	HBB:c.170_183dup	β0
	Codons 57/58 (+C); AAC CCT(Asn Pro)->AAC C CCT	HBB:c.174_175insC	β0
	Codon 59 (AAG>TAG)	HBB:c.178A>T	β0

Mutation position in *HBB* gene	Name of the mutations	HGVS nomenclature	Phenotype
	Codon 59 (-A); AAG(Lys)->-AG beta0	HBB:c.179delA	β0
	Codon 61 (A->T); AAG(Lys)->TAG(stop codon)	HBB:c.184A>T	β0
	HBB:c.187_251dup	HBB:c.187_251dup	β0
	Codon 64 (-G); GGC(Gly)->-GC	HBB:c.194delG	β0
	Codon 67 (-TG); GTG(Val)->–G	HBB:c.203_204delTG	β0
	HBB:c.216delT	HBB:c.216delT	β0
	Codons 71/72 (+A); TTT AGT(Phe Ser)->TTT A AGT	HBB:c.216_217insA	β0
	Codon 72/73 (+T)	HBB:c.219_220insT	β (0 or + unclear)
	Codons 74/75 (-C); GGC CTG(Gly Leu)->GG-CTG	HBB:c.226delC	β0
	Cd76 (-GC)	HBB:c.229_230delGC	β0
	Codon 76 (-C); GCT(Ala)->G-T beta0	HBB:c.230delC	β0
	Codon 77/78 (-C)	HBB:c.232delC	β (0 or + unclear)
	Codons 82/83 (-G); AAG GGC(Lys Gly)->AAG -GC	HBB:c.251delG	β0
	Codon 84 (65bp duplication)	HBB:c.252_253insNG_000007.3:g.70911_70975	β0
	Codons 84/85 (+C); ACC TTT(Thr Phe)->ACC C TTT	HBB:c.255_256insC	β0
	Codons 84/85/86 (+T); ACC TTT GCC(Thr Phe Ala)->ACC TTT T GCC	HBB:c.258_259insT	β0
	Codon 88 (+T); CTG(Leu)->CTTG	HBB:c.266_267insT	β0
	Codons 89/90 (-GT); AGT GAG(Ser Glu)->A–GAG	HBB:c.270_271delTG	β0

DOI: http://dx.doi.org/10.5772/intechopen.109999

Mutation position in *HBB* gene	Name of the mutations	HGVS nomenclature	Phenotype
	Codon 90 (G->T); GAG(Glu)->TAG(stop codon)	HBB:c.271G>T	β0
	Codon 95 (+A); AAG(Lys)->AAAG	HBB:c.287_288insA	β0
	Codon 100; -CTT, +TCTGAGAACTT	HBB:c.301_303delinsTCTGAGAACTT	β0
III. Exon-3	Codon 104 (-G)	HBB:c.314delG	β0
	Codon 106 (-CTGGGCAACGTG)	HBB:c.319_330delCTGGGCAACGTG	β (0 or + unclear)
	Codons 106/107 (+G); CTG GGC(Leu Gly)->CTG G GC	HBB:c.321_322insG	β0
	Codons 108/109/110/111/112 (-12 bp)	HBB:c.326_337delACGTGCTGGTCT	β0
	Codon 112 (T->A); TGT(Cys)->TGA(stop codon)	HBB:c.339T>A	β0
	Codon 114 (+TGTGCTG)	HBB:c.345_346insTGTGCTG	β (0 or + unclear)
	Codon 116 (+TGAT)	HBB:c.349_350insTGAT	β0
	Codon 117 (-C)	HBB:c.354delC	β (0 or + unclear)
	Codons 120/121 (+A); AAA GAA(Lys-Glu)->AAA A GAA	HBB:c.363_364insA	β0 (mild/ dominant β)
	Codon 121 (G->T); GAA(Glu)->TAA(stop codon) beta0 (dominant beta-thal trait)	HBB:c.364G>T	β0
	Codon 123/124/125 (-ACCCCACC)	HBB:c.370_378delACCCCACCA	β0
	Codon 124 (-A)	HBB:c.375delA	β0
	Codon 124/125(+A)	HBB:c.375_376insA	β (0 or + unclear)
	Codons 124-126 (+CCA)	HBB:c.378_379insCCA	β0

Mutation position in *HBB* gene	Name of the mutations	HGVS nomenclature	Phenotype
	Codon 125 (-CCAGTG)	HBB:c.376_381delCCAGTG	β (0 or + unclear)
	Codon 125 (-A); CCA(Pro)->CC-	HBB:c.378delA	β0
	Codons 126-131 (Val-Gln-Ala-Ala-Thr-Gln) (-17 bp); GTG CAG GCT GCC TAT CAG->G	HBB:c.380_396delTGCAGGCTGCCTATCAG	β0
	Codon 127 (C->T); CAG(Gln)->TAG(stop codon)	HBB:c.382C>T	β0
	Codon 127 (A->C); CAG(Gln)->CCG(Pro)	HBB:c.383A>C	β+
	Codon 127 (A->G); CAG(Gln)->CGG(Arg)	HBB:c.383A>G	β+
	Codons 127/128 (-AGG); CAG GCT(Gln Ala)->C— CT(Pro)	HBB:c.383_385delAGG	β0
	Codons 128/129 (-4, -GCTG; +5, +CCACA) Codons 132-135 (-11, -AAAGTGGTGGC)	HBB:c.[385_388delinsCCACA;397_407delAAAGTGGTGGC]	β0
	Codon 130 (TAT→TAA)	HBB:c.393T>A	β (0 or + unclear)
	Codon 131 (+A)	HBB:c.394_395insA	β (0 or + unclear)
	Codons 131/132 (-GA)	HBB:c.396_397delGA	β0
	Codon 132A>T	HBB:c.397A>T	β0
	Codons 134-137 [-(G)TGGCTGGTGT(G) and +(G)GCAG(G)]	HBB:c.404_413delinsGCAG	β0
	-7719 bp del	U01317:g.71551_79269del7719	β0
	619 bp deletion	NG_000007.3:g.71609_72227del619	β0
IVS-I	IVS-I (-1) or codon 30 (G->A) AG^GTTGGT->AA^GTTGGT	HBB:c.92G>A	β0
	IVS1-1(G>A); AG^GTTGGT->AGATTGGT	HBB:c.92+1G>A	β0

Mutation position in *HBB* gene	Name of the mutations	HGVS nomenclature	Phenotype
	IVS-I-1 (G->T); AG^GTTGGT->AGTTTGGT	HBB:c.92+1G>T	β0
	IVS-I-2(T>C); AG^GTTGGT->AGACTGGT	HBB:c.92+2T>C	β0
	IVS-I-2 (T->A); AG^GTTGGT->AGGATGGT	HBB:c.92+2T>A	β0
	IVS-I-2 (T->G); AG^GTTGGT->AGGGTGGT	HBB:c.92+2T>G	β0
	IVS-I-5 (G->T)	HBB:c.92+5G>T	β+(severe)
	IVS-I-5 (G->A) plus the Corfu deletion	HBB:c.92+5G>A	β+
	IVS-I-5 (G->A)	HBB:c.92+5G>A	β+(severe)
	IVS-I-5 (G->C)	HBB:c.92+5G>C	β+(severe)
	IVS-I-6 (T->C); the Portuguese	HBB:c.92+6T>C	β+
	IVS I-7 (A>T)	HBB:c.92+7A>T	β+
	IVS-I-110 (G->A) beta+; the mutation is 21 nucleotides 5' to the acceptor splice site AG^GC	HBB:c.93-21G>A	β+
	IVS-I-116 (T->G)	HBB:c.93-15T>G	β0
	IVS-I-128 (T->G); TTAG^GCTG->TGAG^GCTG	HBB:c.93-3T>G	β+
	IVS-I-129 (A>G)	HBB:c.93-2A>G	β0
	IVSI-129 (A>C)	HBB:c.93-2A>C	β (0 or + unclear)
	IVS-I-130 (G->A); TTAG^GCTG->TTAA GCTG	HBB:c.93-1G>A	β0
	IVS-I-130 (G->C); TTAG^GCTG->TTAC GCTG	HBB:c.93-1G>C	β0
IVS-II	IVS II-1 (G>T)	HBB:c.315+1G>T	β0
	IVS-II-1 (G->C)	HBB:c.315+1G>C	β0
	IVS-II-1 (G->A)	HBB:c.315+1G>A	β0

Mutation position in *HBB* gene	Name of the mutations	HGVS nomenclature	Phenotype
	IVS II-2 (T>C)	HBB:c.315+2T>C	β0
	IVS-II-2 (T>A)	HBB:c.315+2T>A	β (0 or + unclear)
	IVS-II-2 (-TGAGTCTATGGG)	HBB:c.315+2_315+13delTGAGTCTATGGG	β (0 or + unclear)
	IVS-II-4,5 (-AG)	HBB:c.315+4_315+5delAG	β (0 or + unclear)
	IVS-II-5 (G->C)	HBB:c.315+5G>C	β+(severe)
	IVS-II-654 (C->T); AAGGCAATA->AAG^GTAATA	HBB:c.316-197C>T	β+(severe)
	IVS-II-705 (T->G); GATGTAAGA->GAG^GTAAGA	HBB:c.316-146T>G	β+
	IVS II-726 (A>G)	HBB:c.316-125A>G	β+
	IVS-II-745 (C->G); CAGCTACCAT->CAG^GTACCAT	HBB:c.316-106C>G	β+
	IVS II-761 A>G	HBB:c.316-90A>G	β (0 or + unclear)
	IVS2-781 C>G	HBB:c.316-70C>G	β (0 or + unclear)
	IVS-II-837 (T->G)	HBB:c.316-14T>G	β+/β0
	IVS-II-843 (T->G)	HBB:c.316-8T>G	β+
	IVS-II-844 (C->G)	HBB:c.316-7C>G	β+
	IVS-II-848 (C->G)	HBB:c.316-3C>G	β+
	IVS-II-848 (C->A)	HBB:c.316-3C>A	β+
	IVS-II-849 (A->G)	HBB:c.316-2A>G	β0
	IVS-II-849 (A->C)	HBB:c.316-2A>C	β0
	IVS-II-850 (G->A)	HBB:c.316-1G>A	β0

DOI: http://dx.doi.org/10.5772/intechopen.109999

Mutation position in *HBB* gene	Name of the mutations	HGVS nomenclature	Phenotype
	IVS-II-850 (G->T)	HBB:c.316-1G>T	β0
	IVS-II-850 (G->C)	HBB:c.316-1G>C	β0
	IVS-II-2,3 (+11, -2)	HBB:c.315+2_315+3delinsACGTTCTCTGA	β0
	IVS-II-765 L1	HBB:c.316-86_316-85insCTGCTTTTATTTT	β+
	IVS-I, 3' end; -17 bp	HBB:c.93-17_93-1delTATTTTCCCACCCTTAG	β0
	IVS-II-850 (-G)	HBB:c.316-1delG	β0
	+1480 (C->G)	HBB:c.*6C>G	β+
(E) 3'- UTR region and poly A signalling	3'UTR (-GCATCTGGATTCT)	HBB:c.*91_*103delGCATCTGGATTCT	β (0 or + unclear)
	Poly A (T->C) AATAAA->AACAAA	HBB:c.*110T>C	β+
	Poly A (A->G) AATAAA->AATGAA	HBB:c.*111A>G	β+
	Poly A (A→T) AATAAA>AATATA	HBB:c.*112A>T	β (0 or + unclear)
	Poly A (A->G); AATAAA->AATAGA	HBB:c.*112A>G	β+
	Poly A (A->G); AATAAA->AATAAG	HBB:c.*113A>G	β+
	Poly A (-AATAA); AATAAA->———A	HBB:c.*108_*112delAATAA	β+
	Poly A (-AT or -TA); AATAAA->A–AAA	HBB:c.[*109_*110delAT or *110_*111delTA]	β+

Author details

Amrita Panja[1], Brahmarshi Das[2], Tuphan Kanti Dolai[3]* and Sujata Maiti Choudhury[1]*

1 Biochemistry, Molecular Endocrinology, and Reproductive Physiology Laboratory, Department of Human Physiology, Vidyasagar University, Paschim Medinipore, West Bengal, India

2 Department of Biochemistry, Midnapore Medical College, Paschim Medinipore, West Bengal, India

3 Department of Haematology, Nilratan Sircar Medical College and Hospital, Kolkata, West Bengal, India

*Address all correspondence to: tkdolai@hotmail.com, sujata_vu@mail.vidyasagar.ac.in and sujata.vu2009@gmail.com

References

[1] Origa R. β-Thalassemia. Genetics in Medicine. 2017;**19**(6):609-619. DOI: 10.1038/gim.2016.173

[2] Muncie HL Jr, Campbell J. Alpha and beta thalassemia. American Family Physician. 2009;**80**(4):339-344 PMID: 19678601

[3] Malagù M, Marchini F, Fiorio A, Sirugo P, Clò S, Mari E, et al. Atrial fibrillation in β-thalassemia: Overview of mechanism, significance and clinical management. Biology (Basel). 2022;**11**(1):148. DOI: 10.3390/biology11010148

[4] Williams TN, Weatherall DJ. World distribution, population genetics, and health burden of the hemoglobinopathies. Cold Spring Harbor Perspectives in Medicine. 2012;**2**(9):a011692. DOI: 10.1101/cshperspect.a011692

[5] Colah R, Italia K, Gorakshakar A. Burden of thalassemia in India: The road map for control. Pediatric Hematology Oncology Journal. 2017;**2**(4):79-84. DOI: doi.org/10.1016/j.phoj.2017.10.002

[6] MOHFW (2016) National Health Mission - Guidelines on hemoglobinopathies in India: Prevention and control of hemoglobinopathies in India [Internet]. Available from: https://nhm.gov.in/images/pdf/programmes/RBSK/Resource_Documents/Guidelines_on_Hemoglobinopathies_in India.pdf

[7] Lee JS, Cho SI, Park SS, Seong MW. Molecular basis and diagnosis of thalassemia. Blood Research. 2021;**56**(S1):S39-S43. DOI: 10.5045/br.2021.2020332

[8] Kountouris P, Lederer CW, Fanis P, Feleki X, Old J, Kleanthous M. IthaGenes: An interactive database for haemoglobin variations and epidemiology. PLoS One. 2014;**9**(7): e103020. DOI: 10.1371/journal.pone.0103020

[9] Thein SL. Molecular basis of β thalassemia and potential therapeutic targets. Blood Cells, Molecules & Diseases. 2018;**70**:54-65. DOI: 10.1016/j.bcmd.2017.06.001

[10] Giardine B, Borg J, Viennas E, Pavlidis C, Moradkhani K, Joly P, et al. Updates of the HbVar database of human hemoglobin variants and thalassemia mutations. Nucleic Acids Research. 2014;**42**(Database issue): D1063-D1069. DOI: 10.1093/nar/gkt911

[11] Modell B, Darlison M. Global epidemiology of haemoglobin disorders and derived service indicators. Bulletin of the World Health Organization. 2008; **86**(6):480-487. DOI: 10.2471/blt.06.036673

[12] Weatherall DJ, Clegg JB. The Thalassaemia Syndromes. 4th ed. Oxford, UK: Blackwell Science Ltd; 2001. DOI: 10.1002/9780470696705

[13] Angastiniotis M, Modell B. Global epidemiology of hemoglobin disorders. Annals of the New York Academy of Sciences. 1998;**850**:251-269. DOI: 10.1111/j.1749-6632.1998.tb10482.x

[14] Apidechkul T, Yeemard F, Chomchoei C, Upala P, Tamornpark R. Epidemiology of thalassemia among the hill tribe population in Thailand. PLoS One. 2021;**16**(2):e0246736. DOI: 10.1371/journal.pone.0246736

[15] Kishore B, Khare P, Gupta RJ, Bisht S, Majumdar K. Hemoglobin E disease in North Indian population: A report of 11 cases. Hematology. 2007;**12**(4):343-347. DOI: 10.1080/10245330701255247

[16] Saha, S., Ghosh, S., Basu, K. Bhattacharyya, M. Prevalence of β-haemoglobinopathies in Eastern India and development of a novel formula for carrier detection. Journal of Hematopathology 2020; 13: 159–164. https://doi.org/10.1007/s12308-020-00407-7

[17] Nigam N, Kushwaha R, Yadav G, Singh PK, Gupta N, Singh B, et al. A demographic prevalence of β thalassemia carrier and other hemoglobinopathies in adolescent of Tharu population. Journal of Family Medicine and Primary Care. 2020;**9**(8):4305-4310. DOI: 10.4103/jfmpc.jfmpc_879_20

[18] Fucharoen S, Weatherall DJ. The hemoglobin E thalassemias. Cold Spring Harbor Perspectives in Medicine. 2012;**2**(8):a011734. DOI: 10.1101/cshperspect.a011734

[19] Roca X, Sachidanandam R, Krainer AR. Intrinsic differences between authentic and cryptic 5′ splice sites. Nucleic Acids Research. 2003;**31**(21):6321-6333. DOI: 10.1093/nar/gkg830

[20] Brancaleoni V, Di Pierro E, Motta I, Cappellini MD. Laboratory diagnosis of thalassemia. International Journal of Laboratory Hematology. 2016;**38**(Suppl 1):32-40. DOI: 10.1111/ijlh.12527

[21] Fucharoen S, Sanchaisuriya K, Fucharoen G, Panyasai S, Devenish R, Luy L. Interaction of hemoglobin E and several forms of alpha-thalassemia in Cambodian families. Haematologica. 2003;**88**(10):1092-1098 PMID: 14555303

[22] Traivaree C, Boonyawat B, Monsereenusorn C, Rujkijyanont P, Photia A. Clinical and molecular genetic features of Hb H and AE Bart's diseases in central Thai children. The Application of Clinical Genetics. 2018;**11**:23-30. DOI: 10.2147/TACG.S161152

[23] Hariharan P, Gorivale M, Sawant P, Mehta P, Nadkarni A. Significance of genetic modifiers of hemoglobinopathies leading towards precision medicine. Scientific Reports. 2021;**11**(1):20906. DOI: 10.1038/s41598-021-00169-x

[24] Angastiniotis M, Eleftheriou A, Galanello R, Harteveld CL, Petrou M, Traeger-Synodinos J, Giordano P, Jauniaux E, Modell B, Serour G. Prevention of Thalassaemias and Other Haemoglobin Disorders: Volume 1: Principles [Internet]. Old J, editor. 2nd ed. Nicosia (Cyprus): Thalassaemia International Federation; 2013. PMID: 24672827.

[25] Tyagi S, Pati HP, Choudhry VP, Saxena R. Clinico-haematological profile of HbE syndrome in adults and children. Hematology. 2004;**9**(1):57-60. DOI: 10.1080/10245330310001638983

[26] Old J, Harteveld CL, Traeger-Synodinos J, Petrou M, Angastiniotis M, Galanello R. Prevention of Thalassaemias and Other Haemoglobin Disorder: Volume 2: Laboratory Protocols [Internet]. 2nd ed. Nicosia (Cyprus): Thalassaemia International Federation; 2012. PMID: 24672828

[27] Premawardhena A, Fisher CA, Olivieri NF, de Silva S, Arambepola M, Perera W, et al. Haemoglobin E beta thalassaemia in Sri Lanka. Lancet. 2005;**366**(9495):1467-1470. DOI: 10.1016/S0140-6736(05)67396-5

[28] Olivieri NF, Muraca GM, O'Donnell A, Premawardhena A, Fisher C, Weatherall DJ. Studies in haemoglobin E beta-thalassaemia. British Journal of Haematology. 2008;**141**(3):388-397. DOI: 10.1111/j.1365-2141.2008.07126.x

[29] Olivieri NF, Pakbaz Z, Vichinsky E. HbE/β-thalassemia: Basis of marked clinical diversity. Hematology/Oncology Clinics of North America. 2010;**24**(6):

1055-1070. DOI: 10.1016/j.hoc.2010.08.008

[30] Weatherall DJ. Phenotype-genotype relationships in monogenic disease: Lessons from the thalassaemias. Nature Reviews. Genetics. 2001;**2**(4):245-255. DOI: 10.1038/35066048

[31] George E. HbE β thalassemia in Malaysia: Revisited. Journal of Hematology and Thromboembolic Diseases. 2013;**1**(1):1-3. DOI: 10.4172/2329-8790.1000101

[32] Winichagoon P, Thonglairoam V, Fucharoen S, Wilairat P, Fukumaki Y, Wasi P. Severity differences in beta-thalassaemia/haemoglobin E syndromes: Implication of genetic factors. British Journal of Haematology. 1993;**83**(4):633-639. DOI: 10.1111/j.1365-2141.1993.tb04702.x

[33] Panigrahi I, Marwaha RK. Mutational spectrum of thalassemias in India. Indian Journal of Human Genetics. 2007;**13**(1):36-37. DOI: 10.4103/0971-6866.32034

[34] Shrivastava M, Bathri R, Chatterjee N. Mutational analysis of thalassemia in transfusion-dependent beta-thalassemia patients from central India. Asian Journal of Transfusion Science. 2019;**13**(2):105-109. DOI: 10.4103/ajts.AJTS_115_18

[35] Sherva R, Sripichai O, Abel K, Ma Q, Whitacre J, Angkachatchai V, et al. Genetic modifiers of Hb E/beta-thalassemia identified by a two-stage genome-wide association study. BMC Medical Genetics. 2010;**11**:51. DOI: 10.1186/1471-2350-11-51

[36] Winichagoon P, Fucharoen S, Chen P, Wasi P. Genetic factors affecting clinical severity in beta-thalassemia syndromes. Journal of Pediatric Hematology/Oncology. 2000;**22**(6):573-580. DOI: 10.1097/00043426-200011000-00026

[37] Olivieri NF, Pakbaz Z, Vichinsky E. Hb E/beta-thalassaemia: A common & clinically diverse disorder. The Indian Journal of Medical Research. 2011;**134**(4):522-531 PMID: 22089616

[38] Panigrahi I, Agarwal S, Gupta T, Singhal P, Pradhan M. Hemoglobin E-beta thalassemia: Factors affecting phenotype. Indian Pediatrics. 2005;**42**(4):357-362 PMID: 15876597

[39] Sripichai O, Munkongdee T, Kumkhaek C, Svasti S, Winichagoon P, Fucharoen S. Coinheritance of the different copy numbers of alpha-globin gene modifies severity of beta-thalassemia/Hb E disease. Annals of Hematology. 2008;**87**(5):375-379. DOI: 10.1007/s00277-007-0407-2

[40] Sharma V, Saxena R. Effect of alpha-gene numbers on phenotype of HbE/beta thalassemia patients. Annals of Hematology. 2009;**88**(10):1035-1036. DOI: 10.1007/s00277-009-0723-9

[41] Bashir S, Mahmood S, Mohsin S, Tabassum I, Ghafoor M, Sajjad O. Modulatory effect of single nucleotide polymorphism in Xmn1, BCL11A and HBS1L-MYB loci on foetal haemoglobin levels in β-thalassemia major and Intermedia patients. The Journal of the Pakistan Medical Association. 2021;**71**(5):1394-1398. DOI: 10.47391/JPMA.1351

[42] Jaing TH, Chang TY, Chen SH, Lin CW, Wen YC, Chiu CC. Molecular genetics of β-thalassemia: A narrative review. Medicine (Baltimore). 2021;**100**(45):e27522. DOI: 10.1097/MD.0000000000027522

[43] Menzel S, Garner C, Gut I, Matsuda F, Yamaguchi M, Heath S, et al. A QTL

influencing F cell production maps to a gene encoding a zinc-finger protein on chromosome 2p15. Nature Genetics. 2007; **39**(10):1197-1199. DOI: 10.1038/ng2108

[44] Thein SL, Menzel S, Peng X, Best S, Jiang J, Close J, et al. Intergenic variants of HBS1L-MYB are responsible for a major quantitative trait locus on chromosome 6q23 influencing fetal hemoglobin levels in adults. Proceedings of the National Academy of Sciences of the United States of America. 2007;**104** (27):11346-11351. DOI: 10.1073/pnas.0611393104

[45] Favero ME, Costa FF. Alpha-hemoglobin-stabilizing protein: An erythroid molecular chaperone. Biochemistry Research International. 2011;**2011**:373859. DOI: 10.1155/2011/373859

[46] Bosma PJ, Chowdhury JR, Bakker C, Gantla S, de Boer A, Oostra BA, et al. The genetic basis of the reduced expression of bilirubin UDP-glucuronosyltransferase 1 in Gilbert's syndrome. The New England Journal of Medicine. 1995;**333**(18):1171-1175. DOI: 10.1056/NEJM199511023331802

[47] Premawardhena A, Fisher CA, Fathiu F, de Silva S, Perera W, Peto TE, et al. Genetic determinants of jaundice and gallstones in haemoglobin E beta thalassaemia. Lancet. 2001;**357**(9272): 1945-1946. DOI: 10.1016/s0140-6736 (00)05082-0

[48] Rees DC, Duley J, Simmonds HA, Wonke B, Thein SL, Clegg JB, et al. Interaction of hemoglobin E and pyrimidine 5′ nucleotidase deficiency. Blood. 1996;**88**(7):2761-2767 PMID: 8839873

[49] Merryweather-Clarke AT, Pointon JJ, Jouanolle AM, Rochette J, Robson KJ. Geography of HFE C282Y and H63D mutations. Genetic Testing. 2000;**4**(2): 183-198. DOI: 10.1089/109065700 50114902

[50] Pointon JJ, Viprakasit V, Miles KL, Livesey KJ, Steiner M, O'Riordan S, et al. Hemochromatosis gene (HFE) mutations in South East Asia: A potential for iron overload. Blood Cells, Molecules & Diseases. 2003;**30**(3):302-306. DOI: 10.1016/s1079-9796(03)00041-x

[51] Jones E, Pasricha SR, Allen A, Evans P, Fisher CA, Wray K, et al. Hepcidin is suppressed by erythropoiesis in hemoglobin E β-thalassemia and β-thalassemia trait. Blood. 2015;**125**(5): 873-880. DOI: 10.1182/blood-2014-10-606491

[52] Ha J, Martinson R, Iwamoto SK, Nishi A. Hemoglobin E, malaria and natural selection. Evolution, Medicine, and Public Health. 2019;**2019**(1):232-241. DOI: 10.1093/emph/eoz034

[53] Yuthavong Y, Butthep P, Bunyaratvej A, Fucharoen S. Inhibitory effect of beta zero-thalassaemia/ haemoglobin E erythrocytes on *Plasmodium falciparum* growth in vitro. Transactions of the Royal Society of Tropical Medicine and Hygiene. 1987;**81** (6):903-906. DOI: 10.1016/0035-9203 (87)90344-0

[54] O'Donnell A, Premawardhena A, Arambepola M, Samaranayake R, Allen SJ, Peto TE, et al. Interaction of malaria with a common form of severe thalassemia in an Asian population. Proceedings of the National Academy of Sciences of the United States of America. 2009;**106**(44):18716-18721. DOI: 10.1073/pnas.0910142106

[55] Mettananda S, Pathiraja H, Peiris R, Bandara D, de Silva U, Mettananda C, et al. Health related quality of life among

children with transfusion dependent β-thalassaemia major and haemoglobin E β-thalassaemia in Sri Lanka: A case control study. Health and Quality of Life Outcomes. 2019;**17**(1):137. DOI: 10.1186/s12955-019-1207-9

[56] Lal A, Wong T, Keel S, Pagano M, Chung J, Kamdar A, et al. The transfusion management of beta thalassemia in the United States. Transfusion. 2021;**61**(10):3027-3039. DOI: 10.1111/trf.16640

[57] Sari TT, Gatot D, Akib AA, Bardosono S, Hadinegoro SR, Harahap AR, et al. Immune response of thalassemia major patients in Indonesia with and without splenectomy. Acta Medica Indonesiana. 2014;**46**(3):217-225 PMID: 25348184

[58] Rachmilewitz EA, Giardina PJ. How I treat thalassemia. Blood. 2011;**118**(13): 3479-3488. DOI: 10.1182/blood-2010-08-300335

[59] Entezari S, Haghi SM, Norouzkhani N, Sahebnazar B, Vosoughian F, Akbarzadeh D, et al. Iron chelators in treatment of iron overload. Journal of Toxicology. 2022;**2022**:4911205. DOI: 10.1155/2022/4911205

[60] Jaiswal S, Hishikar R, Khandwal O, Agarwal M, Joshi U, Halwai A, et al. Efficacy of deferasirox as an oral iron chelator in paediatric thalassaemia patients. Journal of Clinical and Diagnostic Research. 2017;**11**(2):FC01-FC03. DOI: 10.7860/JCDR/2017/22650.9395

[61] Olivieri NF, Sabouhanian A, Gallie BL. Single-center retrospective study of the effectiveness and toxicity of the oral iron chelating drugs deferiprone and deferasirox. PLoS One. 2019;**14**(2): e0211942. DOI: 10.1371/journal.pone.0211942

[62] Ali S, Mumtaz S, Shakir HA, Khan M, Tahir HM, Mumtaz S, et al. Current status of beta-thalassemia and its treatment strategies. Molecular Genetics & Genomic Medicine. 2021;**9**(12):e1788. DOI: 10.1002/mgg3.1788

[63] Hider RC, Hoffbrand AV. The role of deferiprone in iron chelation. The New England Journal of Medicine. 2018;**379**(22):2140-2150. DOI: 10.1056/NEJMra1800219

[64] Bayanzay K, Alzoebie L. Reducing the iron burden and improving survival in transfusion-dependent thalassemia patients: Current perspectives. Journal of Blood Medicine. 2016;**7**:159-169. DOI: 10.2147/JBM.S61540

[65] Taher AT, Cappellini MD. How I manage medical complications of β-thalassemia in adults. Blood. 2018;**132**(17):1781-1791. DOI: 10.1182/blood-2018-06-818187

[66] Davis BA, Porter JB. Long-term outcome of continuous 24-hour deferoxamine infusion via indwelling intravenous catheters in high-risk beta-thalassemia. Blood. 2000;**95**(4):1229-1236 PMID: 10666195

[67] Tanner MA, Galanello R, Dessi C, Smith GC, Westwood MA, Agus A, et al. A randomized, placebo-controlled, double-blind trial of the effect of combined therapy with deferoxamine and deferiprone on myocardial iron in thalassemia major using cardiovascular magnetic resonance. Circulation. 2007;**115**(14):1876-1884. DOI: 10.1161/CIRCULATIONAHA.106.648790

[68] De Domenico I, Ward DM, Kaplan J. Specific iron chelators determine the route of ferritin degradation. Blood. 2009;**114**(20):4546-4551. DOI: 10.1182/blood-2009-05-224188

[69] Majolino I, Othman D, Rovelli A, Hassan D, Rasool L, Vacca M, et al. The start-up of the first hematopoietic stem cell transplantation center in the Iraqi Kurdistan: A Capacity-Building Cooperative Project by the Hiwa Cancer Hospital, Sulaymaniyah, and the Italian Agency for Development Cooperation: An Innovative Approach. Mediterranean Journal of Hematology and Infectious Diseases. 2017;**9**(1):e2017031. DOI: 10.4084/MJHID.2017.031

[70] Jeengar R K, Upadhyaya A, Agarwal N, Mehta A. Red cell alloimmunization in repeatedly transfused children with beta thalassemia major. International Journal of Contemporary Pediatrics, 2017;4(3): 775–779. https://doi.org/10.18203/2349-3291.ijcp20171486.

[71] Bernardo ME, Piras E, Vacca A, Giorgiani G, Zecca M, Bertaina A, et al. Allogeneic hematopoietic stem cell transplantation in thalassemia major: Results of a reduced-toxicity conditioning regimen based on the use of treosulfan. Blood. 2012;**120**(2): 473-476. DOI: 10.1182/blood-2012-04-423822

[72] Cario H. Hemoglobinopathies: Genetically diverse, clinically complex, and globally relevant. European Medical Oncology2018;11(3): 235–240. https://doi.org/10.1007/s12254-018-0402-4.

[73] Morgan RA, Gray D, Lomova A, Kohn DB. Hematopoietic stem cell gene therapy: Progress and lessons learned. Cell Stem Cell. 2017;**21**(5):574-590. DOI: 10.1016/j.stem.2017.10.010

[74] Yang J, Li S, He XB, Cheng C, Le W. Induced pluripotent stem cells in Alzheimer's disease: Applications for disease modeling and cell-replacement therapy. Molecular Neurodegeneration. 2016;**11**(1):39. DOI: 10.1186/s13024-016-0106-3

[75] Lino CA, Harper JC, Carney JP, Timlin JA. Delivering CRISPR: A review of the challenges and approaches. Drug Delivery. 2018;**25**(1):1234-1257. DOI: 10.1080/10717544.2018.1474964

[76] Li H, Yang Y, Hong W, Huang M, Wu M, Zhao X. Applications of genome editing technology in the targeted therapy of human diseases: Mechanisms, advances and prospects. Signal Transduction and Targeted Therapy. 2020;**5**(1):1. DOI: 10.1038/s41392-019-0089-y

[77] Zivot A, Lipton JM, Narla A, Blanc L. Erythropoiesis: Insights into pathophysiology and treatments in 2017. Molecular Medicine. 2018;**24**(1):11. DOI: 10.1186/s10020-018-0011-z

[78] Alebouyeh M, Moussavi F, Haddad-Deylami H, Vossough P. Hydroxyurea in the treatment of major beta-thalassemia and importance of genetic screening. Annals of Hematology. 2004;**83**(7):430-433. DOI: 10.1007/s00277-003-0836-5

[79] Dixit A, Chatterjee TC, Mishra P, Choudhry DR, Mahapatra M, Tyagi S, et al. Hydroxyurea in thalassemia intermedia – a promising therapy. Annals of Hematology. 2005;**84**(7):441-446. DOI: 10.1007/s00277-005-1026-4

[80] Cao H. Pharmacological induction of fetal hemoglobin synthesis using histone deacetylase inhibitors. Hematology. 2004;**9**(3):223-233. DOI: 10.1080/10245330410001701512

[81] Gambari R, Fibach E. Medicinal chemistry of fetal hemoglobin inducers for treatment of beta-thalassemia. Current Medicinal Chemistry. 2007;**14**(2):199-212. DOI: 10.2174/092986707779313318

[82] Suwanmanee T, Sierakowska H, Fucharoen S, Kole R. Repair of a splicing

defect in erythroid cells from patients with beta-thalassemia/HbE disorder. Molecular Theory. 2002;**6**:718-726. DOI: 10.1006/mthe.2002.0805

[83] Shaeffer JR, Cohen RE. Ubiquitin aldehyde increases adenosine triphosphate-dependent proteolysis of hemoglobin alpha-subunits in beta-thalassemic hemolysates. Blood. 1997;**90** (3):1300-1308

[84] Hashemieh M, Saadatmandi ZAS, Azarkeivan A, Najmabadi H. The Effect of Xmn -1 Polymorphism and Coinheritance of Alpha Mutations on Age at First Blood Transfusion in Iranian Patients with Homozygote IVSI-5 Mutation. Int J Hematol Oncol Stem Cell Res. 2022;**16**(1):47-54. DOI: 10.18502/ijhoscr.v16i1.8441

[85] Cao A, Galanello R. Beta-thalassemia. Genetics in Medicine. 2010; **12**(2):61-76. DOI: 10.1097/GIM.0b013e3181cd68ed

[86] de Dreuzy E, Bhukhai K, Leboulch P, Payen E. Current and future alternative therapies for beta-thalassemia major. Biomedical Journal. 2016;**39**(1):24-38. DOI: 10.1016/j.bj.2015.10.001

[87] Ben Salah N, Bou-Fakhredin R, Mellouli F, Taher AT. Revisiting beta thalassemia intermedia: Past, present, and prospects. Hematology. 2017;**22**(10): 607-616. DOI: 10.1080/10245332.2017.1333246

[88] Cighetti G, Duca L, Bortone L, Sala S, Nava I, Fiorelli G, et al. Oxidative status and malondialdehyde in beta-thalassaemia patients. European Journal of Clinical Investigation. 2002;**32**(1):55-60. DOI: 10.1046/j.1365-2362.2002.0320s1055.x

[89] Dissayabutra T, Tosukhowong P, Seksan P. The benefits of vitamin C and vitamin E in children with beta-thalassemia with high oxidative stress. Journal of the Medical Association of Thailand. 2005;**88**(4):S317-S321

Chapter 5

Interaction of Thalassemia and Hb Variants in Southeast Asia: Genotype-Phenotype Relationship

Manit Nuinoon

Abstract

Thalassemia and hemoglobinopathies are characterized by globin gene mutations affecting the production of quantitative and structural defects of the globin chain. α-Thalassemia, β-thalassemia, hemoglobin E (Hb E), and hemoglobin Constant Spring (Hb CS) are very common in Southeast Asian countries. Complex interactions of thalassemia and Hb variants are also common and affect the thalassemia diagnosis with several techniques including Hb typing and DNA analysis. A family study (family pedigree) is required in the proband with a complex interaction of several globin gene defects with rare types. Homozygous β-thalassemia, Hb E/β-thalassemia, and Hb Bart's hydrops fetalis are severe thalassemia and these diseases have been concerned and included in the prevention and control program in several countries. Understanding the genotype-phenotype could help with the proper laboratory tests, genetic counseling, and effective treatment for the patients.

Keywords: thalassemia, Hb variants, southeast Asian countries, thalassemia interaction, genotype-phenotype, DNA analysis

1. Introduction

Southeast Asia (SEA) is composed of 11 countries such as Burma (Myanmar), Laos, Thailand, Cambodia, Vietnam, Malaysia, Singapore, Brunei, Indonesia, the Philippines, and Timor-Leste (**Figure 1**). As of 2021, around 676 million people live in the region [1]. The ethnic origins of people living in SEA countries are very heterogeneous according to religion, culture, and history. This chapter focused on the genotype-phenotype relationship between thalassemia and hemoglobinopathies in the Southeast Asian population. Both common and rare types of thalassemia and Hb variant are demonstrated in homozygous, double heterozygous, and compound heterozygous states for clinical and red blood cell phenotypes.

IntechOpen

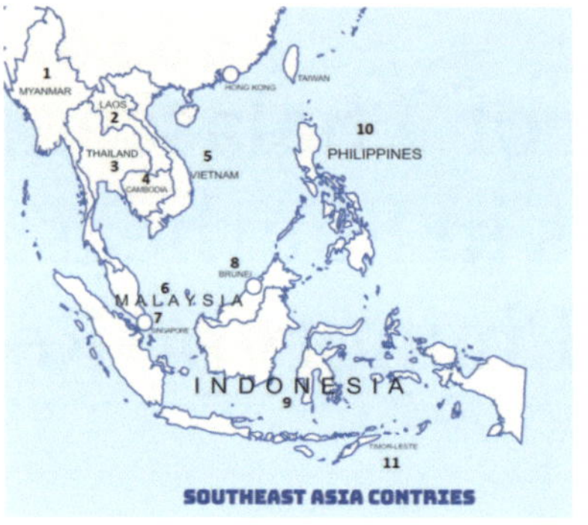

Figure 1.
The map of southeast Asian countries [2].

2. Globin gene cluster, functional globin genes, and normal adult hemoglobin

In humans, two globin gene clusters are responsible for hemoglobin synthesis in all developmental stages, including embryonic, fetal, and adult stages (**Figure 2**). The α-like gene cluster contains three functional genes, including the ζ2, α2, and α1 globin genes in chromosome 16 (16p13.3), and encoded to form the ζ- and α-globin chains which consist of 141 amino acids. In addition, the β -like gene cluster contains 5 functional genes including the ε, $^{G}\gamma$, $^{A}\gamma$, δ, and β-globin genes, in chromosome 11 (11p15.5), and encoded to form the ε, γ, δ, and β-globin chains which consist of 146 amino acids. During normal humans, each globin gene from 2 globin gene clusters is activated and expressed according to the specific developmental stage such as the embryonic stage (Hb Portland, Hb Gower I, and Hb Gower II), fetal stage (Hb F or fetal hemoglobin), and adult stage (Hb A and Hb A_2) [3, 4].

Hemoglobin (Hb), an iron-containing protein in erythrocytes (red blood cells), is responsible for transporting oxygen (O_2) from the lungs to tissues and to transporting carbon dioxide (CO_2) from tissues. In adult life, Hb A ($\alpha_2\beta_2$), or adult hemoglobin is the major component of normal adult hemoglobin (more than 95% of the total hemoglobin). Hb A_2 ($\alpha_2\delta_2$) is the second component about less than 3.5% in normal adults. Hb F ($\alpha_2\gamma_2$) or fetal hemoglobin with 1–2% is found in normal individuals [5].

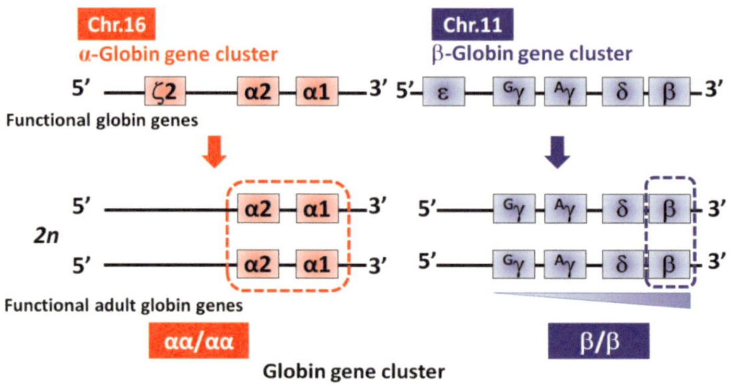

Figure 2.
Schematic representation of the globin gene cluster.

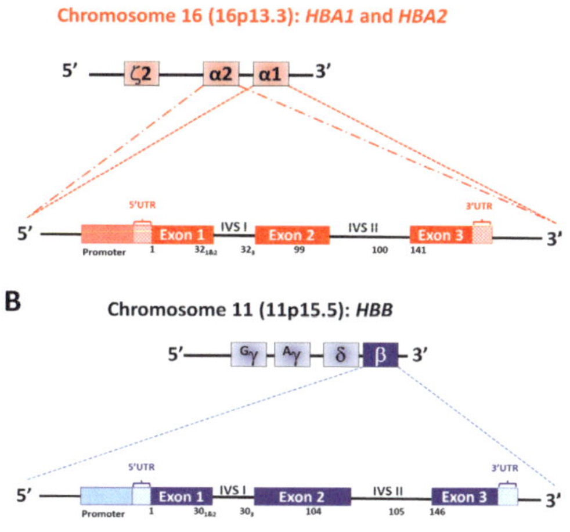

Figure 3.
General structure functional α -globin genes (A)and the β-globin gene (B).

According to Hb A ($\alpha_2\beta_2$) is the major component of total hemoglobin and contributes to gas transport in the human body. In the adult stage, α and β-globin genes are the two most important for globin chain synthesis and build up to form the tetramerization of 2 α-globin chains and 2 β-globin chains and each globin chain bound heme group (an iron atom bound within a protoporphyrin IX ring) [6]. Therefore, α and β-globin gene mutations were the most considered condition in the adult for thalassemia or Hb variants. An approximate 50 bp of the 5′ untranslated region (5'UTR) and codons for amino acid sequences 1–31 in the *HBA1*(or *HBA2*) and 1–30 in the *HBB* genes are represented as the first exon. The second exon encodes amino acids 32–99 and 31–104, respectively. The third exon encodes amino acids 101–141 for the α-globin gene and 105–146 for the β-globin gene, together with about 100 bp of 3′UTR (**Figure 3**) [3].

3. Genotype-phenotype relationship

In the human globin gene clusters, the α-globin gene cluster is located at the short arm of chromosome 16 (two copies of the α-globin gene per chromatid, *HBA2*, and *HBA1* genes) whereas the β-globin gene cluster is located at the short arm of chromosome 11 (one copy of each β-globin gene per chromatid, *HBB* gene). Both chromosomes 11 and 16 are autosomal chromosomes (*2n*, diploid cell). Therefore, a total of four genes per diploid cell of the α-globin genotype (αα/αα) and a total of two genes per diploid cell for the β -globin genotype (β^A/β^A). The mutations of the human globin gene can inherit from the parent ranging from 1 allele to 4 alleles of α- and β-globin genes and resulting in various forms of the carrier or thalassemia disease. α- and β-Globin genotyping can be characterized by several PCR-based methods [7]. In the context of globin gene defects, phenotype refers to the observable hematological (red blood cell morphology, osmotic fragility test, abnormal Hb screening, and Hb analysis) or clinical characteristics of the carriers or patients. Recently, the clinical classification of thalassemia is divided into two phenotypes according to the patient's clinical severity and transfusion requirements such as non-transfusion-dependent thalassemia (NTDT) and transfusion-dependent thalassemia (TDT) [8]. Therefore, genotype-phenotype correlation is a relationship between specific globin mutations and hematological profiles or clinical symptoms. The red blood cell phenotypes and other related screening methods are the primary results for predicting a possible type of thalassemia carrier or disease [9, 10]. However, globin genotyping is required for a definitive and precise diagnosis of thalassemia for proper management and treatment [11].

4. Thalassemia and hemoglobinopathy

Thalassemia, a quantitative defect of globin chain synthesis, is caused by globin gene mutation and characterized by the absence (designed with a "0" superscript) or reduced (designed with a "+" superscript) synthesis of one or more of the normal globin chains. The α- and β-thalassemia are major types during the adult stage. In contrast, hemoglobinopathy is characterized by a qualitative or structural defect of globin chain synthesis. Thalassemic hemoglobinopathy is the combination of quantitative and qualitative features of globin chain synthesis such as Hb Constant Spring (Hb CS, α^+-thalassemia-like effect) and hemoglobin E (Hb E, β^+-thalassemia) [12]. Hereditary persistence of fetal hemoglobin (HPFH) and δβ-thalassemia are characterized by elevated fetal hemoglobin (Hb F) levels in adult life. There are no morphological changes to the red blood cells and red cell indices in HPFH whereas more abnormal red blood cells are observed in δβ-thalassemia [13]. In Southeast Asia α-thalassemia, β-thalassemia, Hb E, and Hb CS are prevalent and the gene frequencies vary in different countries. In Thailand, the carrier frequencies of 10–30% for α-thalassemia, 3–9% for β-thalassemia, and 10–53% for Hb E [14, 15]. The combinations of different globin gene mutations lead to over 60 different thalassemia syndromes and the most complex thalassemia genotypes were found among Southeast Asians [15]. According to common globin gene mutations found in the Southeast Asian population, the four major thalassemia diseases are Hb Bart's hydrops fetalis (−−/−−), homozygous β-thalassemia (β^*/β^*), Hb E/β-thalassemia (β^E/β^*), and Hb H diseases (deletional Hb H disease, −−/−α; non-deletional Hb H disease, $--/\alpha^T\alpha$) [15–17]. Only the first three thalassemia diseases were concerned with prevention and control programs for severe thalassemia in Thailand and other Southeast Asian countries [18–21]. Clinical manifestations of thalassemia range from asymptomatic with mild microcytic hypochromic red blood cells to the totally lethal Hb Bart's hydrops fetalis [16, 22]. Moreover, the interaction of the thalassemias and hemoglobin variants from multiple globin gene mutations may not be uncommon in Southeast Asians. The hematological and complex hemoglobin profile has been reported in several publications and DNA analysis is required to characterize disease-causing mutation [7, 21]. Therefore, understanding the genotype-phenotype relationship is very useful for precise diagnosis with proper laboratory tests and economic benefits [23]. In Southeast Asia α-Thalassemia is associated with variable numbers of α-globin gene deletions by combining 2 alleles such as $-\alpha^{3.7}$, $-\alpha^{4.2}$, $-(\alpha)^{-20}$, $--^{SEA}$, $--^{THAI}$, $--^{FIL}$, and $--^{CR}$ with other alleles such as normal (αα) or α-globin chain variants ($\alpha^T\alpha$ or $\alpha\alpha^T$) [15, 24–27]. The clinical phenotype of α-thalassemia relates to the number of affected α-globin genes ranging from no clinical symptom (hypochromic and microcytic red cells without anemia) to lethal thalassemia disease [16, 28]. β-Thalassemias are very heterogenous and various β-globin gene mutations have been characterized. β-Thalassemia mutations could be classified as β^{++}, β^+, or β^0 thalassemia phenotypes according to different molecular mechanisms [11, 29–31]. In addition, several Hb chain variants of α-globin genes

(*HBA1* and *HBA2*), β-globin gene (*HBB*), and δ-globin gene (*HBD*) have been found among the Southeast Asian population which are summarized in **Table 1**.

5. Interaction of common thalassemia and hemoglobin variants

α- and β-globin genes can be inherited independently by the next generation. There are 4 possible genotypes of the α-globin gene and 4 possible genotypes of the β -globin gene. Therefore, the maximum genotypes of α- and β-globin genes are 16 possible genotypes. This model is useful for the prediction of severe thalassemia for the child in preconception counseling or prenatal diagnosis (PND) process (**Figure 4**).

In Southeast Asian countries, the complex interaction of thalassemia and the Hb variant is common. The dihybrid cross with the mutations in both α- and β-globin genes from the father (CS EA Bart's disease) and mother (double heterozygosity for β^0-thalassemia and α^0-thalassemia) is used to give an example for the reader. All globin genotypes obtained from the parent are essential information for evaluating the risk ratio of being severe thalassemia. The list of possible α-globin genotypes are 4 distinct genotypes as follows; $\alpha^{CS}\alpha/\alpha\alpha$ (Hb Constant Spring heterozygote), $--^{SEA}/\alpha\alpha$ (α^0-thalassemia heterozygote), $--^{SEA}/\alpha^{CS}\alpha$ (Hb H-Constant Spring), and $--^{SEA}/--^{SEA}$ (Hb Bart's hydrops fetalis or homozygous α^0-thalassemia). In addition, the list of possible β-globin genotypes are 4 distinct genotypes as follows; β^A/β^A (normal genotype), β^A/β^0 (β^0-thalassemia heterozygote), β^E/β^A (Hb E heterozygote), and β^E/β^0 (Hb E/β^0-thalassemia). According to 4 possible α- and 4 possible β-globin genotypes, 16 distinct combinations are obtained. In this case, Hb Bart's hydrops fetalis and Hb E/β^0-thalassemia are concerned and 7 combined genotypes (1, 2, 3, 4, 7, 11, and 15) are risk genotypes and this couple is a true risk couple with 7/16 (43.75%) for being severe thalassemia in the child (**Figure 5**).

Because of the high frequency of thalassemias and Hb variants, the interactions of thalassemias and Hb variants especially in two major globin chains (α- and β-globin) were observed in the Southeast Asian population. Hb E and Hb CS are the two most common Hb variants represented for β- and α-globin genes. Commonly, interactions of Hb E with other thalassemias or Hb variants resulting in Hb E-related syndromes such as Hb E/β-thalassemia with or without α-thalassemia interaction, AE Bart's disease, EF Bart's disease, etc. (**Table 2**). In an area where Hb E, β-thalassemia, and α-thalassemia are prevalent, the interaction of Hb E with several types of thalassemia is frequently observed. Among Hb E heterozygotes, a proportion of Hb A_2/E lower than 25% has been used for suspecting α-thalassemia interaction and confirmed by DNA analysis [9]. Various forms of α-thalassemia are common and interaction of thalassemia with heterozygous Hb E can result in a reduced Hb A_2/E level and hematological changes [35]. In contrast, the interaction of homozygous Hb E with α-thalassemia could not be differentially diagnosed by red cell indices and Hb-HPLC analysis [36]. Hb analysis by capillary electrophoresis can separate Hb A_2 from Hb E and Hb A_2 could be reported in the presence of Hb E [37, 38]. Interestingly, an increased Hb A_2 level is a useful biomarker for differentiation of Hb E homozygote with or without α^0-thalassemia [39]. The combination of heterozygous Hb E and Hb H disease or Hb H-Constant Spring disease has a marked decrease of Hb E (13–15%) with thalassemia intermedia, which is called AE Bart's disease [22]. Co-inheritance of Hb H disease with homozygous Hb E resulted in EF Bart's disease with mild anemia and increased Hb F levels and Hb

Gene	HGVS nomenclature	Mutation
α-Globin chain variants		
Hb Q-India	*HBA1*:c.193G>C	alpha1 64(E13) Asp>His
Hb Q-Thailand	*HBA1*:c.223G>C	alpha1 74(EF3) Asp>His
Hb Grey Lynn (Hb Vientiane)	*HBA1*:c.274C>T	alpha1 91(FG3) Leu>Phe
Hb St. Luke's-Thailand	*HBA1*:c.287C>G	alpha1 95(G2) Pro>Arg
Hb O-Indonesia	*HBA1*:c.349G>A	alpha1 116(GH4) Glu>Lys
Hb Phnom Penh	*HBA1*:p.Phe118_Thr119insI	I- inserted between codons 117(GH5) and 118(H1) of alpha1
Hb Dunn	*HBA2*:c.19G>A (or *HBA1*)	alpha2 or alpha1 6(A4) Asp>Asn
Hb J-Wenchang-Wuming	*HBA2*:c.34A>C (or *HBA1*)	alpha2 or alpha1 11(A9) Lys>Gln
Hb Siam (Hb Ottawa)	*HBA2*:c.46G>C (or *HBA1*)	alpha2 or alpha1 15(A13) Gly>Arg
Hb I	*HBA2*:c.49A>G	alpha2 16(A14) Lys>Glu
Hb Beijing	*HBA2*:c.[51G>C (or *HBA1*) or 51G>T (or HBA1)]	alpha2 or alpha1 16(A14) Lys>Asn
Hb Shenyang	*HBA2*:c.80C>A (or *HBA1*)	alpha2 or alpha1 26(B7) Ala>Glu
Hb Hekinan	*HBA2*:c.84G>C	alpha2 27(B8) Glu>Asp
Hb G-Honolulu	*HBA2*:c.91G>C (or *HBA1*)	alpha2 or alpha1 30(B11) Glu>Gln
Hb Prato	*HBA2*:c.[96G>C (or *HBA1*) or 96G>T (or *HBA1*)]	alpha2 or alpha1 31(B12) Arg>Ser
Hb Queens	*HBA2*:c.104T>G (or *HBA1*)	alpha2 or alpha1 34(B15) Leu>Arg
Hb Wiangpapao	*HBA1*:c.133C>T	alpha1 44(CE2) Pro>Ser
Hb Kawachi	*HBA2*:c.134C>G (or *HBA1*)	alpha2 or alpha1 44(CE2) Pro>Arg
Hb Thailand	*HBA2*:c.170A>C (or *HBA1*)	alpha2 or alpha1 56(E5) Lys>Thr
Hb J-Norfolk	*HBA2*:c.173G>A (or *HBA1*)	alpha2 or alpha1 57(E6) Gly>Asp
Hb Adana	*HBA2*:c.179G>A (or *HBA1*)	alpha2 or alpha1 59(E8) Gly>Asp
Hb Nakhon Ratchasima	*HBA2*:c.191C>T	alpha2 63(E12) Ala>Val
Hb Westmead	*HBA2*:c.369C>G	alpha2 122(H5) His>Gln
Hb Quong Sze	*HBA2*:c.377T>C	alpha2 125(H8) Leu>Pro
Hb Constant Spring (Hb CS)	*HBA2*:c.427T>C	alpha2 142, Stop>Gln; modified C-terminal sequence: (142)Gln-Ala-Gly-Ala-Ser-Val-Ala-Val-Pro-Pro-Ala- Arg-Trp-Ala-Ser-Gln-Arg-Ala-Leu-Leu-Pro- Ser-Leu-His-Arg-Pro-Phe-Leu-Val-Phe-(172) Glu-COOH
Hb Pakse	*HBA2*:c.429A>T	alpha2 142, Stop>Tyr; modified C-terminal sequence: (142)Tyr-Ala-Gly-Ala-Ser-Val-Ala-Val-Pro-Pro-Ala- Arg-Trp-Ala-Ser-Gln-Arg-Ala-Leu-Leu-Pro- Ser-Leu-His-Arg-Pro-Phe-Leu-Val-Phe-(172) Glu-COOH

Gene	HGVS nomenclature	Mutation
β-Globin chain variants		
Hb Raleigh	*HBB*:c.5T>C	beta 1(NA1) Val>Ala
Hb C	*HBB*:c.19G>A	beta 6(A3) Glu>Lys
Hb G-Makassar	*HBB*:c.20A>C	beta 6(A3) Glu>Ala
Hb S	*HBB*:c.20A>T	beta 6(A3) Glu>Val
Hb G-Siriraj	*HBB*:c.22G>A	beta 7(A4) Glu>Lys
Hb Malay	*HBB*:c.59A>G	beta 19(B1) Asn>Ser
Hb E-Saskatoon	*HBB*:c.67G>A	beta 22(B4) Glu>Lys
Hb E	*HBB*:c.79G>A	beta 26(B8) Glu>Lys
Hb Henri Mondor	*HBB*:c.80A>T	beta 26(B8) Glu>Val
Hb Athens-Georgia	*HBB*:c.122G>A	beta 40(C6) Arg>Lys
Hb J-Bangkok	*HBB*:c.170G>A	beta 56(D7) Gly>Asp
Hb Dhofar	*HBB*:c.176C>G	beta 58(E2) Pro>Arg
Hb J-Kaohsiung	*HBB*:c.179A>C	beta 59(E3) Lys>Thr
Hb Phimai	*HBB*:c.218G>C	beta 72(E16) Ser>Thr
Hb Korle Bu (Hb G-Accra)	*HBB*:c.220G>A	beta 73(E17) Asp>Asn
Hb Pyrgos	*HBB*:c.251G>A	beta 83(EF7) Gly>Asp
Hb D-Punjab (Hb D-Los Angeles)	*HBB*:c.364G>C	beta 121(GH4) Glu>Gln
Hb Tende	*HBB*:c.374C>T	beta 124(H2) Pro>Leu
Hb Dhonburi	*HBB*:c.380T>G	beta 126(H4) Val>Gly
Hb Cook	*HBB*:c.398A>C	beta 132(H10) Lys>Thr
Hb Hope	*HBB*:c.410G>A	beta 136(H14) Gly>Asp
Hb Tak	*HBB*:c.441_442insAC	beta 147(+AC); modified C-terminal sequence: (147)Thr-Lys-Leu- Ala-Phe-Leu-Leu-Ser-Asn-Phe-(157)Tyr-COOH
δ-Globin chain variants		
Hb A_2-Melbourne	*HBD*:c.130G>A	delta 43(CD2) Glu>Lys
Hb A_2-Lampang	*HBD*:c.142G>A	delta 47(CD6) Asp>Asn
Hb A_2-Walsgrave	*HBD*:c.157G>C	delta 52 (D3) Asp>His
Hemoglobin A_2-Mae Phrik	*HBD*:c.158A > G	delta 52(D3) Asp > Gly
Hb A_2-Kiriwong	*HBD*:c.233A>G	delta 77(EF1) His>Arg
Hb Lepore-Hollandia	NG_000007.3:g.63290_70702del	delta-beta hybrid (delta through 22; beta from 50)
Hb Lepore-Washington-Boston	NG_000007.3:g.63632_71046del	delta-beta hybrid (delta through 87; beta from 116)

Table 1.
Hb variants in southeast Asian countries [32–34].

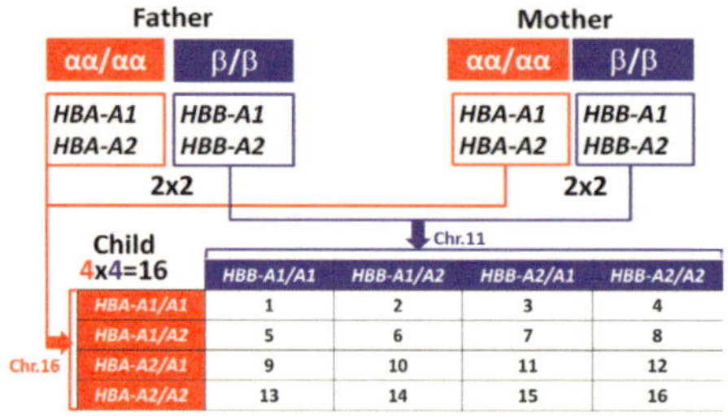

Figure 4.
The model of the dihybrid cross of α- and β-globin genotypes.

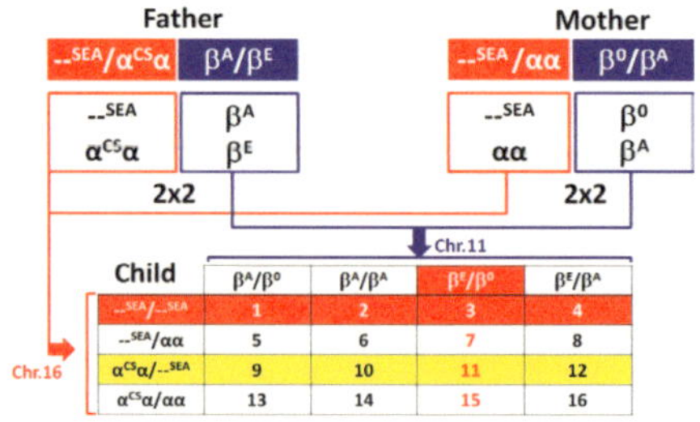

Figure 5.
The model of dihybrid cross of CS EA Bart's disease and double heterozygosity for β^0-thalassemia and α^0-thalassemia.

Bart's [22]. The compound heterozygous state for β-thalassemia and Hb E namely Hb E-β-thalassemia is variable disease severity ranging from transfusion-dependent thalassemia to thalassemia intermedia. An ameliorating effect of α-thalassemia interactions and high Hb F determinants has been well studied [40–42]. Moreover, the interaction of thalassemia and Hb variants has been reported in several publications in the Thai population such as compound heterozygosity for Hb Korle-Bu and Hb E with α^+-thalassemia, complex interactions between Hb Lepore-Hollandia and Hb E with α^+-thalassemia and interaction between Hb E and Hb Yala resulting in Hb E/β^0-thalassemia, double heterozygosity of Hb Hope and α^0-thalassemia and compound heterozygotes for Hb Hope and β^0-thalassemia [43–46]. Hereditary persistence (HPFH) and δβ-thalassemia are characterized by elevated fetal hemoglobin levels in adult life. There are several mutations reported in the Thai population such as ${}^G\gamma{}^A\gamma\ (\delta\beta)^0$-thalassemia, deletional HPFH-6, and deletion-inversion ${}^G\gamma({}^A\gamma\delta\beta)^0$-thalassemia [47–49].

6. Conclusions

The understanding of the genotype-phenotype relationship is essential for proper laboratory testing, genetic counseling, and treatments. The concept of thalassemia interaction could be applied in a country with high frequency and heterogeneity of thalassemia and hemoglobinopathies. DNA analysis is very important for definitive diagnosis, as well as the family study, and could be helped in complex thalassemia with a rare hemoglobin variant. Characterization of globin

DOI: http://dx.doi.org/10.5772/intechopen.110001

Type	Genotype	Disease/clinical phenotype	Hb type*
Homozygous conditions			
α^+-thal	$-\alpha/-\alpha$	No clinical symptoms	A_2A
α^+-thal (Hb variant)	$\alpha^T\alpha/\alpha^T\alpha$ ($\alpha^{CS}\alpha/\alpha^{CS}\alpha$)	Hb H disease	(CS) A_2A Bart's H
α^0-thal	$--/--$	Hb Bart's hydrops fetalis	Bart's
β^0 or severe β^+ thal	β^0/β^0	Thal major (TM) or TDT	A_2F
Mild β^+ or β^{++} thal	β^+/β^+	Thal intermedia (TI) or NTDT	A_2FA
Hb E (β^+ thal)	β^E/β^E	No clinical symptoms	EE or E(F)
Compound heterozygous conditions			
α^0-thal/α^+-thal	$--/-\alpha$	Deletional Hb H disease	A_2A Bart's H
α^0-thal/α^+-thal (Hb variants)	$--/\alpha^T\alpha$ ($--/\alpha^{CS}\alpha$)	Non-deletional Hb H disease (severe)	(CS) A_2A Bart's H
Severe β^+ thal/β^0 thal	β^+ (severe form)/β^0	Thal major (TM) or TDT	A_2F
Mild β^+/β^0 thal	β^+ (mild form)/β^0	Variable disease severity	A_2FA
Hb E/β^+ thal	β^E/β^+	Thal intermedia (TI)	EFA
Hb E/β^0 or severe β^+ thal	β^E/β^0 or β^E/β^+ (severe)	Variable disease severity	EF
Hb E/Hb C	β^E/β^C	No clinical symptoms (mild anemia)	EC
Hb E/$(\delta\beta)^0$ thal	$\beta^E/(\delta\beta)^0$	Thal intermedia	EF
Hb E/HPFH	β^E/HPFH	Mild thal intermedia	EF
Hb E-related syndromes			
Heterozygous Hb E + α^0-thal heterozygote	$\beta^E/\beta^A + --/\alpha\alpha$	Double heterozygotes for Hb E and α^0-thal, no clinical symptoms	EA (reduced Hb E levels)
Heterozygous Hb E + α^0-thal/α^+-thal	$\beta^E/\beta^A + --/-\alpha$	AE Bart's disease, thal intermedia	EA Bart's
Heterozygous Hb E + α^0-thal/α^+-thal (Hb variants)	$\beta^E/\beta^A + --/\alpha^T\alpha$ ($\alpha^T\alpha = \alpha^{CS}\alpha$ or $\alpha^{PS}\alpha$)	CS/PS AE Bart's disease, thal intermedia	(CS) EA Bart's
Homozygous Hb E + α^0-thal/α^+-thal	$\beta^E/\beta^E + --/-\alpha$	EF Bart's disease, thal intermedia	EF Bart's
Homozygous Hb E + α^0-thal/α^+-thal (Hb variants)	$\beta^E/\beta^E + --/\alpha^T\alpha$ ($\alpha^T\alpha = \alpha^{CS}\alpha$ or $\alpha^{PS}\alpha$)	CS/PS EF Bart's disease, thal intermedia	(CS) EF Bart's
Hb E/β^0 thal+α^0-thal/α^+-thal	$\beta^E/\beta^0 + --/-\alpha$	EF Bart's disease, thal intermedia	EF Bart's
Hb E/β^0 thal+α^0-thal/α^+-thal (Hb variants)	$\beta^E/\beta^0 + --/\alpha^T\alpha$ ($\alpha^T\alpha = \alpha^{CS}\alpha$ or $\alpha^{PS}\alpha$)	CS EF Bart's disease, thal intermedia	(CS) EF Bart's

*CS, Constant Spring; PS, Pakse; HPFH, hereditary persistence of fetal hemoglobin; NTDT, non-transfusion-dependent thalassemia; TDT, transfusion-dependent thalassemia; Thal, Thalassemia; TI, thalassemia intermedia; TM, thalassemia major. *Hb type is based on HPLC technique.*

Table 2.
Phenotypes of thalassemias, Hb variants and interaction of thalassemia and Hb variants in the southeast Asian population.

gene mutations in the population is important and a globin gene mutation database in each country is required for improving prevention and control program for severe thalassemia.

Conflict of interest

The author declares no conflict of interest.

Author details

Manit Nuinoon[1,2]

1 Hematology and Transfusion Science Research Center, Walailak University, Nakhon Si Thammarat, Thailand

2 School of Allied Health Sciences, Walailak University, Nakhon Si Thammarat, Thailand

*Address all correspondence to: manit.nu@wu.ac.th

References

[1] Southeast Asian. Available from: https://en.wikipedia.org/wiki/Southeast_Asia

[2] Map chart. Available from: https://www.mapchart.net/index.html

[3] Weatherall DJ. Globin Genes, Human. In: Maloy S, Hughes K, editors. Brenner's Encyclopedia of Genetics. 2nd ed. San Diego: Academic Press; 2013. pp. 337-339

[4] Higgs D, Thein S, Wood W, Human haemoglobin. The Thalassaemia Syndromes. Oxford: Blackwell Science Ltd; 2001. pp. 65-120

[5] Otto CN. 7 - Hemoglobin metabolism. In: Keohane EM, Otto CN, Walenga JM, editors. Rodak's Hematology. 6th ed. St. Louis (MO): Elsevier; 2020. pp. 91-103

[6] Steinberg MH, Benz EJ, Adewoye AH, Ebert BL. Chapter 33 - Pathobiology of the Human erythrocyte and its Hemoglobins. In: Hoffman R, Benz EJ, Silberstein LE, Heslop HE, Weitz JI, Anastasi J, et al., editors. Hematology. 7th ed. Philadelphia (PA): Elsevier; 2018. pp. 447-457

[7] Munkongdee T, Chen P, Winichagoon P, Fucharoen S, Paiboonsukwong K. Update in laboratory diagnosis of thalassemia. Frontiers in Molecular Biosciences. 2020;**7**:74

[8] Viprakasit V, Ekwattanakit S. Clinical classification, screening and diagnosis for thalassemia. Hematology/Oncology Clinics of North America. 2018;**32**(2):193-211

[9] Fucharoen G, Sanchaisuriya K, Sae-ung N, Dangwibul S, Fucharoen S. A simplified screening strategy for thalassaemia and haemoglobin E in rural communities in south-East Asia. Bulletin of the World Health Organization. 2004;**82**(5):364-372

[10] Savongsy O, Fucharoen S, Fucharoen G, Sanchaisuriya K, Sae-Ung N. Thalassemia and hemoglobinopathies in pregnant Lao women: Carrier screening, prevalence and molecular basis. Annals of Hematology. 2008;**87**(8):647-654

[11] Danjou F, Anni F, Galanello R. β-thalassemia: From genotype to phenotype. Haematologica. 2011;**96**(11):1573-1575

[12] Steinberg MH, Adams JG. Thalassemic hemoglobinopathies. The American Journal of Pathology. 1983;**113**(3):396-409

[13] Forget BG. Molecular basis of hereditary persistence of fetal hemoglobin. Annals of the New York Academy of Sciences. 1998;**850**:38-44

[14] Fucharoen S, Winichagoon P, Siritanaratkul N, Chowthaworn J, Pootrakul P. α- and β-thalassemia in Thailand. Annals of the New York Academy of Sciences. 1998;**850**:412-414

[15] Fucharoen S, Winichagoon P. Haemoglobinopathies in Southeast Asia. The Indian Journal of Medical Research. 2011;**134**(4):498-506

[16] Vichinsky EP. Clinical manifestations of α-thalassemia. Cold Spring Harbor Perspectives in Medicine. 2013;**3**(5):a011742

[17] Farashi S, Najmabadi H. Diagnostic pitfalls of less well recognized HbH disease. Blood Cells, Molecules, and Diseases. 2015;**55**(4):387-395

[18] Yamsri S, Sanchaisuriya K, Fucharoen G, Sae-Ung N, Ratanasiri T, Fucharoen S. Prevention of severe thalassemia in Northeast Thailand: 16 years of experience at a single university center. Prenatal Diagnosis. 2010;**30**(6):540-546

[19] Fucharoen S, Winichagoon P. Prevention and control of thalassemia in Asia. Asian Biomedicine. 2007;**1**:1-6

[20] Fucharoen S, Winichagoon P. Thalassemia in SouthEast Asia: Problems and strategy for prevention and control. The Southeast Asian Journal of Tropical Medicine and Public Health. 1992;**23**(4):647-655

[21] Nopparatana C, Nopparatana C, Saechan V, Karnchanaopas S, Srewaradachpisal K. Prenatal diagnosis of α- and β-thalassemias in southern Thailand. International Journal of Hematology. 2020;**111**(2):284-292

[22] Fucharoen S, Weatherall DJ. The hemoglobin E thalassemias. Cold Spring Harbor Perspectives in Medicine. 2012;**2**(8):a011734

[23] Cao A, Galanello R, Rosatelli MC. Genotype-phenotype correlations in β-thalassemias. Blood Reviews. 1994;**8**(1):1-12

[24] Tritipsombut J, Sanchaisuriya K, Phollarp P, Bouakhasith D, Sanchaisuriya P, Fucharoen G, et al. Micromapping of thalassemia and hemoglobinopathies in diferent regions of Northeast Thailand and Vientiane, Laos People's Democratic Republic. Hemoglobin. 2012;**36**(1):47-56

[25] Charoenkwan P, Taweephon R, Sae-Tung R, Thanarattanakorn P, Sanguansermsri T. Molecular and clinical features of Hb H disease in northern Thailand. Hemoglobin. 2005;**29**(2):133-140

[26] Tangvarasittichai O, Jeenapongsa R, Sitthiworanan C, Sanguansermsri T. Laboratory investigations of Hb constant spring. Clinical and Laboratory Haematology. 2005;**27**(1):47-49

[27] Nittayaboon K, Nopparatana C. Molecular characterization of Hb H diseaseinsouthernThailand. International Journal of Hematology. 2018;**108**(4):384-389

[28] Piel FB, Weatherall DJ. The α-Thalassemias. New England Journal of Medicine. 2014;**371**(20):1908-1916

[29] Yamsri S, Singha K, Prajantasen T, Taweenan W, Fucharoen G, Sanchaisuriya K, et al. A large cohort of β^{+}-thalassemia in Thailand: Molecular, hematological and diagnostic considerations. Blood Cells, Molecules & Diseases. 2015;**54**(2):164-169

[30] Abdullah UYH, Ibrahim HM, Mahmud NB, Salleh MZ, Teh LK, Noorizhab M, et al. Genotype-phenotype correlation of β-thalassemia in Malaysian population: Toward effective genetic Counseling. Hemoglobin. 2020;**44**(3):184-189

[31] Yamsri S, Sanchaisuriya K, Fucharoen G, Sae-Ung N, Fucharoen S. Genotype and phenotype characterizations in a large cohort of β-thalassemia heterozygote with different forms of α-thalassemia in Northeast Thailand. Blood Cells, Molecules & Diseases. 2011;**47**(2):120-124

[32] Giardine B, Borg J, Viennas E, Pavlidis C, Moradkhani K, Joly P, et al. Updates of the HbVar database of human hemoglobin variants and thalassemia mutations. Nucleic Acids Research. 2014;**42**(Database issue):D1063-D1069

[33] Saechan V, Nopparatana C, Nopparatana C, Fucharoen S. Molecular basis and hematological features of

hemoglobin variants in southern Thailand. International Journal of Hematology. 2010;**92**(3):445-450

[34] Srivorakun H, Singha K, Fucharoen G, Sanchaisuriya K, Fucharoen S. A large cohort of hemoglobin variants in Thailand: Molecular epidemiological study and diagnostic consideration. PLoS One. 2014;**9**(9):e108365

[35] Sanchaisuriya K, Fucharoen G, Sae-ung N, Jetsrisuparb A, Fucharoen S. Molecular and hematologic features of hemoglobin E heterozygotes with different forms of α-thalassemia in Thailand. Annals of Hematology. 2003;**82**(10):612-616

[36] Fucharoen G, Trithipsombat J, Sirithawee S, Yamsri S, Changtrakul Y, Sanchaisuriya K, et al. Molecular and hematological profiles of hemoglobin EE disease with different forms of α-thalassemia. Annals of Hematology. 2006;**85**(7):450-454

[37] Sangkitporn S, Sangkitporn SK, Tanjatham S, Suwannakan B, Rithapirom S, Yodtup C, et al. Multicenter validation of fully automated capillary electrophoresis method for diagnosis of thalassemias and hemoglobinopathies in Thailand. The Southeast Asian Journal of Tropical Medicine and Public Health. 2011;**42**(5):1224-1232

[38] Hafiza A, Malisa MY, Khirotdin RD, Azlin I, Azma Z, Thong MC, et al. HbA_2 levels in normal, β-thalassaemia and haemoglobin E carriers by capillary electrophoresis. The Malaysian Journal of Pathology. 2012;**34**(2):161-164

[39] Singha K, Srivorakun H, Fucharoen G, Fucharoen S. Co-inheritance of α^0-thalassemia elevates Hb A_2 level in homozygous Hb E: Diagnostic implications. International Journal of Laboratory Hematology. 2017;**39**(5):508-512

[40] Sripichai O, Munkongdee T, Kumkhaek C, Svasti S, Winichagoon P, Fucharoen S. Coinheritance of the different copy numbers of α-globin gene modifies severity of β-thalassemia/Hb E disease. Annals of Hematology. 2008;**87**(5):375-379

[41] Winichagoon P, Fucharoen S, Chen P, Wasi P. Genetic factors affecting clinical severity in β-thalassemia syndromes. Journal of Pediatric Hematology/Oncology. 2000;**22**(6):573-580

[42] Winichagoon P, Thonglairoam V, Fucharoen S, Wilairat P, Fukumaki Y, Wasi P. Severity differences in β-thalassaemia/haemoglobin E syndromes: Implication of genetic factors. British Journal of Haematology. 1993;**83**(4):633-639

[43] Pornprasert S, Panyasai S, Kongthai K. Comparison of capillary electrophoregram among heterozygous Hb Hope, Hb Hope/α-thalassemia-1 SEA type deletion and Hb Hope/ β^0-thalassemia. Clinical Chemistry and Laboratory Medicine. 2012;**50**(9):1625-1629

[44] Ekwattanakit S, Riolueang S, Viprakasit V. Interaction between Hb E and Hb Yala (HBB:c.129delT); a novel frameshift β globin gene mutation, resulting in Hemoglobin E/ β^0-thalassemia. Hematology. 2018;**23**(2):117-121

[45] Viprakasit V, Pung-Amritt P, Suwanthon L, Clark K, Tanphaichtr VS. Complex interactions of δβ hybrid haemoglobin (Hb Lepore-Hollandia) Hb E (β(26G-->A)) and α^+ thalassaemia in a Thai family. European Journal of Haematology. 2002;**68**(2):107-111

[46] Changtrakun Y, Fucharoen S, Ayukarn K, Siriratmanawong N, Fucharoen G, Sanchaisuriya K. Compound heterozygosity for Hb Korle-Bu (beta(73); Asp-Asn) and Hb E (beta(26); Glu-Lys) with a 3.7-kb deletional α-thalassemia in Thai patients. Annals of Hematology. 2002;**81**(7):389-393

[47] Svasti S, Paksua S, Nuchprayoon I, Winichagoon P, Fucharoen S. Characterization of a novel deletion causing (δβ)0-thalassemia in a Thai family. American Journal of Hematology. 2007;**82**(2):155-161

[48] Panyasai S, Fucharoen S, Surapot S, Fucharoen G, Sanchaisuriya K. Molecular basis and hematologic characterization of δβ-thalassemia and hereditary persistence of fetal hemoglobin in Thailand. Haematologica. 2004;**89**(7):777-781

[49] Fucharoen S, Pengjam Y, Surapot S, Fucharoen G, Sanchaisuriya K. Molecular and hematological characterization of HPFH-6/Indian deletion-inversion Gγ(Aγδβ)^0-thalassemia and Gγ(Aγδβ)^0-thalassemia/HbE in Thai patients. American Journal of Hematology. 2002;**71**(2):109-113

Section 3

Treatment Modalities in Beta Thalassemia

Chapter 6

The Thalassemia Syndromes: New Insights

Saksham Singh, Chittala Kiran Sri and Atish Bakane

Abstract

Thalassemia is characterized by impaired synthesis of globin chains in hemoglobin. Supportive care for this condition includes regular transfusions and adequate iron chelation. Hemopoietic stem cell transplant (HSCT) is the only curative option available at present to most of the patients. The currently accepted indication for allogenic HSCT is transfusion dependency. For patients with available HLA-matched siblings or related or unrelated donors, a transplant should be offered as soon as possible to avoid transfusion-associated complications. The three risk factors are the presence of hepatomegaly >2 cm, the presence of liver/portal fibrosis and a history of inadequate chelation. Stem cells for HSCT can be obtained from bone marrow, peripheral blood and cord blood. In the majority, all the transplant centres across the world use bone marrow as a stem cell source as it is associated with a lesser incidence of GVHD (especially chronic) as compared to peripheral blood because of the high concentration of T lymphocytes in the latter. Conditioning regimen is being evolved from myeloablative to reduced intensity conditioning to reduced toxicity myeloablative conditioning regimens. Post-transplant management includes monitoring of engraftment and chimerism. It also aims at infection prophylaxis, prevention of GVHD, hematopoietic support and management of iron overload post-transplant.

Keywords: thalassemia, Hsct, conditioning, GVHD, mixed Chimerism

1. Introduction

Thalassemia is an inherited blood disorder characterized by impaired synthesis of globin chains in hemoglobin. It is a recessive monogenic disorder and 5% of population globally are carrier of this disease [1]. The estimated global prevalence of severe beta thalassemia is 288,000 per annum [2]. Transfusion-dependent thalassemia is associated with severe anemia and its complications, iron overload affecting multiple organs due to frequent transfusions, extramedullary hematopoiesis and hepatosplenomegaly. Supportive care for this condition includes regular transfusions and adequate iron chelation. However, hemopoietic stem cell transplant (HSCT) is the only curative option available at present [2].

Allogenic stem cell transplant in thalassemia as a cure was first reported in 1982 from a human leukocyte antigen (HLA) identical sibling donor [3]. Following this, more than 3000 successful transplants in thalassemia have been done [4]. In the 1980s and early 1990s, the Pesaro group in Italy pioneered the therapeutic approach to

IntechOpen

transplant in thalassemia [5–11]. This was later accepted worldwide. Since then, there has been gradual improvement in outcomes over the past 20 years due to improved strategies of conditioning, risk stratification and better control of complications. Overall survival (OS) and Thalassemia free survival (TFS) rates of thalassemia have improved to around 90% and 80%, respectively [12, 13]. The best available donor for HSCT is a full HLA-matched sibling donor (MSD) or family member. However, such donors are not easily available and hence strategies are coming up to use matched unrelated and mismatched donors as a source of stem cells for transplant. Till now their outcomes are inferior to matched related donors [14, 15]. Hence case to case basis discussions among transplant physicians and parents are required to choose between transplant or supportive therapies as part of the management of the disease when matched related donors are not available.

2. Indication of transplant and risk stratification

The currently accepted indication for allogenic HSCT is transfusion dependency. For patients with available HLA-matched siblings or related or unrelated donors, a transplant should be offered as soon as possible to avoid transfusion-associated complications [16]. HSCT is not chosen for patients with severe organ damage e.g. uncompensated cirrhosis.

In the early 1990s, the Pesaro group identified three patient-related risk factors which can affect the outcomes of transplants. These three risk factors were incorporated to stratify three classes of patients with the best outcomes available from class1 and the worst from class 3 [11].

The three risk factors were presence of hepatomegaly >2 cm, the presence of liver/portal fibrosis and a history of inadequate chelation. The quality of chelation was characterized as regular when deferoxamine therapy was initiated no later than 18 months after the first transfusion and was administered subcutaneously for 8–10 h continuously for at least 5 days/week. Any deviation from this regimen was defined as irregular chelation.

Class 1 had no risk factors, class 2 had one or two risk factors, and class 3 had three risk factors. The 3-year overall survival (OS) for class 1 was 94% and dropped to 61% for class 3. Class 3 also contained a group of very high-risk (HR) patients, typically aged ≥7 years and with liver size ≥5 cm from the costal arch.

Age older than 14 years is an independent risk factor. If MSD HSCT is performed before 14 years of age, procedure-related mortality is <10%. This decreases to <5% when performed before 5 years of age [17].

3. Pretransplant evaluation

In addition to classical pre-HSCT evaluation, the following tests need to be done:

Liver iron concentration: Assessment of liver Iron is done by liver biopsy or liver MRI, this can be avoided in patients with age less than 3 years. Compensated Cirrhosis (e.g. Child-Pugh class A) can have an impact on the prognosis and outcome of the transplant. It is not a contraindication to transplant but it should be weighed as a factor to choose HSCT on a case-to-case basis. Liver histology—with particular attention to the degree of fibrosis (for this purpose liver biopsy remains the preferred tool, over liver elastography) should be done. For the evaluation of liver fibrosis by biopsy, Knodell's numerical scoring system should be used [18].

Viral hepatitis tests: Viral hepatitis is not a contraindication to HSCT but tests should be done and appropriate antiviral drugs should be started and viral load should be lowered before starting of transplant.

Cardiac assessment: Electrocardiography or Echocardiography are appropriate tests to assess cardiac functions and then T2* MRI can be done to assess cardiac iron concentration in selected cases. A fully recovered case of iron-related heart failure is not a contraindication to transplant provided that the patient has received adequate iron chelation therapy.

Endocrine function: Fasting blood glucose levels, thyroid function tests, and growth-hormone-releasing hormone (GHRH) stimulation tests can be performed in children with age more than 10 years to rule out iron-related damage to endocrine organs. These evaluations do not impact transplant outcomes or procedures but can be very useful for long-term post-transplant follow up care.

Fertility assessment: Post pubertal males and females should be encouraged for sperm banking and ovarian tissue preservation respectively as temporary or permanent hypogonadism is common following allogeneic HSCT.

4. Donor selection

The ideal donor for HSCT is HLA-matched/HLA-identical sibling i.e. a sibling who shares the same HLA haplotype at six of six (or eight of eight) HLA loci (HLA—A, B and DR or HLA—A, B, C and DR respectively). The probability of availability of such a donor is 25% and that of a donor without thalassemia major is 18.5%.

5. Evolution of strategies of HSCT in Thalassemia

Over the last 20 years, the probability of thalassemia-free survival in MSD-HSCT has improved from 73% to 80–90% [19]. A survey of 1061 patients who underwent MSD-HSCT in the last 10 years, conducted by EBMT showed two years of overall survival (OS) as 91% [20]. The factors which helped in getting better survival were improved HLA typing, better maintenance of asepsis, more effective prophylaxis and treatment of various infections with the availability of broad-spectrum higher antibiotics, better prophylaxis of graft vs. host disease (GVHD), improved iron chelation before transplant and evolved strategies to deal with Pesaro class 3 transplant. **Table 1**, highlights the recent evidence from MSD-HSCT in thalassaemic children.

Different centres have come up with strategies for improving outcomes in Pesaro Class 3 patients as can be figured out in **Table 1**.

1. Hyper transfusion along with effective iron chelation to keep hemoglobin more than 13 g/dl and keep ferritin less than 2000 ng/ml.

2. Reducing the dose of cyclophosphamide (≤160 mg/kg), and adding fludarabine in the conditioning regimen to decrease treatment-related mortality (reduced intensity conditioning; RIC regimens).

3. Adding anti thymocyte globulin (ATG)/total lymphocyte irradiation (TLI)/total body irradiation (TBI) helps in achieving similar survival rates with RIC when compared with myeloablative conditioning regimens (MAC).

4. Pretransplant additional therapies with immunosuppression with azathioprine (Aza) and suppression of erythropoiesis with hydroxyurea (Hu). Sodani et al. [19] reported **Protocol 26** which combines RIC regimens with Aza and Hu improving survival to 93% and decreasing graft rejection to 6%

5. Using intravenous (i.v.) busulfan

6. Targeted i.v. busulfan

7. New drugs like treosulfan, thiotepa, and fludarabine (TTF regimen or adding thiotepa individually to the conditioning regimen), as well as intensive pretransplant transfusion-chelation regimens.

8. Gaziev et al. [20] reported **Modified Protocol 26**. It was similar to that of Sodani et al. but with a higher dose of Fludarabine (150 mg/kg) and the addition of thiotepa (10 mg/kg). This was used in MSD-HSCT with results of 92% OS and no graft rejection.

9. Anurathapan et al. [21] reported a novel reduced toxicity conditioning regimen (RTC) regimen involving sequential administration of Hu (to suppress erythropoiesis) followed by two cycles of Pre transplant immunosuppression (PTIS) including Fludarabine and dexamethasone (to suppress recipient T cells) followed by RTC with Fludarabine, Busulfan and Anti thymocyte globulin along with administration of a relatively high number of hematopoietic progenitor cells (>5 × 106 CD34+ cells/kg of recipient weight). This regimen was used in MSD and unrelated donors and resulted in overall survival of 94% in both groups (**Figure 1**).

Authors	No. of patients	Patient cohort/ overall survival Pesaro risk category	Thalassemia free survival	Treatment related mortality	Comments
Galambrun et al.	108	Children all categories 15 years of risk 86.8%	15 years	15 years	96 sibling donor
			69.40%	12%	Regimen: Bu-Cy ± ATG
Li et al.	82	Children all risk categories 3 years	3 years	3 years	52 MUD, 30 sibling
		91%	87%	8%	Regimen Bu-Cy-Thiotepa, Fludarabine
Bernardo et al.	60	Low: 275 years	5 years	7%	20 sibling donor, 40 MUD
		Intermediate: 17, high: 4 93%	84%		Regimen Treosulfan
		Adults: 12			Thiotepa-Fludarabine
Sabloff et al.	179	Low: 2% 5 years	5 years	Intermediate risk	Bu-Cy + ATG in 77

Authors	No. of patients	Patient cohort/ overall survival Pesaro risk category	Thalassemia free survival	Treatment related mortality	Comments
		Intermediate: Intermediate risk	Intermediate risk	May-75	Bu-Cy in 102
		42% 91%	88%	High risk	
		High: 36% High risk: 64%	High risk: 62%	23/64	
Irfan et al.	56	Children 5 years	5 years	100 days:	29 BM, 27 PBSCs
		Low: 20 BM: 73%	BM: 67%	Oct-56	Lower risks: Bu-Cy
		Intermediate: 20 PBSCs: 65%	PBSCs: 55%		High risk: Hydroxyurea-
		High: 16			Azathioprine-Fludarabune-
					Bu-Cy
Locatelli et al.	259	Median age 8 years (range 1–24) 6 years	6 years	4%	Multicentric retrospective
		Low: 86 95%	86%		Registry study.
		Intermediate: 122			Regimens: Bu-Cy,
		High: 51			Bu-Cy_Fludarabine, Bu-Cy-
					Thiotepa ±ATG.
Mathews et al.	50	High Risk: 48%	79%	12%	Treo based conditioning with PBSC graft in 74%
Anurathapan et al.	18	NA	89%	5%	Conditioning regimen with Flu and Iv Bu, Preconditioning Immunosuppression with Fludrabine and dexamethasone for one months.
Gaziev et al.	68	6 low risk 3 years	3 years	100 days	Intravenous Busulfan
		23 intermediate risk 91%	87%	3%	Based regimen
		39 high risk			

OS, overall survival; TFS, thalassemia free survival; TRM, transplant related survival; NR, not reported; Bu, busulfan; Cy, cyclophosphamide; ATG, antithymocyte globulin; BM, bone marrow; PBSC, peripheral blood stem cells; CB, cord blood.

Table 1.
Recent results of matched sibling donor transplant in children with thalassemia major [16].

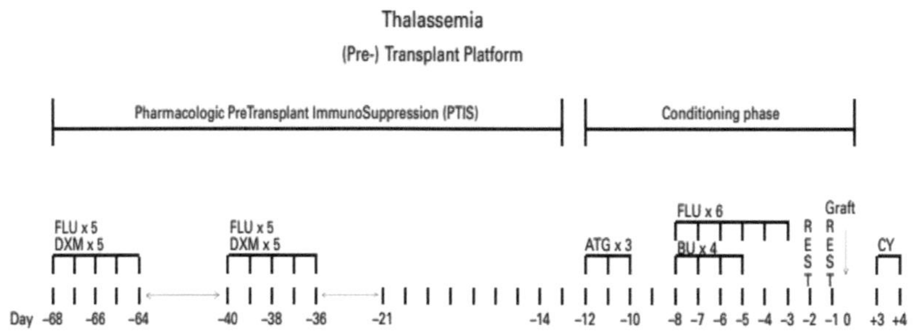

Figure 1.
Depiction of the transplant program with first pharmacological PTIS, followed by RTC with ATG, Flu and IV Bu. For the haplo-identical donors, we used post-Cy-based GvHD prophylaxis and delayed-calcineurin inhibitor-/sirolimus therapy, and short-course mycophenolate mofetil, the latter two starting on day SCT +5. Please see Patients and Methods section for details.

6. Alternative donors

HLA matched sibling as an option for the donor is available only in a quarter of cases. Because of its curative potential, the spectrum of the donor has been extended to alternative donors also. The experience of various types of the donor is as followed:

7. Matched unrelated donor (MUD) transplant

MUD transplant has been reported to be an acceptable strategy for the cure of thalassemia as an alternative option for MSD-HSCT if matched sibling donor is not available. An Italian bone marrow transplant group conducted a study in 2005 regarding MUD transplant using molecular typing in 68 patients with a median age of 15 years. The thalassemia-free survival for 30 patients in Pesaro classes 1 and 2 at a median follow-up of 3.4 years was 97%. However, for the other 38 class 3 patients, the survival was 65% [22]. Experience from several centres suggested that survival can be improved if there is high-resolution molecular typing at both HLA class I and II loci (HLA—A, B, C, DR B1 and DQB1). A recent study has demonstrated that the risk of thalassemia recurrence after unrelated bone marrow transplantation is associated with the presence of nonpermissive HLA-DPB1 mismatches in the host-versus-graft direction [23]. A novel conditioning regimen (WZ-14-TM protocol) based on reduced dose cyclophosphamide, i.v. Busulfan, fludarabine and addition of ATG, used by Chinese group Lan Sun et al. in 48 children of 2–11 years of age with beta-thalassemia major who underwent MUD peripheral blood transplant reported OS and TFS of 100% [24]. In 2021, Kharya et al. reported their experience of using modified PTIS protocol (Apollo Protocol) in 3 thalassemia patients who underwent MUD transplants. Along with Hu, and Aza, they gave 2 cycles of modified PTIS involving decreased cumulative dose of fludarabine as compared to that of Anurathapan et al. along with the addition of cyclophosphamide followed by augmented John Hopkins conditioning and subsequently Post-transplant cyclophosphamide (PtCy). At a median follow-up of 307.5 days, all patients were alive and disease free [23]. The limitations with MUD transplants are limited experience with lesser studies across the globe and the limited number of registries available for searching for matched donors.

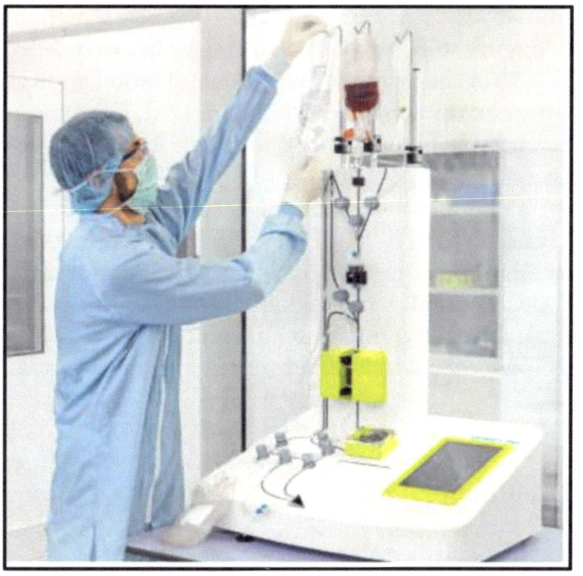

Figure 2.
T cell depletion.

8. Mismatched related donor (MMRD)/haploidentical transplant (haploidentical-HSCT)

MMRD/haploidentical transplants are considered experimental strategies to be taken as therapy for Thalassemia. Reports from such transplants are limited but with novel strategies, the outcomes are improving over the years. In 2018, Gaziev et al. reported their experience of using T cell receptor alpha-beta+/CD 19+ depleted grafts (**Figure 2**) for haplo-HSCT in 14 patients. At the median follow-up of 3.9 years, the five years probability of overall survival was 84%. The incidence of graft failure was 14%. Anurathapan et al. [21] used their Ric protocol (flu-i.v. blu) with PTIS along with ATG, PtCy, tacrolimus and mycophenolate mofetil (MMF) in 83 patients who underwent haplo HSCT. Six patients developed severe acute Graft vs. host disease (GVHD). Projected OS at 3 years was 96%. Experience with haplo-HSCT is very limited and more trials are required in this area.

9. Stem cell source

Stem cells for HSCT can be obtained from bone marrow, peripheral blood and cord blood. In the majority, all the transplant centres across the world use bone marrow as a stem cell source as it is associated with a lesser incidence of GVHD (especially chronic) as compared to peripheral blood because of the high concentration of T lymphocytes in the latter. Overall survival has been better with bone marrow stem cells in some studies. The incidence of graft failure has been similar to all the sources 2014 expert panel guidelines recommend bone marrow as a source of stem cells over peripheral blood [16].

Ghavamzadeh et al. in a 2007 study reported chronic GVHD in 19% of bone marrow HSCT and 48% of peripheral blood HSCT involving 183 children who underwent

MSD HSCT [25]. Similar results were seen in a 2010 study which involved 52 children with thalassemia belonging to Pesaro Class 3. They underwent MSD-HSCT. The chronic GVHD was 40% in the group with peripheral blood stem cell transplant and 16% in that with bone marrow stem cell transplant [26]. Cord blood (CB) as a source of stem cells has been tried to extend the donor pool. Also, the rates of acute and chronic GVHD are theoretically less with cord blood. However, the survival rates were similar between cord blood and bone marrow [27]. With unrelated cord blood, high rates of graft failure and delayed hematopoietic recovery were the major concerns [28]. This limitation might be mitigated by using ≥1 CB donor unit or by giving CB together with T cell-depleted HLA-haploidentical CD34 with cells. Current recommendations for CB transplant suggest using units containing at least 3.5×10^7 total nucleated cell/kg recipient body weight before cryopreservation, and with less than 2 HLA disparities.

10. Conditioning regimen

The conditioning regimen for HSCT requires two conditions to be fulfilled. First, ablation of expanded erythropoietic marrow and second immunosuppression of the host for effective engraftment of graft cells. The first condition is fulfilled by Busulfan and its derivative. However, for the second condition busulfan is not that effective and hence cyclophosphamide is incorporated into the backbone as an effective immunosuppressive agent. The myeloablative conditioning derived from this principle was busulfan at the dose of 14–16 mg/kg and cyclophosphamide at the dose of 200 mg/kg. This conditioning regimen has evolved over the years to improve graft survival and overall survival with a lesser incidence of treatment-related toxicities and mortalities. With Busulfan the idea evolved from using it intravenously for effective bioavailability then infusing it with therapeutic drug monitoring [29], then using its derivative treosulfan as in Thiotepa-Treosulfan-Fludarabine (TTF) regimen [30–32]. With cyclophosphamide, the idea evolved from decreasing its dose from 200 mg/kg to 160 mg/kg [33], which improved survival but increased the graft rejection rate also followed by the addition of fludarabine (RIC regimen) as another immunosuppressive agent followed by the use of pretransplant immunosuppression [21] (Protocol 26, as described above) followed by addition of thiotepa and increasing the dose of fludarabine (modified Protocol 26, as described above), a type of Reduced toxicity Myeloblative (RTM) regimen [34]. As mentioned above Anurathapan et al. [24] and Kharya et al. [23] came up with the novel idea of Pretransplant Immunosuppression and reported optimal survival rates.

11. Graft versus host disease prophylaxis

An international expert panel in 2014 recommended the use of cyclosporine and methotrexate (on days +1, +3, +6, +11 post-transplant) as standard of prophylaxis for GVHD. Cyclosporine is continued for one year [16]. Anti-thymocyte globulin (ATG) has been shown to improve the GVHD rates in MSD, MUD and Haplo-HSCT [35, 36]. It is recommended for use in alternative donor transplants and when using peripheral blood as the source of stem cells. For haploidentical transplants post-transplant cyclophosphamide (PtCy) has also been incorporated for GVHD prophylaxis to get better results [37–39].

12. Mixed chimerism

Mixed chimerism is defined by the presence of >5% recipient cells at any time post-transplant. The severity is graded as levels 1, 2, 3 depending on the percentage of recipient cells as <10%, 10–25%, and >25% respectively. Andreani et al. [39] showed that engraftment with day +60 chimerism more than 90%, also called bulk engraftment is required for achieving stable complete chimerism or mixed chimerism. Aby Abraham et al. [35] reported the management of mixed chimerism. Initially, they tapered immunosuppression (tapering of dose of cyclosporine by 30% every two weeks) until there was stable mixed chimerism or complete donor chimerism. If there was progressive loss of donor chimerism leading to level 2 or level 3 chimerism on two consecutive occasions despite the tapering of immunosuppression and absence of GVHD, Donor Lymphocyte Infusion (DLI) was given. In their study, 80% of the patients with level II chimerism responded to DLI and 31.2% of those with level III chimerism showed the response. 40% of patients achieved stable mixed chimerism or complete donor chimerism with DLI.

13. Post-transplant management

Post-transplant management includes monitoring of engraftment and chimerism. It also aims at infection prophylaxis, prevention of GVHD, hematopoietic support and management of iron overload post-transplant. Patients are kept at antibacterial, antiviral and antifungal prophylaxis with special attention to protection against Cytomegalovirus (CMV) and Pneumocystis Carini. Transfusion support is given as per needs. GVHD prophylaxis is given as discussed above. Patients should be monitored for organ functions, growth and gonadal functions also. Regarding iron overload, the aim is to keep serum ferritin <2000 ng/ml and liver iron <7.5 mg/g of dry weight. To achieve this a phlebotomy of 5–6 ml/kg every two weeks or four weeks is done until patients are on immunosuppression [40]. After a patient is free of immunosuppression and has stable engraftment, the patient can be kept on iron chelators according to the dosing schedule. Deferiprone should be used with caution as it may cause agranulocytosis.

Author details

Saksham Singh[1], Chittala Kiran Sri[2] and Atish Bakane[1*]

1 Centre for BMTCT, Indraprastha Apollo Hospital, New Delhi, India

2 MAMC, New Delhi, India

*Address all correspondence to: atishalways2000@gmail.com

References

[1] Angelucci E, Baronciani D. Allogeneic stem cell transplantation for thalassemia major. Haematologica. 2008;**93**(12):1780-1784. DOI: 10.3324/haematol.2008.001909

[2] Porter J. Beyond transfusion therapy: New therapies in thalassemia including drugs, alternate donor transplant, and gene therapy. Hematology American Social Hematological Education Program. Dec 2008;**93**(12):1780-1784

[3] Lucarelli G, Galimberti M, Polchi P, Angelucci E, Baronciani D, Giardini C. Bone marrow transplantation in patients with thalassemia. The New England Journal of Medicine. 1990;**322**:417-421

[4] Lucarelli G, Polchi P, Izzi T, Manna M, Agostinelli F, Delfini C. Allogeneic marrow transplantation for thalassemia. Experimental Hematology. 1984;**12**:676-681

[5] Lucarelli G, Polchi P, Galimberti M, Izzi T, Delfini C, Manna M. Marrow transplantation for thalassaemia following busulphan and cyclophosphamide. Lancet. 1985;**1**:1355-1357

[6] Lucarelli G, Galimberti M, Polchi P, Giardini C, Politi P, Baronciani D. Marrow transplantation in patients with advanced thalassemia. The New England Journal of Medicine. 1987;**316**:1050-1055

[7] Lucarelli G, Weatherall DJ. For debate: Bone marrow transplantation for severe thalassaemia (1). The view from Pesaro (2). To be or not to be. British Journal of Haematology. 1991;**78**:300-303

[8] Lucarelli G, Galimberti M, Polchi P, Angelucci E, Baronciani D, Durazzi SM. Bone marrow transplantation in adult thalassemia. Blood. 1992;**80**:1603-1607

[9] Lucarelli G, Galimberti M, Polchi P, Angelucci E, Baronciani D, Giardini C. Marrow transplantation in patients with thalassemia responsive to iron chelation therapy. The New England Journal of Medicine. 1993;**329**:840-844

[10] Choudhary D, Divya S, Sanjeev K, Vipin S, Rasika H. Allogenic hematopoietic cell transplantation in Thalassemia major: A single-center retrospective analysis from India. Journal of Pediatric Hematology/Oncology. 2019;**41**(5):e296-e301. DOI: 10.1097/MPH.0000000000001475

[11] Huang K, Zhou D-H, Li Y, et al. Modified conditioning regimen improves outcomes of unrelated donor peripheral blood stem cell transplantation for patients with β-thalassaemia major. Pediatric Blood & Cancer. 2018;**65**:e27026

[12] Li C, Mathews V, Kim S, George B, Hebert K, Jiang H, et al. Related and unrelated donor transplantation for β-thalassemia major: Results of an international survey. Blood Advances. 2019;**3**(17):2562-2570

[13] John MJ, Mathew A, Philip CC, Singh S, Tanuja T, Kakkar N. Unrelated and related donor transplantation for beta-thalassemia major: A single-center experience from India. Pediatric Transplantation. 2018;**22**:e13209

[14] Angelucci E, Matthes-Martin S, Baronciani D, Bernaudin F, Bonanomi S. Cappellini stem cell transplantation in thalassemia major and sickle cell disease: Indications and management recommendations from an international expert panel. Haematologica. 2014;**99**(5):811-820. DOI: 10.3324/haematol.2013.099747

[15] Baronciani D, Angelucci E, Potschger U, et al. Hemopoietic stem cell transplantation in thalassemia: A report from the European Society for Blood and Bone Marrow Transplantation Hemoglobinopathy Registry, 2000-2010. Bone Marrow Transplantation. 2016;**51**(4):536-541

[16] Knodell RG, Ishak KG, Black WC, Chen TS, Craig R, Kaplowitz N, et al. Formulation and application of a numerical scoring system for assessing histological activity in asymptomatic chronic active hepatitis. Hepatology. 1981;**1**(5):431-435. DOI: 10.1002/hep.1840010511

[17] Angellucci E, Srivastava A, Usai S. Haemopoietic stem cell transplantation. In: Cappellini MD, Cohen A, Porter J, et al., editors. Guidelines for the Management of Transfusion Dependent Thalassaemia (TDT). 3rd ed. Nicosia (CY): Thalassaemia International Federation; 2014 Chapter 12

[18] Baronciani D, Pilo F, Lyon-Caen S, Poetschger U, Dini G, Peters C. Hematopoietic Stem Cell Transplantation in Thalassemia Major. Report from the EBMT Hemoglobinopathy Registry. ASH Annual Meeting; 2011

[19] Sodani P, Gaziev D, Polchi P, Erer B, Giardini C, Angelucci E. New approach for bone marrow transplantation in patients with class 3 thalassemia aged younger than 17 years. Blood. 2004;**104**(4):1201-1203. DOI: 10.1182/blood-2003-08-2800

[20] Gaziev J, Isgrò A, Sodani P, et al. Optimal outcomes in young Class 3 patients with thalassemia undergoing HLA-identical sibling bone marrow transplantation. Transplantation. 2016;**100**(4):925-932

[21] Anurathapan U, Pakakasama S, Mekjaruskul P, Sirachainan N, Songdej D, Chuansumrit A, et al. Outcomes of thalassemia patients undergoing hematopoietic stem cell transplantation by using a standard myeloablative versus a novel reduced-toxicity conditioning regimen according to a new risk stratification. Biology of Blood and Marrow Transplantation. 2014;**20**(12):2066-2071

[22] Sun L, Wang N, Chen Y, Tang L, Xing C, Nina L. Unrelated donor peripheral blood stem cell transplantation for patients with β-thalassemia major based on a novel conditioning regimen. Biology of Blood and Marrow Transplantation. 2019;**25**(8):1592-1596

[23] Kharya G, Bakane AN, Rauthan AM. Pretransplant myeloid and immune suppression, reduced toxicity conditioning with posttransplant cyclophosphamide: Initial outcomes of novel approach for matched unrelated donor hematopoietic stem cell transplant for hemoglobinopathies. Pediatric Blood & Cancer. 2021;**68**:e28909

[24] Anurathapan U, Hongeng S, Pakakasama S, Songdej D, Sirachainan N, Pongphitcha P. Hematopoietic stem cell transplantation for severe thalassemia patients from haploidentical donors using a novel conditioning regimen. Biology of Blood and Marrow Transplantation. 2020;**26**(6):1106-1112. DOI: 10.1016/j.bbmt.2020.01.002

[25] Locatelli F, Kabbara N, Ruggeri A, et al. Outcome of patients with hemoglobinopathies given either cord blood or bone marrow transplantation from an HLA-identical sibling. Blood. 2013;**122**(6):1072-1078

[26] Ruggeri A, Eapen M, Scaravadou A, Cairo MS, Bhatia M, Kurtzberg J, et al.

Umbilical cord blood transplantation for children with thalassemia and sickle cell disease. Biology of Blood and Marrow Transplantation. 2011;**17**(9):1375-1382

[27] Gaziev J, Nguyen L, Puozzo C, et al. Novel pharmacokinetic behavior of intravenous busulfan in children with thalassemia undergoing hematopoietic stem cell transplantation: A prospective evaluation of pharmacokinetic and pharmacodynamic profile with therapeutic drug monitoring. Blood. 2010;**115**(22):4597-4604. DOI: 10.1182/blood-2010-01-265,405

[28] Casper J, Knauf W, Kiefer T, et al. Treosulfan and fludarabine: A new toxicity-reduced conditioning regimen for allogeneic hematopoietic stem cell transplantation. Blood. 2004;**103**:725

[29] Bernardo ME, Zecca M, Piras E, et al. Treosulfan-based conditioning regimen for allogeneic hematopoietic stem cell transplantation in patients with thalassaemia major. British Journal of Haematology. 2008;**143**:548

[30] Bernardo ME, Piras E, Vacca A, et al. Allogeneic hematopoietic stem cell transplantation in thalassemia major: Results of a reduced-toxicity conditioning regimen based on the use of treosulfan. Blood. 2012;**120**:473

[31] Lucarelli G, Clift R, Galimberti M, et al. Marrow transplantation for patients with thalassemia: Results in class 3 patients. Blood. 1996;**87**:2082-2088

[32] Sauer M, Bettoni C, Lauten M, Ghosh A, Rehe K, Grigull L, et al. Complete substitution of cyclophosphamide by fludarabine and ATG in a busulfan-based preparative regimen for children and adolescents with beta-thalassemia. Bone Marrow Transplantation. 2005;**36**(5):383-387

[33] Goussetis E, Peristeri I, Kitra V, Vessalas G, Paisiou A, Theodosaki M, et al. HLAmatched sibling stem cell transplantation in children with beta-thalassemia with antithymocyte globulin as part of the preparative regimen: The Greek experience. Bone Marrow Transplantation. 2012;**47**(8):1061-1066

[34] La Nasa G, Argiolu F, Giardini C, et al. Unrelated bone marrow transplantation for beta-thalassemia patients: The experience of the Italian Bone Marrow Transplant Group. Annals of the New York Academy of Sciences. 2005;**1054**:186

[35] Abraham A, Edison E, Korula A, Fouzia N, Alok S, Biju G, et al. Donor lymphocyte infusion in patients with thalassemia major who have mixed chimerism following allogeneic stem cell transplant. Blood. 2015;**126**:1965-1965. DOI: 10.1182/blood.V126.23.1965.1965

[36] Andreani M, Nesci S. Lucarelli G. Long-term survival of ex-thalassemic patients with persistent mixed chimerism after bone marrow transplantation. Bone Marrow Transplantation. 2000;**25**: 401-404

[37] Fleischhauer K, Locatelli F, Zecca M, et al. Graft rejection after unrelated donor hematopoietic stem cell transplantation for thalassemia is associated with nonpermissive HLA-DPB1 disparity in host-versus graft direction. Blood. 2006;**107**:2984-2992

[38] Ghavamzadeh A, Iravani M, Ashouri A, et al. Peripheral blood versus bone marrow as a source of hematopoietic stem cells for allogeneic transplantation in children with class I and II beta thalassemia major. Biology of Blood and Marrow Transplantation. 2008;**14**:301

[39] Iravani M, Tavakoli E, Babaie MH, et al. Comparison of peripheral blood stem cell transplant with bone marrow transplant in class 3 thalassemic patients. Experimental and Clinical Transplantation. 2010;**8**:66

[40] Angelucci E, Muretto P, Lucarelli G. Phlebotomy to reduce iron overload in patients cured of thalassemia by bone marrow transplantation. Italian Cooperative Group for Phlebotomy Treatment of Transplanted Thalassemia Patients. Blood. 1997;**90**:994-998

Section 4

Blood and Blood Components Transfusion Modalities

Chapter 7

Optimizing Blood Transfusion Service Delivery across the West African Sub-Region

Osaro Erhabor, Josephine O. Akpotuzor, Edward Yaw Afriyie, Godswill Chikwendu Okara, Tosan Erhabor, Donald Ibe Ofili, Teddy Charles Adias, Idris Ateiza Saliu, Evarista Osime, Alhaji Bukar, Oyetunde B. Akinloye, Zakiya Abdul-Mumin, John Ocquaye-Mensah Tetteh, Edwin G. Narter-Olaga, Andrews Yashim-Nuhu, Folashade Aturamu, Ayodeji Olusola Olayan, Adeyinka Babatunde Adedire, Oyeronke Suebat Izobo, Kolawole A. Fasakin, Onyeka Paul, Collins Ohwonigho Adjekuko, Elliot Eli Dogbe and Uloma Theodora Ezeh

Abstract

The sub-continent of West Africa is made up of 16 countries: Benin, Burkina Faso, Cape Verde, Ghana, Guinea, Guinea-Bissau, Ivory Coast, Liberia, Mali, Mauritania, Niger, Nigeria, Senegal, Sierra Leone, The Gambia and Togo. As of 2018, the population of the sub-continent was estimated at about 381 million. The main challenge associated with blood transfusion service delivery across the sub-region concerns adequacy and safety. In this chapter, we highlighted the challenges associated with the delivery of a quality blood transfusion service in countries in the sub-region including: implementation of component therapy rather than whole blood transfusion, effective cold chain management of blood and blood products, alloimmunization prevention, implementation of column agglutination and automation rather than the convention manual tube method in blood transfusion testing, effective management of major haemorrhage, optimization of screening for transfusion transmissible infections, optimizing blood donation, implementation of universal leucodepletion of blood and blood products, effective management of transfusion-dependent patients, pre-operative planning and management of surgical patients, management of Rhesus D negative pregnancy and women with clinically significant alloantibodies, implementation of haemovigilance system, implementation of alternatives to allogenic blood, availability

IntechOpen

and use of specialized blood products, optimizing safe blood donation, enhancing blood transfusion safety, operating a quality management system-based blood transfusion service and implementation of non-invasive cell-free foetal DNA testing. There is the urgent need for the implementation of evidence-based best practices in blood transfusion service delivery across the sub-region to allow for excellent, safe, adequate and timely blood transfusion service delivery across the sub-region.

Keywords: blood transfusion, service delivery, West Africa, optimization, sub region

1. Introduction

Blood transfusion has life-saving potential and can improve the wellbeing and quality of life of anaemic and bleeding patients [1]. However, the major challenge to blood transfusion service delivery across the West African sub region is access to adequate, safe and timely blood transfusion service [2]. Effective blood transfusion requires that blood sourced from the right voluntary non-remunerated blood donor, is rightly screened, processed, stored and distributed. It is the right blood given to the right patient in the right quantity, in the right condition, at the right time, in the right place, for the right clinical indication and that is effective [3, 4]. There are several challenges associated with blood transfusion service delivery across the West African sub-region. In 2016, WHO global status report on blood safety and availability indicated that an insignificant 5.6 million units of blood (4% of the global supply) were collected in Africa with 38 African countries collecting <10 whole-blood donations per 1,000 populations [5]. The West African sub-region and other developing countries have a significantly increased need for blood and constitute a significant part of the global population, yet it contributes an insignificant number of units to the global allogenic blood pool. The rate of blood donation across the sub-region and other developing countries is significantly lower and often from less safe family replacement and commercial remunerated donor rather than from safer, benevolent and altruistic voluntary non-remunerated blood donors. There are 4.6, 11.7 and 33.1 donations per 1000 population in low- income developing, middle -income and high-income countries respectively [5]. In addition, there is a significant variation in the groups that are most frequently transfused in developing and developed countries. In West Africa and other developing countries, a significant 65% of transfusions are given to children <5 years and to manage pregnancy-related complications including ante and post-partum bleeding compared to 76% of blood transfused to patients >65 years of age in developed countries.

The provision of safe, adequate, and timely blood should ideally be the responsibility of the National blood transfusion service (NBTS) and should be an essential part of every nation's national health care policy. The WHO recommends that every nation should have a centrally coordinated and regionally based National Blood Transfusion Service governed by national blood policy and legislative framework to allow for the maintenance of standards and consistency in the quality and safety of blood and blood products [6]. The NBTS sole responsibility is to coordinate all activities related to blood collection, testing, processing, storage and distribution blood collected from safe voluntary non-remunerated blood donors who form a reliable, safe, assured and stable base of blood donors [7]. Although the national blood transfusion services are present in member countries across the sub region, they have not been able to solve the challenge of ensuring the safety, adequacy and timely blood transfusion service delivery [8, 9].

Blood supply across the sub region is still predominantly dependent on family/ replacement and some commercial remunerated donors. Only few donors across the region donate blood voluntarily. The West African sub-region does not seem to be as altruistic as their counterpart in the developed world regarding voluntary blood donation [10].

WHO recommends that all blood donations should be screened mandatorily for transfusion transmissible diseases including, HIV, hepatitis B, hepatitis C and syphilis and that such screening should meet quality management system requirements. The prevalence of TTIs is considerably higher in the West African sub region compared to the high-income developed nations. In the West African sub region, the challenge has been the availability of screening measures, adequately trained personnel and relevant infrastructure that is required to reduce the risk of introducing potentially infected blood from donor in the window phase of infection in the allogenic blood pool. Use of antibody-based screening with its limitation is prevalent for screening of blood donors for HIV and HCV. Blood donor screening most times is not monitored through external quality assessment (EQA) schemes, there is irregular supply and sometimes stock out of screening kits and other consumables [11, 12].

Suboptimal utilization of the limited allogenic bloodstock is another a major challenge. Whole blood transfusion rather than universally leucodepleted component therapy is prevalent across the sub region [13, 14]. National haemovigilance systems and Hospital Transfusion Committees (HTC) required to monitor, improve, and ensure the rational use and by extension the safety of the blood transfusion process are often non-existent in many setting across the sub region [15]. Adverse events, reactions and near misses are not reported and investigated properly. The root causes are not determined neither are the corrective and preventive action implemented in a timely and action-planned format. Clinical audits are seldom implemented and unnecessary non-clinically indicated and unsafe transfusion practices that expose patients to the risk of serious adverse transfusion reactions and TTIs and that reduces the availability of blood products for patients in whom it is clinically indicated are prevalent. There is absence of indication coding tool required to guide the safe, appropriate, and clinical use of blood across the sub region [16]. The decision to transfuse a patient across the sub region should ideally be based on clinical judgement, laboratory-based evidence and the patient's risk/benefit ratio including risks associated with transfusion and anaemia [17]. There is need to ensure that all transfusion across the region is clinically effective, prevent mortality in acute situations, ensure the reversal of a physiological transfusion trigger, restores adequate tissue perfusion and ensures maintenance of optimum coagulation [18]. There is an urgent need to solve the challenges associated with timely access to a safe and adequate supply of blood products. The aim of this chapter is to highlight the challenges associated with blood transfusion service delivery in the West African sub region and advocate for the implementation of realistic, pragmatic and evidence-based best practices required to optimize blood transfusion service ensuring that there is universal access to safe blood and blood products.

2. Urgent need for the implementation of component therapy in the West African sub-region

Traditionally, blood can be transfused either as whole blood or as one of its components. Blood components include red cell concentrates (RCCs), fresh frozen plasma (FFP), platelet concentrates (PCs) and cryoprecipitate. However, global safety initiatives and evidence-based best practice advocate that donation be separated into components for safety reasons and to facilitate optimal utilization of scarce allogenic blood stock [19]. Blood component therapy (BCT) is the therapeutic use of blood components rather than the wasteful use of whole blood to manage patients. Patients seldom need all the components of in whole blood. Anaemic patients require red cell concentrate, coagulopathy patients with raised international normalized ration (INR) above 1.5 require fresh frozen plasma, thrombocytopenic patients require platelet concentrate while bleeding patients with significantly low fibrinogen level (< 2 g/L for obstetric haemorrhage and < 1 g/L in non-obstetrics haemorrhage) requires cryoprecipitate. BCT involves whole blood being leucodepleted, divided into individual components, and delivered separately. It often requires that a patient receives the specific blood component required to treat their specific deficiency or condition [20]. Component separation was first developed in 1960 aimed at separating blood products from a unit of whole blood using refrigerated centrifuges and controlled conditions of gravitational force and temperature [19]. A considerable number of literatures has accumulated over the past decade indicating that leukocytes present in allogeneic cellular blood components, intended for transfusion, are associated with adverse effects to the recipient [21]. These include the development of febrile transfusion reactions, graft-versus-host disease, alloimmunization to leukocyte antigens and the immunomodulatory effects that might influence the prognosis of patients with malignancy and HIV. Moreover, it has become evident that leukocytes present in whole blood may be the vector of infectious agents such as cytomegalovirus (CMV), Human T-Lymphotrophic Virus 1/11 (HTLV-I/II), and Epstein Barr (EBV) as well as other viruses. Effective stewardship of blood ensuring that several patients potentially benefit from components derived from one unit of donated whole blood is important for economic, supply/demand reasons and to protect the national inventory at times of national blood shortage [22]. Blood safety in developing countries can be improved by more appropriate use of blood components rather than whole blood transfusion and the provision of alternatives such as oral and intravenous iron, erythropoietin, saline and colloids to manage anaemic and bleeding patients. This will facilitate the optimal use of the limited blood supply. Political will and open-mindedness to innovative ways to improve supply, appropriateness, optimal use and safety of blood from blood donors are essential to promote more evidence-based approaches to blood transfusion practice in sub-Saharan Africa. A recent review on blood transfusion in sub-Saharan Africa highlights the gaps in the area of quality, safety, supply and efficacy of blood and plasma products [23]. BCT is evidence-based best practice and constitutes effective stewardship in the management of our scarce blood resource. BCT allows for targeted therapy and maximum utilization of donated whole blood ensuring that several patients potentially benefit from components derived from the unit. It makes economic, supply/demand sense to implement BCT across the West African sub region- a region where there is high demand, but little supply coupled with the challenge of safety of blood and blood products [24, 25]. BCT can potentially protect regional inventory at times of national blood shortage [20]. Evidence-based clinical decision is crucial in ensuring appropriate transfusion practice. Education, training, and competency testing of all healthcare personnel involved in the blood transfusion process is vital in ensuring effective and appropriate clinical use of blood and components. In countries across the West African sub-region, non-leucodepleted whole blood transfusion thrives rather than component derived from leucodepleted whole blood [26]. Previous report indicates that the utility of cryoprecipitate platelet concentrate and other plasma products is low in many settings in sub-Saharan Africa. This is often due to multiple factors; unavailability due to lack of equipment in NBTS for blood product preparation [27] and lack of education and knowledge among physicians on evidence-based best practices on blood management principles. Other factors include logistical issues and lack of laboratory infrastructure to produce blood components. A previous report that investigated the knowledge and practices of physicians on blood component therapy in two tertiary hospitals in Nigeria indicated that although majority of the physicians have a good knowledge concerning BCT, there is however a knowledge-practice mismatch attributable to the unavailability of the various blood components thus limiting optimal practice of BCT [28]. In each country across the sub region, the blood collection service should have the technical capabilities and financial resources required to facilitate the supply of a range of safe blood products adapted to the specific clinical needs in the country, in particular and for labile therapeutic cellular components. Use of blood products should rely on evidence-based clinical practice, a concept which requires a well- structured and operational clinical interface between blood establishments and care centres. Transfusion committees are an operational tool to monitor and record transfusion epidemiology, patient blood management and blood product use within hospitals. A previous report that investigated the clinical utility of component therapy in sub-Saharan Africa indicated that a total of 40 out of the 43 countries studied reported that they have capacity to produce blood components with red cell concentrates being prepared in 35 of the 40 countries while platelets and fresh frozen plasma were prepared in 27 and 30 countries respectively. In most countries in West Africa an insignificant proportion of blood collection is separated into components; Benin 39.2%, Cameroon 2.8%, Burkina Faso 98.4, Central African Republic100, Congo 20.5, Côte d'Ivoire 86.2, DRC45.0, Sao Tome and Principe 85.2, Senegal 20.5, Mauritius 47.6, Gambia0.0, Ghana 2.6, Nigeria 0.0, Guinea 0.4, Madagascar 38.6, Mali 30.4, Togo 72.2, Mauritania 100, Niger 7.2, Tanzania 1.7 and Sierra Leone 0.0 [29]. In Burkina Faso, the blood transfusion centre produces red cell concentrates (RCC) from whole blood by centrifugation or simple gravity to meet the blood component demand for patients suffering from severe anaemia, such as pregnant women and children with malaria [30]. Separating blood into red cell concentrates, platelet concentrates, plasma and cryoprecipitate is a tool that can be implemented across the West African sub region along with universal leucodepletion and possibly virus inactivation treatments. It is vital that the preparation of blood components be guided by clinical requirements, especially to prevent unnecessary wastage of recovered plasma. One practical way to avoid wasting plasma would require cost-effective and tightly controlled processing of qualified plasma from throughout the West Africa sub region to produce polyvalent and hyperimmune immunoglobulins, VIII (to treat patients with haemophilia A and albumin [31]. Fractionation of plasma can generate a range of purified, virally inactivated, protein therapeutics that can potentially reduce some adverse effects (fevers, chills, transfusion-transmitted infections like CMV, HTLV-1 and 2 as well as prevent volume overload) while providing a better treatment for people suffering from haemophilia or immunodeficiency and other diseases that requires plasma derived proteins for the management. The plasma derived from blood component can be fractionated to produce various Plasma-derived Medicinal Products (PDMPs) of significant economic and therapeutic value [32, 33]. The effective implementation of BCT across the West African region is a huge but surmountable technological challenge hindered in many cases by the lack of a fit for purpose and structured national blood transfusion service, suboptimal number of qualified and skilled health workers, uninterrupted power supply challenges and challenge associated with cold-chain management of blood components. These challenges, although daunting, is surmountable and will require the political will by government of ECOWAS countries working together as a team and taking bold steps to implement BCT (**Figures 1–6**).

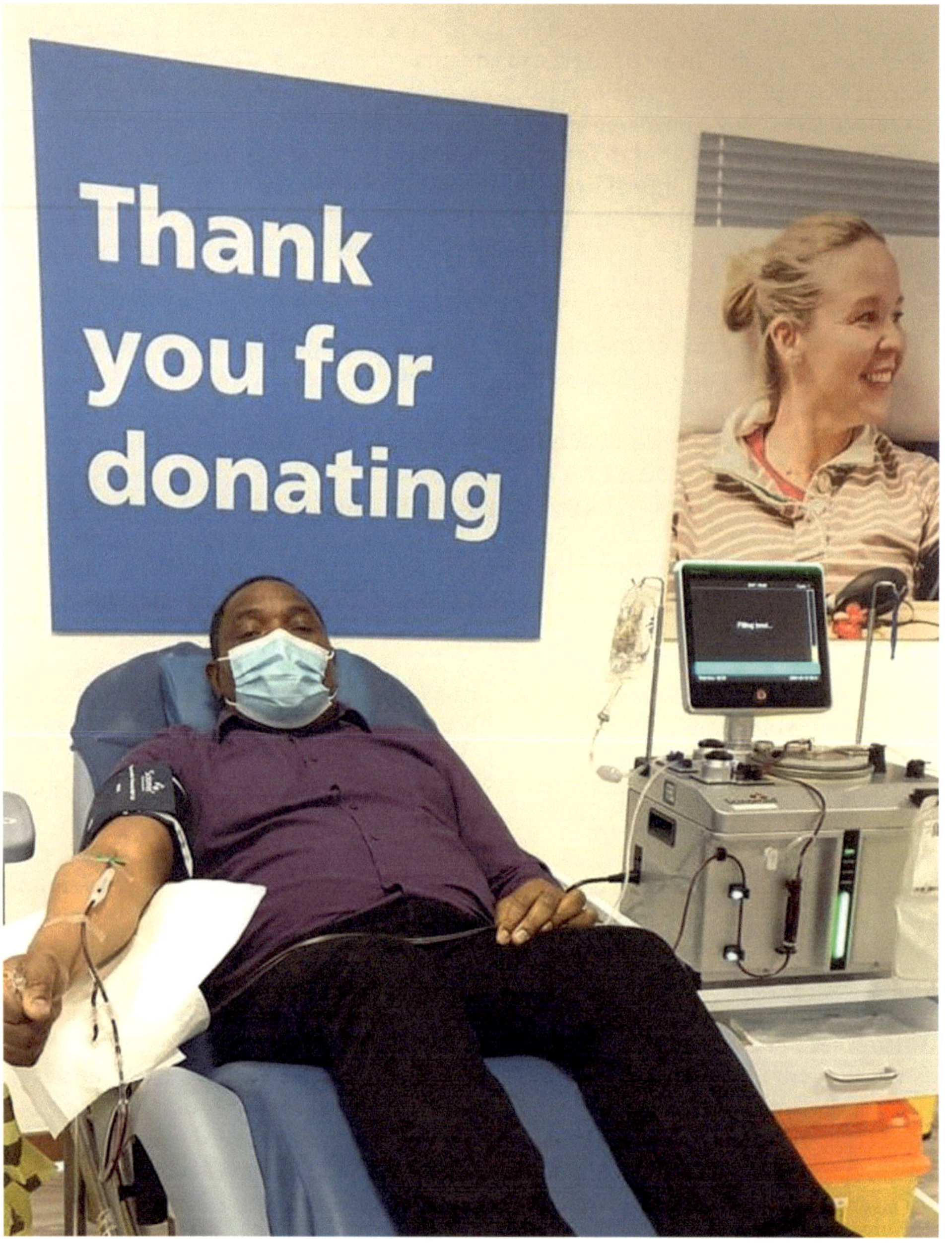

Figure 1.
Donation of plasma by apheresis.

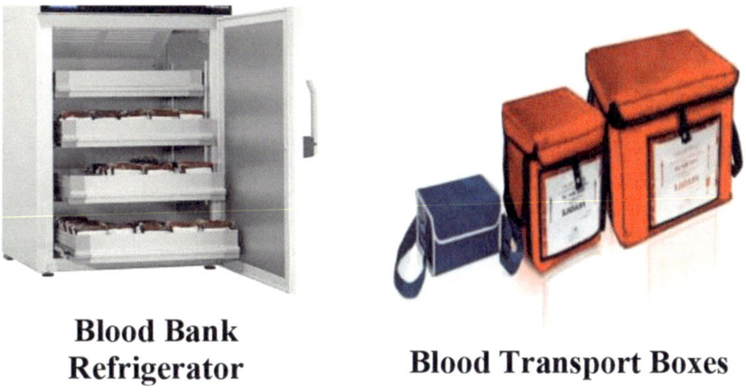

Figure 2.
Cold chain management of blood and blood products.

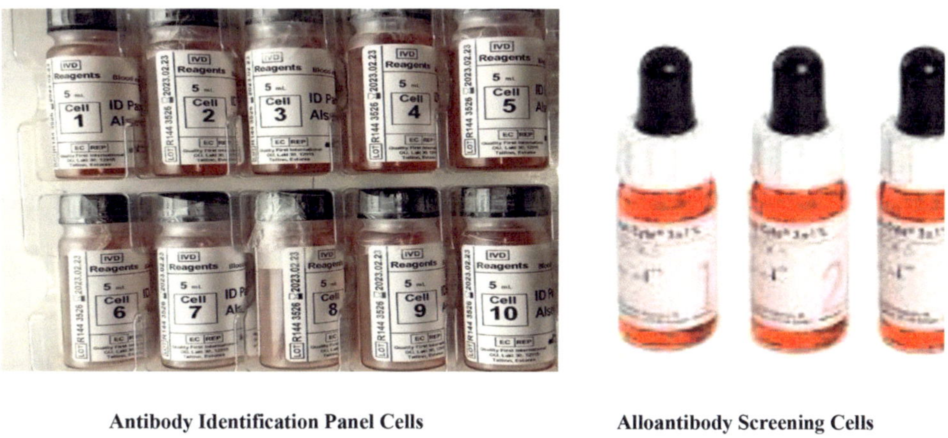

Figure 3.
Alloantibody screening and panel cells.

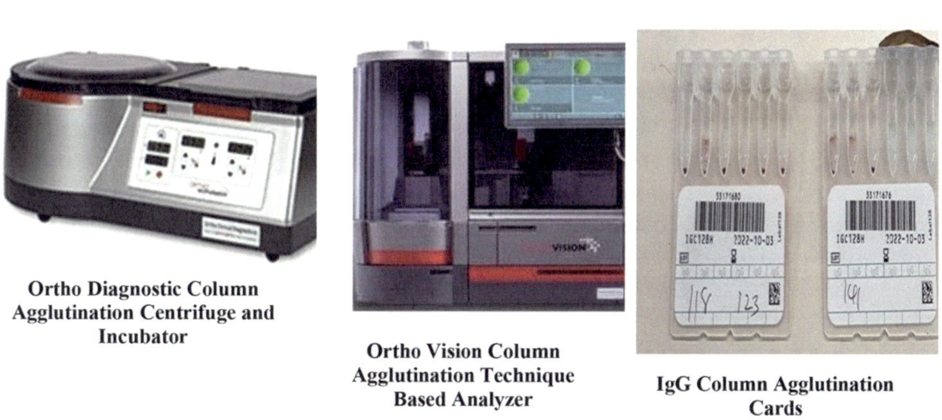

Figure 4.
Column agglutination technique.

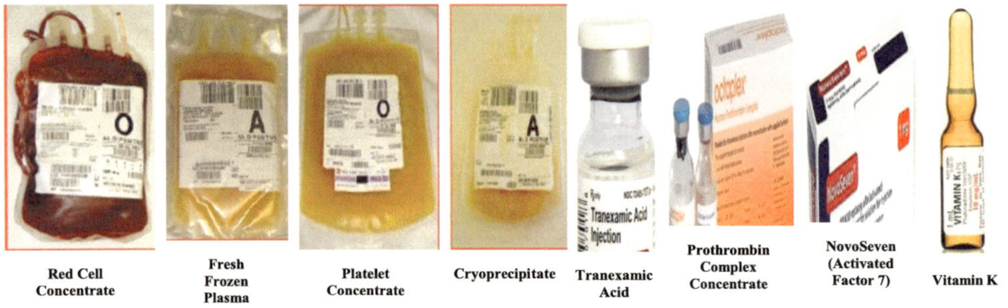

Figure 5.
Blood products and pharmacologic agent used to manage major haemorrhage.

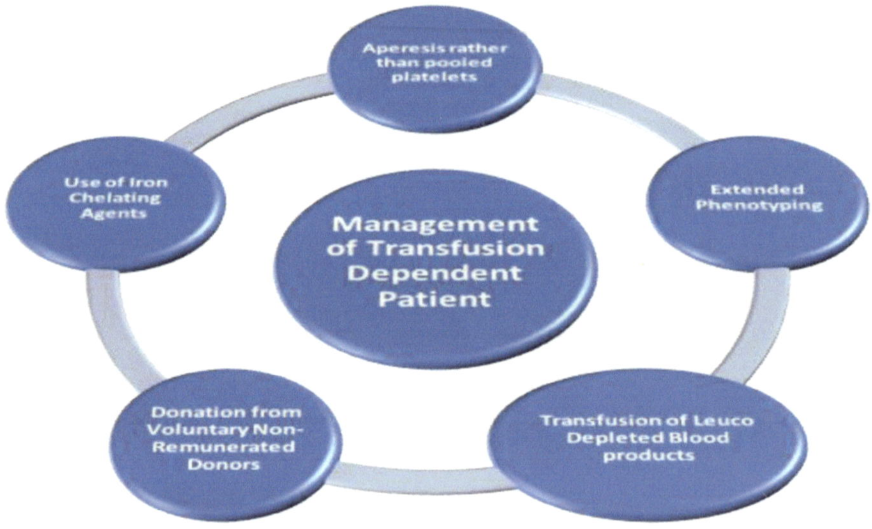

Figure 6.
Evidence-based best practice in the management of transfusion-dependent patients.

2.1 Getting cold chain management of blood and blood products right across the West African sub-region

Blood transfusion is an indispensable part of modern medicine. The efficient and effective use of appropriately stored blood has lifesaving potential. Effective transfusion requires the implementation of several integrated strategies for blood safety including effective cold chain of blood and blood products. A cold chain is a temperature-controlled supply chain of perishable products such as blood, medicines, vaccines that are sensitive to temperature fluctuations and for which a break in the cold chain can affect its clinical effectiveness and potentially cause harm to the patient. The cold chain for the hospital transfusion laboratory is 24 hours a day, 7 days a week and 365 days a year projects that starts from the receipt of the blood from the blood centre to the time the unit is transfused to the patients or otherwise disposed. Good Distribution Practice (GDP) requires that optimum storage conditions

DOI: http://dx.doi.org/10.5772/intechopen.108628

are always observed, including during transportation. The ambient temperatures should be measured continually (24 hours, 7-days a week and 365-days a year) for temperature alarm conditions [34]. The optimum storage temperature for red cell concentrate, plasma and platelet concentrate in blood bank refrigerator, freezers and platelet incubator are 2–6°C, −35°C and 20–24°C respectively. In countries with restricted economies including setting across the West African sub region, the poor practice of using domestic refrigerators and freezers for the storage of blood and blood components is prevalent [35]. Although generally affordable, they are not suitable for blood storage because they are not designed for this purpose. The insulation in domestic fridges and freezers are poor and, in the event of power outage, they will not hold temperatures adequately. Furthermore, domestic refrigerators do not have temperature monitoring devices, such as audio-visual alarms for temperatures outside the set limits for the products being stored. In many settings across the West African sub region especially in remote rural areas, hospitals are often dependent on fuel-driven generators for their electricity supplies which may be inadequate to meet their power needs, particularly the special requirements of blood bank refrigerators and freezers that must function round the clock. Frequent power outages sometimes for long duration are prevalent in hospitals that are on the national power grid with a significant negative implication on the quality, safety and wastage of the scarce blood resource. Also, sensitive blood bank refrigerators are often damaged because of power surges that are common in many settings across the sub region. One of the main reasons of ensuring optimum storage of blood and blood products is to minimize the risk of bacterial growth. If blood is kept at temperature higher than the defined limit bacteria that have infiltrated into blood during collection from the blood donor will quickly grow and proliferate [36, 37]. Also, the suboptimum storage of blood at a temperature less than the defined lower limit predisposes the red cell membrane to damage, release of the free radical haemoglobin contained in the cytoplasm with resultant haemolysis that will increase mortality and morbidity [38]. The transportation of blood between and within blood banks and hospitals is often dependent on the availability of cooler boxes that can maintain temperature over long distances and in relatively high ambient temperatures [39]. Across West Africa the use of domestic type (picnic) cooler boxes or other containers that are not validated and are not reliable in maintaining ambient storage temperature is prevalent. The absence of safe validated blood transport boxes can affect the safe movement of blood and blood products and compromise the quality and potentially cause harm to the patient [40]. Scientific evidence exists that indicates that transfusion of RBC units that exceeding defined temperature is associated with a greater degree of haemolysis and septic transfusion reactions [41, 42]. Evidence-based best practice recommend that all boxes used for the transport of blood and blood products be validated with documentary evidence to show that temperature during storage are ambient [34]. Validation is a documented assessment to prove that the requirement for a specific intended use is reliably fulfilled. It is evidence-based best practice that validation of all blood transport boxes be performed in advance to ensure that transport of components is at the right storage conditions and to ensure that the integrity of the blood product is not compromised. Also, the need for regular mapping of blood fridges cannot be overemphasized. The aim for temperature mapping of blood fridges and freezers is to demonstrate by way of documented evidence that the chosen storage area is suitable for the optimum storage of temperature sensitive blood and blood products [43]. There is also the need for blood transfusion laboratories across the sub region to have back up fridges and freezers where products can be transferred in a timely manner (30 minutes' rule is not compromised) when the routine fridges and freezers malfunctions or are not keeping optimum temperature. The prevailing temperature across the West African sub region is high. The time it takes for the temperature of blood to rise above +6°C when the power supply to the equipment is cut off or when the fridge is left open (holdover time) is dependent on the quality of the insulation of the cabinet and the prevailing temperature in the environment. In the West African sub region where there is a high tendency to use domestic refrigerators and freezers with poorer insulated cabinet for storage of blood and blood product, the challenge is even worse. Temperatures in the lowlands of West Africa are high throughout the year, with annual means usually above 18°C. In the Sahel, the maximum temperatures can reach above 40°C. The hold-over time in these hot environments will likely be shorter and could be worse when there are power outages. The hold-over time is however less critical for plasma freezers, since plasma are stored frozen at −35°C and will usually take about 24 hours before it begins to thaw. Cold chain management of blood and blood products is expensive, complicated, comprehensive, and associated with several logistical challenges [44]. There is a need for countries in West Africa sub region to develop a cost-effective blood cold chain programme that is technologically appropriate, affordable and accessible at all levels of the health care delivery (primary, secondary and tertiary) system. The equipment must meet international standards, together with WHO minimum performance specifications and be correctly used and maintained by all personnel involved. The West African sub region is blessed with a vast amount of green renewable energy potential that is adequate to ensure a universal access to uninterrupted electricity. Heads of State and Government of the Economic Community of West African States (ECOWAS) will need to invest in solar energy to enable her to maximize the solar energy potential in the management of critical infrastructure including the cold chain management of blood and blood products.

2.2 Alloimmunization prevention and antenatal management of pregnant women in West Africa

Currently, there are about 400 red blood cell antigens in 33 blood group systems. Of these, there are 50 different antigens that have the capacity to cause maternal alloimmunization and haemolytic disease of the foetus and the newborn (HDFN). The most clinically significant blood group system is the ABO blood group system followed by the Rhesus and then Kell blood group system [45]. Of the antigens of the Rhesus blood group system the D antigen is the most immunogenic. Individuals positive for the Rhesus D antigen are referred to as Rhesus D positive while those who are negative are Rhesus D negative. The prevalence of Rh D negative group varies in different ethnic populations, with approximately 15.8% of Caucasians, 8% of Blacks, and 1% of Asians being RhD negative [46–50]. Alloantibodies are produced because of blood group incompatibility between a mum and her developing foetus or because of the transfusion of a foreign red cell antigen to a patient. These alloantibodies are low molecular weight immunoglobulin G (IgG) that can cross the placenta and causing haemolytic disease of the foetus and the newborn (HDFN) as well as haemolytic transfusion reaction (HTR) if the patient is exposed to a red cell antigen in the donor unit to which the patient has the group specific alloantibody. About 1.5–2% of pregnant show the presence of alloantibodies at booking [51] and a further 0.18% of women who had no alloantibodies at booking become immunized and show the presence of alloantibodies at 28-week gestation [52]. Commonly encountered alloantibodies include the Rhesus (Anti-D, anti-C, anti-c, anti-E, or anti-e), anti-K, anti-Kidd (Jka and b), Duffy (Fya and b) and anti-S. Of all these the most encountered are the Rhesus antibodies with anti-D and c predominating [53]. A previous report among Cameroonian women of reproductive age has indicated an anti-D prevalence of 4% among Rh-negative African women [54]. Evidence-based best practices in the management of pregnant women requires the routine antenatal determination of the ABO and Rh D group of pregnant women and alloantibody screening during antenatal booking. This alloantibody screen facilitates the identification of Rhesus D negative women who have developed alloantibodies. Those that are Rhesus D negative and are previously non-sensitized are enrolled into the routine antenatal anti-D prophylaxis (RAADP) program and are universally administered anti- D prophylaxis at the 28th-week gestation and a postpartum injection of anti-D within 72 hours of delivering an RhD-positive infant. This protects the woman from being sensitized by foetal red cells containing the D antigen during the transplacental bleeding that can potentially occur during pregnancy or delivery [54, 55].

Transplacental or fetomaternal haemorrhage (FMH) that occur during pregnancy or during delivery can predispose the mum to sensitization leading to development of anti-D that can cause haemolytic disease of the foetus and newborn (HDFN) in subsequent D-positive pregnancies [56]. Also evidenced best practices in the West recommend that mass foetal blood group by analysis of cell-free foetal DNA in the maternal plasma should be carried out based on the finding that 38% of Rhesus D negative women are likely to be carrying an RhD-negative foetus and would receive the treatment unnecessarily [57]. There are several advantages associated with this practice, firstly, there would be a substantial reduction in the use of anti-RhD immunoglobulin, an expensive blood product in short supply. Secondly, women with an RhD-negative foetus would be spared unnecessary exposure to this pooled human blood product with its associated pain and perceived risk from viral or prion contamination. Also, these women can be spared FMH that would have been carried out following a potentially sensitizing event that occur during such pregnancy [58]. Evidence-based best practice recommend availability of facilities for the determination of FMH (acid elution method, or the Kleihauer-Betke (KB) or Flow cytometry) to enable the quantification of Rhesus D foetal red cells that potentially enters the maternal circulation of a Rhesus D negative mother following a potentially sensitizing event post 20-week gestation or post-delivery of a Rhesus D positive baby. This is to enable the administration of the adequate dose of anti-D prophylaxis to be issued within 72 hours of the sensitizing event to clear the foetal red cells from the maternal circulation and thus prevent the mother from being sensitized to produce immune anti-D that can cause HDFN in subsequent D positive pregnancy [59]. Previous report indicates that a dose of anti-D of 125iu is required to clear 1 ml of Rhesus D positive foetal cell from maternal circulation. Implementation of preventive screening programs for antenatal care in the West has led to a significant reduction in maternal and infant mortality rates to approximately 1 in 7000 compared to 1 in 23 for women living in parts of Africa where antenatal care is poor or sometimes non-existent [60]. In many settings across the West African sub region these evidence-based best practices are often not available. Other challenges include; the absence of universal access to anti-D immunoglobulin for the Rh-negative women and following potentially sensitizing events [amniocentesis, cordocentesis, antepartum haemorrhage, vaginal bleeding during pregnancy, external cephalic version (ECV), abdominal trauma, intrauterine death and stillbirth, miscarriage, and therapeutic termination of pregnancy (TOP)] [61, 62], unaffordability of anti-D prophylaxis [62, 63], lack of facilities for alloantibody screening and identification during antenatal booking [64, 65], lack of alloimmunization prevention during illegal abortions and poor documentation [66]. Knowledge of anti-D prophylaxis among biomedical scientist, obstetricians, pharmacists, midwives, nurses, and traditional birth attendant across the West African sub region needs to be improved [67]. This will facilitate quality antenatal and postnatal care to be offered to Rh-negative pregnant population as well as pregnant women with alloantibodies and improve perinatal outcomes.

2.3 Paradigm shift from convention tube method to column agglutination technique and automation in blood transfusion service delivery in the West African sub-region

Over the years, the conventional test tube (CTT) was being used for pre-transfusion testing [ABO and Rhesus D blood group, Direct antiglobulin test (DAT) alloantibody screen and identification and compatibility testing]. However, recent scientific development in the field of transfusion has led to the discovery of semi-automated and fully automated equipment using Column agglutination technology (CAT) [68]. This technique often includes the use of column agglutination-based cards, centrifugation, and incubation. Larger laboratories are moving towards automation of all the hitherto manual techniques using CTT. The advantages of these automated techniques include elimination of human associated errors, reduction in the risk of exposure to bio-hazardous samples, allows for better traceability, reliability, improved turnaround time (TAT) and throughput [69–71]. The principle of the CAT is based on the sieving effect of glass microspheres and gel of agglutinated red cells while allowing non-agglutinated cells to filter to the bottom. In principle, the test is performed in a micro column in which red blood cells containing red cell antigens suspended in low ionic strength saline and serum-containing antibodies are pipetted into the microtubes, incubated, and then centrifuged. RBC agglutinates are trapped in the glass bead matrix during centrifugation and the non-agglutinated cells form a pellet at the bottom of the column. The gel or glass microspheres within each column act as a sieve, trapping agglutinated red cells and allowing non-agglutinated red cells to pass through the pores of the gel or glass microspheres to the bottom of the column. A previous report indicated a sensitivity and specificity of 100% with CAT and concluded that the gel technique is better and should be introduced as a replacement to the CTT [72]. The CAT has several advantages compared to the CTT [73]. The antiglobulin testing used for the detection of clinically significant red cell antibodies can be performed using the CAT card impregnated with AHG without the need to wash with the CTT thus eliminating the potential errors associated with suboptimal washing and potential neutralization of anti-human globulin (AHG). Other advantages of this techniques over the CTT is that it allows for the detection of Ig and complement in diagnosis of HDFN, it can be used for ABO, Rh, Kell phenotype, DAT, ABs screen and XM, it is paediatric friendly as only a small quantity of cells and serum is required, no washing is required as in CTT, it is not subjective and the results are clear and readable and does not require a microscope, it is easy to automate, the risk of miss-up is minimal, it is more sensitive and specific and can detect weaker antibodies, it reduces the turnaround time to make compatible units available, result is standardized and can be automated [74–77]. The CAT, although more expensive than the CTT, has several advantages. Many Blood transfusion laboratories across the West African sub region still rely on the less sensitive CTT. It is highly recommended that government of West African countries should implement the CAT for routine pretransfusion testing across the region to enhance the quality of blood transfusion service delivery.

2.4 Implementing evidence-based best practices in the management of major haemorrhage across the West African sub-region

Haemorrhage from post-traumatic bleeding, intra and post-operative, gastrointestinal, ante and post-partum remains a leading cause of potentially preventable death particularly in the West African sub region. Major haemorrhage is defined as: loss of more than one blood volume within 24 hours (around 70 mL/kg, >5 litres in a 70 kg adult), loss of 50% of total blood volume in less than 3 hours and bleeding more than 150 mL/minute [78]. Experience has shown that early recognition and intervention is critical for survival. In major haemorrhage situation the immediate priorities include prompt arrest or control of bleeding (use of surgical and interventional radiology), ensure optimum tissue perfusion by transfusing red cells concentrate and maintaining optimum blood volume to prevent hypovolaemic shock. A protocol-driven multidisciplinary team approach involving trained, and competency tested major stakeholders (medical, anaesthetic, surgical, transfusion staff and porters) reinforced by clear and effective communication between clinicians, transfusion laboratory and porters. Availability of safe, adequate, and promptly delivered blood components is a key factor in the effective management of MH. Major obstetric haemorrhage (MOH) is prevalent and is a leading cause of maternal mortality accounting for one-third of maternal deaths in Africa [79]. Sub Saharan Africa ranks first in the incidence of maternal mortality globally [80]. Postpartum haemorrhage (PPH) is a common factor responsible for 30 to 50% of Maternal mortality in sub-Saharan Africa [81]. PPH is defined as blood loss ≥500 mL during vaginal delivery and ≥ 1000 mL during caesarean section [82]. It is advocated that low income developing countries can reduce PPH related mortality by approximately 30% if the antifibrinolytic agent (tranexamic acid) is administered promptly at the commencement of bleeding [83]. This treatment is simple and relatively inexpensive and can have a significant effect of survival of women in the West African region [84]. There are several factors that complicates the effective management of haemorrhages (ante- and post-partum) in pregnant women across west Africa; medical records are often incomplete and does not have information on haemorrhage risk and past haemorrhage-related risk associated with patients, absence of routine coagulation test to identify patient that are coagulopathic and are prone to bleeding, absence of blood and products (red cell concentrate, fresh frozen plasma, cryoprecipitate and platelet concentrate), pharmacologic (vitamin K, Prothrombin complex concentrate, tranexamic acid) and non-pharmacologic (surgical and explorative) measures to management haemorrhage, poor management of bleeding- related anaemia in an environment of pre-existing anaemia, timely access to emergency interventions, availability of trained healthcare staff, financial and infrastructural factors, absence and lack of awareness of massive transfusion and major haemorrhage protocols, poor collaborations and communication between local teams responsible for the management of haemorrhage (haematology, blood banking, obstetrics and porters), suboptimal training of obstetricians, nurses, anaesthetists and other relevant health workers on the evidence-based management of obstetrics haemorrhage especially in rural clinics [85–90]. The three main causes of major obstetrics haemorrhage (MOH) are placental abruption, complications during or after Caesarean Section (CS) and uterine atony [91]. The availability, appropriate cold chain management and appropriate and consistent use of oxytocin as an effective, affordable, and safe drug of first choice in the prevention and treatment for Post-Partum Haemorrhage (PPH) particularly in the third stage of labour is advocated [92]. The biggest obstacle to oxytocin quality is storage and handling before patient use. The storage condition of oxytocin has been widely reported as inappropriate. Oxytocin is a heat-sensitive medicine and should be kept between 2 and 8°C. Challenges associated with the effective use of oxytocin in developing countries include procurement issues, poor supply chain, logistics, suboptimal cold chain management during transport and storage and lack of stable electricity). There is need to optimize the haemorrhage management training for all stakeholders involved in the management of obstetric haemorrhage across the West African sub-region as a way of significantly reducing the detrimental effects of obstetric haemorrhage in the sub-region. Correction of pre-existing anaemia among pregnant women should be incorporated in the strategy for preventing deaths from PPH across the sub region. An enabling environment (human and infrastructural) needs to be created across the sub-region in urban and rural areas that facilitate regular attendance to antenatal clinics to curb the attendant dangers associated with home deliveries. The need to optimize the number of skilled birth attendants (SBA) and community midwives cannot be overemphasized. Government of West African states must take objective, strategic and effective steps to ensure the prevention, early diagnosis and improved clinical management of MOH in furtherance of achieving the Sustainable Development Goals aimed at reducing maternal mortality. Every minute of every day a woman dies from complications of pregnancy or childbirth with about 99% of deaths occurring in the developing world [93–95]. The maternal mortality ratio of sub-Saharan Africa is more than a hundred times that of the UK with haemorrhage not only accounting for approximately 30% of cases but also the leading cause of maternal death worldwide [96, 97]. PPH is the leading cause of maternal deaths in individual countries in Africa and collectively on the continent [98, 99]. Major haemorrhage protocols (MHP) were introduced to improve the speed and consistency of delivery of red blood cells (RBCs) and other blood components to severely haemorrhaging patients and have been shown in several observational studies to improve outcomes, including mortality providing a clear framework to facilitate a co-ordinated response by a large multi-disciplinary team during the critical time of bleeding [100]. Blood components (red cell concentrate, fresh frozen plasma, cryoprecipitate and platelet concentrate) can play a role in the management of coagulopathy, disseminated intravascular coagulation and thrombocytopenia. For immediate transfusion, group O red cells should be issued after samples are taken for blood grouping and crossmatching. Females less than 50 years of age should receive RhD negative red cells to avoid sensitization. The use of Kell negative red cells is also desirable in this group. Group O red cells must continue to be issued if patient or sample identification is incomplete or until the ABO group is confirmed on a second sample according to local policy. The higher ratio of Fresh Frozen Plasma (FFP): Red blood cells (RBC) is associated with reduced mortality in a major haemorrhage [101, 102] with FFP providing a source of coagulation factors necessary for thrombin generation in the early phase after injury [103]. Cryoprecipitate or fibrinogen concentrate are a good source of fibrinogen. Fibrinogen is critical for effective haemostasis in MOH. Low fibrinogen level is an independent predictor of mortality as well as bleeding [104–106]. Coagulation is also impaired by hypothermia, acidosis and reduced ionized calcium (Ca^{2+}) concentration [107]. Evidence-based best practice indicates that an early and individualized goal-directed treatment improves the outcome among severely injured and bleeding patients [108]. The aim of treatment in major haemorrhage is to rapidly and effectively restores adequate blood volume, prevent hypovolemic shock, allow for adequate haemostasis, optimize the oxygen carrying capacity and blood biochemistry to allow for an early and aggressive correction of coagulopathy, allow for optimal resuscitation and to reduce potentially preventable deaths [109]. The recombinant activated factor VII (FVII, rFVIIa, FXIII), prothrombin complex concentrates (PCC) and antifibrinolytics (tranexamic acid, epsilon aminocaproic acid and aprotinin) have been used for the management of traumatic bleeding [110] and found to produce a reduction in RBC use but not necessarily improvement in mortality. More recently, viscoelastic assays (rotational thromboelastometry – ROTEM or thromboelastography– TEG) have been advocated [111]. Early recognition of a coagulopathy and subsequent monitoring is vital to both initiate and maximize resuscitation therapy. Massive transfusion guidelines use laboratory tests such as prothrombin time (PT), activated partial thromboplastin time (APTT) and fibrinogen to monitor major haemorrhage and guide blood component replacement [112]. Targeting coagulopathy alongside changes to surgical and anaesthetic practices (damage control surgery/damage control resuscitation) has led to a significant reduction in mortality rates [113]. The transfusion of large volumes of red cells and other intravenous fluids that contain no coagulation factors or platelets causes dilutional coagulopathy and hyperfibrinolysis). Non-blood components and non-pharmacologic measures to manage major haemorrhage include; direct pressure/tourniquet if appropriate, stabilization of fractures, surgical interventions (damage control surgery, interventional radiology, use of endoscopic and obstetrics techniques and thromboelastometry [114, 115]. Government of West African States will need to implement evidence-based best practices; implementation of major haemorrhage protocols, availability of coagulation testing to diagnose coagulopathy and to provide evidence-based indication for blood products to manage coagulopathy. Thromboelastometry, use of tranexamic acid and other relevant pharmacologic agents required to effectively manage coagulopathy and fibrinolysis is advocated along with the implementation of component therapy in a bid to reduce the incidence of preventable major haemorrhage-related death in the sub-region.

2.5 Optimizing screening for transfusion transmissible infections (TTI's) in the West African sub-region

Safe appropriately screened and clinically indicated blood transfusion saves lives and improves the quality of life and life expectancy of millions of patients globally [116]. However, donor blood that has not been properly screened is an important mode of transmission of TTI's including HIV, hepatitis B, hepatitis C and syphilis and other transfusion-transmissible infections [117]. Also, these infections can also be transmitted through several different routes; sexual contact, injection practices and cosmetic treatments and rituals (piercing, tattooing, scarification, injections with collagen or botulinum toxoid (botox), electrolysis and semi-permanent make-up). Strict donor selection criteria minimize the risk of transmission of infections from blood donors to recipients [118]. Transfusion safety begins with the recruitment of healthy voluntary non-remunerated blood donors. A fundamental part of preventing TTI is to notify and counsel reactive donors. Donor notification and counselling protect the health of the donor, prevent secondary transmission of infectious diseases to sexual partners, reduces risk of vertical transmission and provide feedback about the effectiveness of donor selection procedures such as pre-donation education and medical history [119]. There is need for government of West African States to implement WHO recommendation to implement holistically across the sub region and as a minimum the screening of all blood donations for TTIs [Viral (HBV, HCV, HIV), Bacteria (syphilis) or Protozoan (malaria)]. The screen of all blood donations should be mandatory using the following markers as a minimum requirement; HIV-1 and HIV-2 (a combination of HIV antigen-antibody or HIV antibodies); Hepatitis B (hepatitis B surface antigen (HBsAg); Hepatitis C (a combination of HCV antigen-antibody or HCV antibodies) and Syphilis (*Treponema pallidum pallidum*): screening for specific treponemal antibodies [120]. Although screening of blood donors is a way to potentially reduce the risk of transmission of TTI's to recipient, however screening process alone irrespective of how high-quality the assays and systems, cannot eliminate the risk of the donor being in the window phase of infection, failure due to assay sensitivity or testing errors. Also, there is the possibility that a blood donor may be infected with an infectious agent for which donations are not routinely screened. Other factors to consider include the timing of infection, the length of the window period (time between exposure to an infective agent and the first detection of a defined marker of infection), the incubation period (time between exposure to an infective agent and the onset of associated symptoms). Screening of blood donors must be implemented as an adjunct to effective donor selection process to further enhance blood transfusion safety. Blood donor selection is the first crucial step in the process of ensuring blood safety as it helps to significantly reduce risk through the deferral process prior to donation, of individuals with identified risks that may be associated with infection [121, 122]. A fundamental part of preventing TTIs is to notify and counsel reactive donors. Donor notification and counselling protect the health of the donor and prevent secondary transmission of infectious diseases [123]. Although transmissions of viruses (HIV-1 and HCV) had occurred as late as 2009 due to nucleic acid testing (NAT) failures because of low level of viraemia and/or suboptimal amplification efficiency [124]. Blood transfusion is safer now than it has ever been through the implementation of evidence-based best practices and continuous improvements in donor recruitment, screening, testing of donated blood using increasingly sensitive and specific assays and by implementing appropriate and safe clinical use of blood [125]. Serologic testing for TTI's had historically been the foundation of blood donor screening, while newer strategies like nucleic acid testing (NAT) have helped to further shorten the challenge of the window period and by extension enhance blood safety [126]. Currently, no technology exists to completely detect all window period donations. No matter how sensitive NAT becomes, we may never be able completely eradicate the risk of exposure-to-seroconversion window period. An ambitious policy for the collection of 100% of blood from safe voluntary non-remunerated donors who donate blood out of altruism should be implemented universally across the sub-region. There is the urgent need for the implementation of the use of the more sensitive NAT testing for transfusion transmissible viral infection across the West African sub region to reduce the risk of potentially introducing donor blood in the window phase of infection and to further improve blood safety. Donors should universally undergo pre-donation counselling to educate them about the risk of infections and the window period. There is an urgent need to formulate a sub-regional policy guideline for notification of all reactive blood donors.

2.6 Changing the narrative about blood donation in the West African sub-region

Urgent concerted efforts are needed in the West African sub region to correct the blood supply deficit and increase the pool of voluntary non-remunerated blood donors. This is expected to significantly improve blood transfusion safety and positively impact the health indices in the sub region [126]. The World Health Assembly in its resolution WHA.63.12 recommended that all countries begin to use only voluntary, non-remunerated blood donors (VNRDs) [127]. The WHO has consistently emphasized blood sourcing from VNRDs, due to their markedly reduced chances of harbouring and transferring TTIs [128]. This recommendation has been reiterated and supported by an increasing body of evidence from researchers in the sub region [129–131]. Unfortunately, several studies in Nigeria in the last couple of years have shown that VNRDs constituted a small fraction of the blood donor pool, this obviously has serious implications for transfusion safety [132, 133]. A previous report [134] chronicled the social demographic information of blood donors in sub-Saharan Africa and reported that commercial blood donors were all males while the median ages of voluntary and family donors were 18 years and 30 years, respectively. Similar studies in Nigeria had equally identified a male dominated donor pool as well as young adults as the predominant donor age group [135]. Unfortunately, this age distribution has also been associated with the highest carriage rates of TTIs (arising most probably from increased involvement in high-risk sexual behaviours and experimentation). This factor poses a huge challenge to the subcontinent's efforts towards attaining blood transfusion safety [136]. VNRD are the safest because they are altruistic and have the highest tendency to self-deferral when they are exposed to a risk of contracting TTIs. In SSA, most blood donors are family replacement donors [137]. Mauritius is one good example nation in the sub-Saharan Africa that has done remarkably well with implementation of the guidelines. About 86.2% of the blood donors in that country were VNRDs as of 2016. Mauritius has also embarked on use of nucleic acid testing as opposed to enzyme-linked immunosorbent assay (ELISA) that was previously in use and since 2010 has embarked on aphaeresis method of blood collection and separation. These developments have made transfusion medicine in Mauritius very safe [138]. Government of countries across the West African sub-region will need to learn from the excellent practice in Mauritius by investing significantly in education, mass mobilization and campaign to facilitate a significant increase in the number of voluntary blood donors in a bid to bridging the wide gap between demand and supply of blood and blood product as well as enhance blood transfusion safety across the sub-region.

2.7 Universal leucodepletion of blood and blood products and prevention of development of anti- leukocyte antibodies

The average content of leucocytes in donated human whole blood is 10^9/unit. Leukoreduction is the reduction to $\leq 1 \times 10^6$ or $< 5 \times 10^6$/ leucocytes per unit after preparation and with a minimum of 85% of red cells still retained [139, 140]. Clinical evidence indicates that the risk of non-haemolytic febrile transfusion reactions is significantly reduced by leucodepletion. This procedure prevents alloimmunization to HLA antigens in transfusion-dependent patients [141]. Leucocyte antibodies due to alloimmunization by a foreign HLA antigen can cause febrile transfusion reaction in subsequent transfusion involving HLA and granulocyte specific antigens [142]. Leucocyte depletion can be achieved by using filters (cotton, cellulose acetate etc.), apheresis, red cell washing, buffy coat removal after centrifugation and freezing and subsequent glycerol removal of red cells [143]. Leucodepletion of donor blood using leucodepletion filters is considered the threshold for reducing the risk of alloimmunization against leucocyte antigens and potentially eliminating transfusion reaction associated with leucocyte antibodies. The importance of transfusion of leucodepleted blood products cannot be over emphasized. Apart from reducing the incidence on non-haemolytic febrile transfusion reaction, it reduces the risk of alloimmunization to platelet antigens that can predispose patients to develop platelet antibodies and becoming refractory to platelet transfusions (critical for MDS and aplastic anaemia patients who requires long- term platelet). It also significantly reduces the risk of transmission of variant Creutzfeldt Jacobs Disease (vCJD) and Cytomegalovirus (CMV) infection. Leucocytes is vector of CMV, HTLV-I/II, EBV & other viruses that can potentially to infection particularly in neonates, pregnant women, HIV patients and organ transplant patients. Leuko reduction is also associated with reduction in the risk of transfusion associated graft versus host disease (TA-GVHD) in immunocompromised patients [142]. Leucocytes in whole blood are believed to have immunomodulatory effects that can potentially influence the prognosis of patients with malignancy, increase the risk of post-operative infection and HIV progression [20]. Government of West African countries need to implement a policy on universal leucodepletion of all blood and blood products transfused across the sub region. This has the potential to prevent primary alloimmunization to HLA antigens and its attendant negative effects and make transfusion safer.

2.8 Optimum management of transfusion dependent patients across the West African sub-region

Transfusion dependence (TD) is a term that usually describes patients receiving regular red cell concentrate and/or platelet concentrate transfusions more frequently than every 8 weeks due to persistent anaemia and thrombocytopenia. Regular transfusion of red cells and platelets are required in these patients to reduce the symptoms of anaemia and thrombocytopenia by increasing the number functional red cells and platelets in the recipient's circulation. Various diseases can lead to transfusion-dependency, most notably myelodysplastic syndromes (MDS), aplastic anaemia and thalassemia). Platelet transfusion is clinically indicated in thrombocytopenic patients with chronic bone marrow failure including patients on low dose oral chemotherapy, to manage patients with chronic bleeding of WHO grade 2, above, or as prophylaxis for patients with low platelet count who are going for invasive procedure that is associated with bleeding [144]. The wellbeing and the quality of life of TD patients across the West African sub region can be optimized by the radical implementation of evidence-based best practices; blood intended for TD patients should be sourced from regular voluntary non-remunerated blood donors; unit should be universally leucodepleted, appropriately screened used sensitive assays and technology to reduce the risk of transfusing donor blood in the window phase; extended red cell phenotyping must be implemented for Rhesus (C, c, E, e) and Kell as a minimum; patients should be transfused ABO, Rhesus and Kell antigen compatible unit; effective pre-transfusion testing including alloantibody screening and a full IAT cross-match particularly for patients with history of alloantibodies as well as implementation of the use of chelating agent to reduce the iron overload related challenges in these patients [145]. Single donor apheresis platelets offer several advantages over random pooled platelets, including the potential for crossmatching, reduction in net donor exposures, maintenance of ABO-compatibility, improved inventory management, diminished rate of alloimmunization and better platelet increments in the recipient [145]. The use of apheresis platelets in TD patients can prevent the incidence of platelet refractoriness often associated with poor post-transfusion platelet increments resulting from the presence of platelet alloantibodies. Evidence-based best practice in preventing alloimmunization to platelet antigens is limiting recipients' exposure to human leukocyte antigen specificities by using single-donor apheresis platelets, filtration to reduce the number of human leukocyte antigen-bearing leukocytes as well as pre-transfusion of gamma irradiation to decrease platelet antigen immunogenicity [146]. Transfusion dependent patients who require platelet transfusion on a regular basis should ideally be transfused apheresis rather than pooled platelets. The advantages are numerous; reduction of donor exposures may decrease the risk of TTIs as well as reduce the risk of developing alloimmunization to foreign platelet antigens in the pooled platelets. The platelet yield from apheresis unit is 6 times higher than from pooled platelets and other transfusion-related complications [2]. Evidence-based best practice from the developed economies recommend the determination of extended phenotyping for TD patients at a minimum for the most clinically significant blood group antigens; Rhesus (C, c, D, E, e) and Kell and where feasible a full red cell phenotype/genotype panel for all clinically significant red cell antigens. For non-transfusion naïve patients, molecular testing rather than serologic testing is indicated. These patients should ideally receive as a minimum requirement ABO, Rhesus (C, c, D, E, e) and Kell compatible red cell product. The aim of this best practice is to reduce the risk of alloimmunization against these clinically relevant red cell antigens [147]. Government of West African States need to urgently develop policies, guidelines as well as promote the implementation of evidence-based best practices that will enhance the management of TD patients and reduce morbidity. Extended phenotype should be carried out prior to commencement of transfusion therapy to ensure that they receive clinically significant antigen negative donor blood that can commonly cause alloimmunization in a particular population. Extended red cell typing is required for the management of TD patients to confirm the identity of suspected alloantibodies or determine the specificity of potential additional antibodies that may be formed in the future [148]. Effective pretransfusion testing including alloantibody screening, panel testing for those whose alloantibody screen is positive and crossmatch of antigen negative units using appropriate technologies (IAT and column agglutination technique) should be implemented universally across the sub region. TD patients who require platelet transfusion on a regular basis should ideally be transfused apheresis instead of pooled platelets.

2.9 Best practices in pre-operative planning and management of the transfusion needs of patients

There are certain priorities in meeting the blood transfusion needs in surgical patients; the need for pre-operative optimization of the haemoglobin level (management of anaemia), pre-operative management of coagulopathy and bleeding predisposition to minimize blood loss intraoperatively and post operatively and avoidance of unnecessary transfusion post operatively [149]. In patients scheduled for elective surgeries, it is critical that blood management is planned even before a patient is referred for surgery at the primary care levels working collaboratively with the preoperative assessment clinic at the hospital. A full blood count should be done at least 6 weeks prior to surgery. If anaemia is identified, effort should be made to identify the cause of anaemia (iron deficiency, chronic kidney disease) and remedial action taken to treat the anaemia and potentially optimize the haemoglobin level using pharmacologic alternatives like oral, IV iron, erythropoietin and in some cased red cell transfusion. Patients who are anaemic pre-operatively are more likely to be transfused with allogenic blood [150]. Evidence has shown that pre-operative anaemia is an independent risk factor for increased morbidity and mortality in surgical patients [151]. In patients with severe anaemia and acute coronary syndromes red cell transfusion is a significant predictor of mortality (there is need to optimize tissue (perfusion to vital organs) when the use of pharmacologic agent will not produce a timely optimization of haemoglobin of the patients). Also, the preoperative assessment clinic should also be able to identify patients who are going for significant bleed prone surgery and those with increased risk of bleeding (patients with liver disease, those on anticoagulants therapy like warfarin, low molecular weight heparins (LMWHs) and direct oral anticoagulants like dabigatran, apixaban and rivaroxaban as well as those on antiplatelet therapy like clopidogrel or aspirin for whom remedial actions such as use of prothrombin complex concentrate (PCC), antifibrinolytic agents, fibrinogen concentrate, fresh frozen plasma, cryoprecipitate, platelet concentrate and temporary withdrawal of haemorrhage prone medication where possible and safe [152, 153]. Patients going for bleeding prone elective surgeries can be identified who potentially can be candidates for Pre-deposit autologous donation (PAD). This is vital particularly in patients who do not accept allogenic blood transfusion based on their religious beliefs, patients that have a rare blood group and those that have alloantibodies against a high incidence antigen for which it may be difficult to source blood for transfusion [154]. It is evidence-based practice to evaluate patient predisposition (coagulopathic status) to bleeding prior to surgery. This is vital to possibly take remedial actions prior to surgery in a bid to minimize significant blood loss during surgery. Basic laboratory testing includes determination of international normalized ratio (INR), activated partial thromboplastin time (APTT) and fibrinogen levels (FIBC). Patients with INR and APTT ratio > 1.5 as well as fibrinogen level < 1 g/L are at a high risk of bleeding during surgery [155]. The results of these laboratory test will provide justification to take remedial steps to correct identified coagulopathic status and clinically indicated pharmacologic (antifibrinolytic agents like tranexamic acid, vitamin K, prothrombin complex concentrate, fibrinogen concentrate) or management with blood products (FFP, cryoprecipitate and platelet concentrate). It is also vital to identify patients that can potentially benefit from blood-sparing techniques like acute nomovolaemic haemodilution (ANH) and perioperative cell salvage (PCS) [156, 157]. It is evidence-based best practice to ensure that patient scheduled for surgery has pre transfusion test for the ABO, Rh D group and alloantibodies screen and that patient meet the 2-sample rule (patients' blood group and alloantibody screen must have been tested on 2 samples taken from two separate venipuncture by two different clinical staff at least a minimum of 15 minutes apart to ensure we have a confirmed group on the patient). By the implementation of this best practice, we can identify patients with rare blood groups and those with alloantibodies for which efforts has to be made in advance to identify the alloantibodies present as well as source antigen negative donor units and possibly crossmatch the units prior to surgery. This is to ensure timely provision of blood if patients begin to bleed intraoperatively or post operatively [158]. It is best practice that we are avoiding unnecessary transfusion post operatively by being conservative and not liberal by the evidence-based use restrictive transfusion triggers ensuring individualized management to prevent unnecessary transfusion particularly in patients that are haemodynamically stable while ensuring safety and effectiveness [159, 160]. This can mean utilizing blood test and presence of symptoms to minimize blood loss and prevent unnecessary transfusion, use of endoscopic radiology and sealants to minimize blood loss, use of post-operative cell salvage and reinfusion if clinically indicated and use of pharmacologic agents (oral or IV iron, and erythropoietin) to optimize the haemoglobin level of patients post operatively and by so doing achieve a reduction in exposure to allogenic blood [161–165]. Patient blood management (PBM) in surgical patients is important for a number of reasons; to optimize the patient's erythropoiesis and haemoglobin level, minimizing blood loss in the patients intra and post-operative and optimizing and exploiting the patients physiological reserve to ability to tolerate anaemia [166]. Many of these best practices are not being implemented in many settings across the West African sub region. This is often the cause of suboptimal management of surgical patients in the subregion that is responsible for preventable deaths from haemorrhage. Government of West African nations will need to implement evidenced best practices to ensure the optimum management of surgical patient, reduce the need for unnecessary transfusion and facilitate the optimum utilization of our limited allogenic bloodstock.

3. Evidence-based management of rhesus negative pregnancy and patients clinically significant alloantibodies

Human red blood cells carry many antigens on their surfaces. The most important of these antigens belong to the ABO system and the Rhesus (Rh) blood group system. The D antigen is the most important antigen of the Rhesus system. People with the Rhesus D (RhD) antigen are referred to as RhD positive, and those without it as RhD negative. A baby inherits its blood type from both parents. Therefore, a mother who is RhD negative can carry a baby who is RhD positive. During pregnancy, because of trans placental bleeding, a small amount of foetal blood can enter the maternal circulation [an event called feto-maternal haemorrhage (FMH)]. The presence of foetal RhD-positive cells in mum's circulation can sensitize the mum triggering an immune response leading to the production of alloantibodies against the RhD antigen (anti-D antibodies). This process is called sensitization or alloimmunization. There are over 600 red cell antigens, which are separated into 30 blood group systems. The presence or absence of these antigens in an individual is important, because they determine the type of blood that should be given if they require a red cell transfusion. If a woman is exposed to red cells containing a foreign red cell antigen which they themselves lacks, it can trigger an immune response leading to the formation against the foreign red cell antigen. Such an antibody can cause extravascular and/or intravascular haemolysis when the recipient is subsequently exposed to the same antigens. Antibodies can either be allo (antibody to an antigen that an individual lacks) or autoantibodies (antibody to an antigen a person has). Alloantibodies are formed in response to pregnancy (blood group incompatibility between the mum and her developing foetus), transfusion (donor red cell containing antigens that are foreign to the recipient), or transplantation (graft containing antigens that are foreign to the recipient). Alloimmunization resulting in the development of one or more clinically significant red cell, leucocyte and platelet antibodies is a vital complication in chronically transfused patients [167–170]. Multiple red cell transfusion could predispose to the formation of clinically significant titres of lytic antibodies, which may cause haemolytic disease of the foetus and newborn (HDFN) or haemolytic transfusion reaction (HTR). Patients with haemoglobinopathies and other TD patients that require regular blood transfusions are particularly at a higher risk of sensitization and development of red cell alloantibodies [2, 171]. The magnitude of red cell sensitization in Nigeria was highlighted in the independent reports by Ugwu and Colleagues (Benin City, Midwestern Nigeria) [172], Kangiwa and Colleagues (Enugu, Southeast

Nigeria) [173], and Jeremiah and Colleagues (Port Harcourt, South-South Nigeria) [174] in which prevalence rates of 9.3, 18.7, and 3.4%, respectively were observed in multiply- transfused patient populations. The presence of these alloantibodies may cause a delay in selecting compatible blood products. Countries in the West African sub region tend to have multiple- ethnic groups, race and genetic heterogeneity. Such multi-ethnic populations are prone to having racial variation in the red cell antigen spectrum that are prevalent with attendant wide variation in commonly identified alloantibodies [65, 175]. Other common factors that facilitate alloantibody formation in persons include: the immune competence, the dose of the antigen the person is exposed to, the route of exposure and how immunogenic the foreign antigen is [176, 177]. Evidence-based best practice in the developed economies requires that alloantibody testing is carried out routinely on all pregnant women presenting to antenatal clinic at booking as well as all patients in whom a red cell transfusion is clinically indicated. The intent of this test is to detect the presence of unexpected red cell antibody in the patient's serum [178, 179]. Once these antibodies are detected during the alloantibody screening, every effort must be made to identify the specificity of the alloantibody by doing a panel test. The purpose of the panel test is to; facilitate the identification of the alloantibody, determine whether the antibody can potentially cause HTR (to allow for the selection of antigen negative red cells for crossmatch) of HDFN (to allow the monitoring of the titre or quantification of the antibody every 4 weeks from booking until 28 weeks' gestation and every 2 weeks thereafter until delivery) [180]. The monitoring of the titre or quantification of the antibody helps to determine to what extent the developing foetus is affected by HDFN, to monitor the baby for anaemia along with Doppler ultrasound determination of the peak systolic velocity of blood through the median cerebral artery, determine whether the baby will require intrauterine transfusion (IUT) and to enable the obstetricians make an informed decision to possibly deliver the baby earlier. These evidence-based best practices are not yet completely implemented in many settings in the West African sub region. Testing of pregnant women and donors for other clinically relevant red cell antigens other than ABO and Rhesus D is not routinely carried out. Also, donor units particularly those intended for transfusion to pregnant women and neonates are also not routinely screened for other blood borne transmissible diseases such as CMV, Hepatitis E virus and others like it is routinely done in more advanced countries of the world.

The clinically significant antibodies are those antibodies that are active at 37°C and/or detected by the indirect antiglobulin (IAT) test. Nine blood group systems (ABO, Rhesus, Kell, Kidd, Duffy, MNS, P, Lewis, and Lutheran) are clinically significant as these are known to cause HTR and HDFN. These antibodies are caused predominantly by maternal alloimmunization to blood group antigens expressed by foetal red blood cells. In severe cases, it may result in foetal anaemia with increased risks of foetal death, severe neonatal hyperbilirubinaemia, and kernicterus, jaundice, intellectual retardation, premature birth, abortion, and stillbirth. Most severe cases of HDFN were attributed to Rh(D) incompatibility between a Rh(D)-negative woman and her Rh(D)-positive foetus, with Rh(D) alloimmunization having occurred during a previous pregnancy [65]. HDFN is an important cause of neonatal morbidity and death [181]. Sensitization can happen at any time during pregnancy but is most common in the third trimester and during childbirth. Sensitizations are commonly associated with events during pregnancy that are associated with FMH, such as medical interventions (chorionic villus sampling, amniocentesis, or external cephalic version), terminations, late miscarriages, antepartum haemorrhage, and abdominal trauma [181]. The risk of sensitization is affected by the ABO blood type of the foetus, with a lower risk if it is compatible with the mother's ABO type. Sensitization depends on the volume of foetal blood entering the mother's circulation, the magnitude of mother's immune response and the immune competence of the mum's immune system. The risk of sensitization is greatest in the first pregnancy and decreases with each subsequent pregnancy. Once sensitization has occurred, it is irreversible. The process of sensitization has no adverse health effects for the mother and usually does not affect the pregnancy during which it occurs. However, if the mother is exposed to the same foreign antigen during a subsequent pregnancy, the immune response is quicker, greater and results in the antibody level being boosted. The anti-D antibodies produced by a Rhesus D negative mother in response to the D positive foetal cells are often low molecular weight IgG antibodies that can cross the placenta and bind to RhD antigen on the surface of foetal red blood cells. These antibody-coated foetal red blood cells are removed from the foetal circulation by the reticuloendothelial system, predominantly the spleen and liver. This is the cause of hepatosplenomegaly commonly seen in babies with HDFN. Foetal anaemia results if the red blood cells are removed faster than they are produced. Severe anaemia can lead to foetal heart failure, fluid retention and swelling (hydrops), and intrauterine death. Before birth, anaemia and hydrops can be managed with intrauterine transfusions, but this carries a 2% risk of foetal loss [182].

Women presenting for antenatal booking are screened for the ABO, Rh D group and for the presence of alloantibodies. The Rh D group categorizes pregnant women into Rh D positive if their red cell contains the Rhesus D antigen and Rh D negative if their red cell lacks the D antigens. The alloantibody screen also determines whether the antibody screen is positive or negative. Those with a positive alloantibody screen are tested for panels to identify the specificity of the alloantibody present. It is evidence-based best practice to recruit all Rhesus D negative non-previously sensitized women into the Routine Antenatal Anti-D Prophylaxis (RAADP) programme and universally offer them universally anti-D prophylaxis at 28-week gestation. The half-life of the anti-D is about 12 weeks, and the aim of the administration is to facilitate the mopping up of all the foetal D positive red cells that enter the maternal circulation as a result of fetomaternal haemorrhage and thus prevent the foreign D positive foetal red cells from sensitizing the mother. By this implementation the risk of anti-D related HDFN in subsequent pregnancy is avoided. This prophylaxis has been used to prevent postpartum disease in Rh D-negative women and has greatly reduced HDFN- related morbidity as well as foetal and neonatal mortality. In the 1960s, studies in the United States and in Great Britain determined that passive immunization of Rh(D)-negative mothers with IgG anti-Rh(D), soon after parturition, could protect women from sensitization against Rh(D) + positive red blood cells of her foetus [183, 184]. This then led to the licensing of IgG anti-Rh(D) for routine post-partum prophylaxis in 1968, however, in 1977 it was demonstrated that, despite adequate post-natal prophylaxis, about 10% of Rh(D)-negative women continued to develop anti-Rh(D) antibodies, presumably due to small, transplacental, foetal-maternal bleed during pregnancy. To manage this challenge, the issue of antenatal administration of IgG anti-Rh (D) preparations was instituted in combination with standard post-partum prophylaxis [185]. Current guidelines recommend that immunoprophylaxis with IgG anti-Rh(D) be given to every non-sensitized Rh(D)-negative woman, as follows; at 28-week gestation during each pregnancy; immediately after delivery of every Rh(D)-positive neonate and following any potentially sensitizing event in pregnancy that could expose the mother to the Rh(D) antigen of the foetus (abortion, miscarriage, abdominal trauma) [186]. The only settings in which antenatal anti-D IgG administration is not necessary is when conception is certain, and the father is also Rh(D)-negative or if the foetus is successfully typed for Rh(D) status by antenatal cell-free DNA testing using maternal plasma [65]. Feto-maternal haemorrhage (FMH) may occur during pregnancy or at delivery. The Kleihauer-Betke (KB) test is a blood test used to measure the amount of foetal red cells that is transferred from a foetus into the maternal circulation [178]. FMH occurs in up to 28% of pregnancies after trauma and the amount of Rh-positive foetal blood required to sensitize the Rh-negative mother is variable, but most patients are sensitized by as little as 0.01 ml of blood [187]. The test utilizes a stain that identifies foetal red blood cells with haemoglobin F in maternal blood. The ratio of foetal: maternal red blood cells can be assessed [188]. The use of flow cytometry for the quantification of haemoglobin F is also available. The aim of the test is to determine the volume of foetal red cells that entered the maternal circuiting following a FMH to facilitate the administration of optimum dose of RhIG required to remove them from the maternal circulation and thus prevent the mother from being sensitized to produce alloantibodies. The Kleihauer-Betke tests have numerous limitations, including low sensitivity, poor reproducibility, and a tendency to overestimate the volume of haemorrhage [188]. An important limitation of the Kleihauer-Betke test is the inability to differentiate between maternal and foetal F cells. This is particularly a challenge in the second trimester of pregnancy when maternal F cells may occasionally reach 5 to 10% as well as in women that hereditary persistence of foetal haemoglobin (HPFH) in whom the count will be falsely raised. Haemoglobin F quantitation by flow cytometry has been reported to be simple, reliable, and more precise than the Kleihauer-Betke test [189]. It is recommended that prophylaxis be within 72 hours of the potential sensitizing event occurring [190]. To prevent sensitization, all D-negative non sensitized women who deliver a D-positive foetus should receive at least a single 300-µg dose of Anti-D within 72 hours of delivery. In addition to the prophylaxis giving during pregnancy, it is recommended that a maternal sample should be obtained post-delivery of a Rhesus D positive baby (approximately1 hour after delivery) and tested for evidence of a FMH [191]. Approximately 17% of Rh D–negative women who deliver Rh D–positive foetus become alloimmunized if Anti- D prophylaxis is not administered appropriately and adequately. Anti- D prophylaxis has been reported to reduce the overall risk of Rh immunization from 13.2 to 0.2%, and testing for large FMH has also further decreased the risk to 0.14% [192]. It is part of modern antenatal care currently in developed countries to offer universally all Rh D-negative pregnant women anti-RhD immunoglobulin IgG injection at about 28- week gestation with a booster at 34-week gestation [193]. However, in countries across the West Africa sub region this evidence-based best practice is not universally implemented due majorly to unaffordability of anti-RhD immunoglobulin [65]. In many of these settings, facility for the effective management of foetuses and babies affected by HDFN such as Doppler ultrasound for diagnosis of foetal anaemia in utero, exchange blood transfusion and ultrasonography guided intrauterine transfusion (IUT) are often unavailable resulting in the preventable deaths of many of the sub region's future generations [194]. Blood meant for exchange and intrauterine transfusion must meet certain requirements (< 5 days old, free from clinically significant irregular blood group antibodies including high-titre anti-A and anti-B, negative for antibodies to CMV, must be gamma irradiated and transfused within 24 hours of irradiation, the donor should be Haemoglobin S screen negative, and the unit must be leucocyte depleted). Many of which are often not available in many settings across the sub region [65]. These implementations will facilitate the effective management of severely anaemic foetuses earlier in gestation and increase the chances of survival of more severely affected foetuses with the potential for poor neurodevelopmental outcome such as cerebral palsy, deafness, and motor and speech delay [187]. This anti-D immunoglobulin which is administered routinely in the third trimester attaches to the Rhesus D positive foetal cells and are promptly removed from the maternal circulation by the reticuloendothelial system (RES) before they can sensitize the mum to produce alloantibodies. This is known as RAADP. RAADP can be given as two doses of anti-D immunoglobulin of 500 IU (one at 28-week and one at 34-week gestation), as two doses of anti-D immunoglobulin of 1000–1650 IU (one at 28-week and one at 34-week gestation), or as a single dose of 1500 IU either at 28 weeks or between 28- and 30-week gestation [195]. There are several technologies, formulations, and doses of anti- D in use in the United Kingdom [196–199]. Anti-D immunoglobulin are produced by deliberating immunizing Rhesus D negative men or women donors without childbearing potential who are carefully screened for transfusion transmissible infections [200]. There is need for the universal access to anti D prophylaxis to be provided for all non-sensitized Rh D negative women across the subregion under the RAADP programme and to cover every potentially sensitizing event that takes place during pregnancy and following the delivery of a Rhesus D positive baby. Facilities for determining fetomaternal haemorrhage should be readily available. Cell free foetal DNA testing should be implemented to determine Rhesus D negative women who are carrying Rhesus D negative babies who could be spared prophylactic anti-D. Facility for non-invasive Doppler ultrasound determination of the peak systolic velocity (PSV) through the median cerebral artery (MCA) of foetuses should be available for the diagnosis of foetal anaemia. Blood that meets the minimum requirement for use for intrauterine (IUT) and exchange transfusion should be readily available. There is also the need to optimize the knowledge of Biomedical Scientists, Obstetricians and Neonatologist in the subregion on the effective management of Rhesus D negative pregnancies as well as the prevention and management of HDFN.

3.1 Haemovigilance implementation in the West African sub-region

Haemovigilance is used to describe a set of surveillance procedures that scrutinizes the entire blood transfusion process from the point of collection of blood and blood components from a blood donor to the point of transfusion in the recipient ensuring that all unexpected or undesirable adverse reactions, events reactions, accidents, errors and near misses are reported, investigated in a timely manner and preventive and corrective actions are implemented to prevent their future occurrence. Haemovigilance system facilitates the delivery of a continually improving blood transfusion service [201, 202]. Haemovigilance encompasses the entire blood transfusion process; blood donation, processing, transfusion, post transfusion monitoring as well as reporting and investigation of all adverse events, reactions and near misses related to the blood donation and transfusion. Haemovigilance is indispensable with relation to safety and quality of blood transfusions, and it cuts across any action in the blood transfusion process that directly harm the blood donor [203] or potentially compromises the quality of the blood taken from the donor that put the recipient potentially at risk [204]. An adverse reaction or event is used to describe any unintended response in a blood donor, or a recipient observed during the collection or transfusion of blood and blood components that is fatal, life-threatening, disabling, incapacitating or results in hospitalization or morbidity [205]. Apart from Japan, many Asian countries do not have a fit for purpose haemovigilance system. Many including India are in the process of establishing a haemovigilance system [206]. Haemovigilance is aimed at improving the quality and safety of blood transfusion. In most developed economies haemovigilance is governed by responsible legal authorities [207, 208]. Many countries including the United Kingdom (Serious Hazards of Transfusion [SHOT]), Canada (Transfusion Transmitted Injuries Surveillance System [TTISS]), Netherlands (Transfusion Reactions in Patients [TRIP]), Japan, Russia, Switzerland and the United States of America have dedicated organizations responsible for haemovigilance with the primary responsibility of improving blood safety. International Haemovigilance Network (IHN) is responsible for developing and maintaining haemovigilance and safety of blood and blood components globally [209]. Blood transfusion services in the West African sub region are not as organized and regulated as it is in the West. This has a negative implication on the adequacy and safety of blood and blood products. There are several challenges militating against an effective haemovigilance system across the sub region; lack of standardized tools for data capturing, poor integrity of data captured, poor governance issues, lack of functional hospital transfusion committee (HTC) in general, specialist and teaching hospitals, suboptimal coordination of the NBTS and lack of relevant policies for transfusion practices, lack of indication coding tool to guide the evidence-based clinical use of blood and blood products, lack of policy in place for clinical use of blood, high incidence and increased risk of TTIs, traceability challenges, training-related challenges, poor culture of documentation, incident reporting and investigation of adverse events, poor implementation of recall and quarantining of suboptimal blood and blood products, reaction and near misses associated with the blood transfusion process [210]. There is need for government across the West African sub region to develop a well-organized haemovigilance system in a bid to enhance transfusion safety. Member States of ECOWAS must take all necessary measures to ensure 100% traceability of all blood and blood components collected, tested, processed, stored, released and transfused across the sub region from vein to vein from the blood donor to the recipient. Effective haemovigilance implementation across the West African sub region will require collaboration, effective communication and cooperation between the National Blood Transfusion Centre and the Health establishment on one hand as well as among all the healthcare professionals involved in blood transfusion service delivery [211]. Haemovigilance practice was observed to be lacking in previous studies on transfusion practice in Africa [212]. There is need to put in place a haemovigilance system across the sub region that facilitate the prompt, accurate, efficient, and provable withdraw from distribution chain of blood or blood components that is suboptimal and has a potential to cause harm to the recipient. This is an urgent need to train health workers across the West African sub region on best practices in various aspects of transfusion medicine; blood donation, screening, transportation, storage and transfusion as well as monitoring and documentation of adverse event and reactions with the hope of reporting, investigating transfusion related incident and implementing corrective action and by so doing learning from mistakes and building a culture of continuous quality improvement in blood transfusion service delivery across sub region.

3.2 Suboptimal use of alternatives to allogenic blood across the West African subregion

Not all anaemic and bleeding patients require allogenic blood. Some can benefit from pharmacologic and non- pharmacologic alternatives. The implementation of these alternatives can potentially reduce the dependence and facilitate the optimum utilization of our scare allogenic blood stock. The need for allogenic blood has continued to increase significantly, particularly in developing countries. There are several factors that affect matching demand with supply in sub-Saharan Africa. Escalating elective surgery, increased fatalities from road traffic accidents, poor management of traumatic injuries, intraoperative, post-operative and obstetric haemorrhage, communal crisis, insurgency, banditry, high incidence of malaria related anaemia, sub-optimal management of bleeding predisposition in surgical patients, pregnancy-related complications, suboptimal national blood transfusion services, appropriate infrastructure, trained personnel, and financial resources to support the running of a voluntary non-remunerated donor transfusion service, high incidence of transfusion-transmitted infection, predominance of family replacement and commercially remunerated blood donors, rather than VNRDs [2]. Evidence has shown that not all anaemic or bleeding patients require blood and blood products. Many can benefit from alternatives. Concerns about adverse events associated with allogenic blood transfusion should prompt a review of transfusion practices and justify the need to search for transfusion alternatives to decrease or avoid the use of allogenic blood. There are pharmacologic alternatives that help to stimulate erythropoiesis (iron, folic acid, erythropoietin) and non-pharmacologic alternatives. Strategies to reduce allogenic blood use include the correction of anaemia using pharmacological agents (oral, IV iron and erythropoietin) and management of coagulopathy and bleeding (use of antifibrinolytics, vitamin K and fibrinogen concentrate). Non-pharmacologic measures including preoperative autologous blood transfusion, perioperative red blood cell salvage and normothermia can help to reduce blood loss in surgical patients. Similarly, the use of surgical and endoscopic technology can minimize blood loss and by extension limit the need for allogenic blood. All these strategies can help countries across the West African sub-region in optimizing the use of our limited allogenic blood stocks [213]. There are several challenges associated with allogenic blood transfusion [risk of TTIs (viral, bacterial, parasitic and prion), non-infectious risks including febrile, allergic/ anaphylactic and haemolytic transfusion reactions, transfusion-related acute lung injury (TRALI) and transfusion-associated circulatory overload (TACO) that warrants the need for the identification and use of transfusion alternatives [214].

3.3 Use of oral and intravenous iron

Iron is an essential micronutrient required for erythropoiesis. Iron deficiency is the most common nutritional deficiency particularly in developing countries. Iron deficiency is the leading cause of anaemia in both men and women [215]. It is a major concern in low-income settings, particularly among children and women of childbearing age. Factors that are responsible for iron depletion are prevalent across the West African sub region [haemorrhage (trauma, surgery, gastrointestinal, ante and postpartum) poor nutrition, age, pregnancy, low socioeconomic status, critical illness, etc.). Treatment of iron deficiency anaemia with oral iron supplements is simple, readily available and affordable. The major limiting factor for oral iron use is the gastrointestinal side-effects and long treatment times needed to resolve anaemia and replenish body iron stores. Non-adherence to therapy is common due to gastrointestinal side effects that limit its efficacy. Intravenous (IV) iron formulations provide a faster replacement, is a safer and effective alternative to oral iron for the treatment of iron deficiency anaemia (IDA) [216–218]. Allogeneic red blood cell transfusion has lifesaving potential in anaemic and haemorrhaging patients. However, a major limiting factor associated with this therapy is the risk of serious adverse events (transfusion reaction, transfusion transmissible disease, alloimmunization and immunomodulatory effect), costs and inadequacy [219]. Its use as an alternative in the management of iron deficiency is for treating critical anaemia (Hb level < 70 g/l), patients with acute myocardial ischaemia and in haemorrhaging patients who are haemodynamically unstable, patients in whom oral and IV iron is contraindicated or in cases of treatment failure nine [220]. Oral iron is a cheap and readily available option in managing patients with iron deficiency anaemia. Its use is however limited by challenge associated with gastrointestinal absorption and compliance [221]. Intravenous iron therapy, though slightly more expensive than oral iron is effective in managing patients with iron deficiency anaemia particularly when oral iron is contraindicated or ineffective [222]. Intravenous iron has the potential to reduce requirement for allogenic red blood cell transfusion [223]. The only limitations associated with the use of IV iron are adverse effects that have been associated with its use: risk of anaphylaxis, increased risk of infections, arthralgia, oxidative stress, hypophosphatemia, hypotension, headache, vomiting, chest tightness, fever, and hot flushes [224, 225]. Free iron has the potential to potentiate bacterial growth in vitro [226]. Intravenous iron therapy is effective in correcting iron deficiency anaemia (IDA) before any major surgery, and it can potentially reduce the need for allogeneic red blood cell transfusion and could help countries across the West African sub region better manage their limited allogenic blood stock for patients in whom oral and IV is contraindicated [227–229]. Oral and IV iron can have broad applicability to many patients particularly in low-income settings. There is need for more advocacy for countries in the West African sub region to promote the use of safe and affordable oral and IV iron more to manage patient with iron deficiency anaemia with the aim of reducing the need for limited allogeneic red blood cell transfusion.

3.4 Erythropoietin use can limit the dependence on allogenic blood across West Africa

Erythropoietin is a glycoprotein cytokine hormone synthesized in the kidney in response to tissue hypoxia. Its primary function is the stimulation of erythropoiesis (stimulate the division and differentiation of erythroid progenitor cells) in the bone marrow [230]. In patients with chronic kidney disease (CKD), there is damage to the kidneys and associated limited EPO production. Erythropoietin stimulating agents (ESAs) are recombinant versions of EPO produced pharmacologically via recombinant DNA technology. Examples of ESAs include epoetin alfa, darbepoetin, and methoxy polyethylene glycol-epoetin beta [231]. In patients with chronic renal failure, cancer, patients who are receiving dialysis, chemotherapy-induced anaemia and those with bone marrow suppression, the use of erythroid stimulating agents is clinically indicated in patients with haemoglobin less than 10 g/dL to increase haemoglobin levels and avoid the need for allogenic blood transfusions [232, 233]. Red blood cell (RBC) transfusion is an independent risk factor for cardiac surgery-associated acute kidney injury (CSA- AKI). Pre-operative administration of EPO may reduce the incidence of CSA-AKI, improve post-operative outcomes, decreasing the length of hospital and reduce the need for allogenic RBC transfusion in patients undergoing cardiac surgery [234]. Previous reports indicate that the administration of erythropoietin before cardiac surgery is associated with a significant reduction in the risk of exposure to allogeneic blood transfusion [235–238]. There are several factors that limit the use of Erythropoietin stimulating agents particularly in low income developing countries; cost [2], its use is contraindicated in patients with hypersensitivity to non-human mammal-derived products [226], it has been shown to increase blood viscosity and may predispose high risk patients to DVT, pulmonary embolism and hypercoagulable state and should be used with caution in patients with history of ischaemic stroke or cardiovascular disease [227]. It is also contraindicated in neonates, peripartum mothers and breastfeeding mothers due to the risk for gasping syndrome in neonates (severe metabolic acidosis and associated gasping respirations, renal failure and neurological deterioration [228].

3.5 Autologous blood transfusion can facilitate the optimum utilization of limited allogenic blood across West Africa

Not all surgical patients require allogenic blood. Some can potentially benefit from autologous blood transfusion (ABT). Forms of ABT include predeposit autologous donation (PAD), acute normovolaemic haemodilution (ANH), and perioperative cell salvage (PCS) [239]. In PAD there is repeated preoperative phlebotomy, 4–5 weeks before surgery, during which time 4 or 5 units of in-date blood can be collected with ease. This technique reduces exposure to allogeneic blood. ANH involves a process where whole blood (1.0–1.5 l) is removed, and simultaneously intravascular volume is replaced with crystalloid or colloid, or both, to maintain blood volume. The anticoagulated blood is then reinfused during or shortly after surgical blood loss has stopped in reverse order of collection. The blood-sparing benefit of haemodilution is the result of the reduced red cell mass lost during surgical bleeding. Intraoperative RBC salvage entails the collection and reinfusion of blood lost during or after surgery. Shed blood is aspirated from the operative field into a specially designed centrifuge. Citrate or heparin anticoagulant is added, and the contents are filtered to remove clots and debris. Centrifuging concentrates the salvaged red cells, and saline washing may be used. This concentrate is then reinfused [239]. ABT is extremely safe, not associated with complications related to allogenic blood transfusion (immunological challenge associated with increase in tumour recurrence after surgical resection, increased postoperative infection rates, increased progression of HIV infection, blood transfusion reaction and multiorgan failure), crossmatching is not required; alloimmunization to foreign red cell antigen can be excluded and the fear of TTIs can be ignored [239–241]. Implementation of pre-operative autologous blood transfusion (PAD and ANH) and perioperative red blood cell salvage are strategies that can help countries in West Africa optimize the use of the limited blood stocks. Intraoperative red blood cell salvage is well recognized as a blood conservation strategy [242, 243] but it has limited applicability in critically ill patients. Postoperative recovery and transfusion of blood from sterile surgical drains in cardiac surgery has shown only marginal reduction in transfusion requirements. The feasibility and effectiveness of blood recovery techniques for other critically ill patients with acute blood loss are more limited. An autologous blood transfusion programme can be implemented as complementary to the established allogenic blood transfusion programme across the West African sub region. It has the potential to help the sub region conserve her allogenic blood stock for patients in whom autologous transfusion is contraindicated and result in more effective use of the limited allogenic blood supplies.

3.6 Implementation of restrictive red cell transfusion triggers

Anaemia is highly prevalent in critically ill and trauma patients. Two-thirds of these patients present with a haemoglobin concentration < 12 g/dl on admission and 97% of them become anaemic by Day 8 on admission [244]. Evidence has shown that critically ill patients with cardiovascular disease risk factors can survive with low haemoglobin than originally thought. Several studies have compared the use of lower haemoglobin thresholds as restrictive transfusion triggers in critically ill patients compared to liberal transfusion triggers. Hébert and Colleagues demonstrated that a restrictive transfusion strategy would reduce transfusion requirements and would be as safe as, and possibly better than, a more liberal strategy for critically ill adults [245]. Similarly, experience from a randomized controlled trial among paediatric ICU patients has shown that a haemoglobin threshold of 70 g/L, compared with a more liberal threshold of 95 g/L, reduced transfusion requirements by 44% [246]. Haemoglobin threshold of 70 g/L seems appropriate for critically ill adult and paediatric and adult patients [247]. Strong evidence exists that shows that a restrictive transfusion strategy with a lowered haemoglobin threshold is safe compared to a liberal strategy with higher haemoglobin threshold particularly in the absence of cardiovascular disease risk factors [248]. Evidence has shown that transfusion at higher haemoglobin thresholds is only beneficial in patients with acute myocardial infarction [249]. A major challenge associated with blood transfusion service delivery across the West African sub region is the challenge of safety and adequacy. Countries across the sub region will need to implement policies on restrictive transfusion triggers to facilitate optimum use of limited allogenic blood stock. Other evidence-based best practices the sub region needs to implement includes; reducing blood loss and the need for blood transfusions, improving the appropriateness of blood transfusion and implementing blood conservation strategies including the use of laboratory test (PT, APTT and fibrinogen) to determine bleeding predisposition in patients scheduled for surgery, evidence-based use of haemostatic agents [antifibrinolytic agents (aprotinin, tranexamic acid and epsilon aminocaproic acid), desmopressin and recombinant activated factor VII), the implementation of diagnostic endoscopy to reduce blood loss as well as maintaining normal pH, temperature and calcium levels to manage coagulopathy [250], blood salvage techniques, use of erythropoietin and use of indication coding or restrictive blood transfusion triggers. These implementations will help to limit the need for transfusion and enable the sub region effectively to manage her limited allogenic blood stock.

3.7 Availability and use of specialized blood products in the West African sub-region

The last 30 years has been associated with a significant development in the field of transfusion medicine particularly with the implementation of blood component therapy and the need to provide specialized blood products to facilitate the effective management of particularly patients with haematological malignancies [251]. Commonly prescribed specialized blood components include antigen negative red cells, gamma irradiated blood products, HLA and HPA matched platelets, washed red cells and CMV negative unit.

3.8 Antigen negative red cells

Red blood cell (RBC) alloimmunization is a significant challenge in blood transfusion practice. Red blood cell alloimmunization often results from antigen disparity between donor and recipient or between a mum and her foetus. The prevalence of alloimmunization ranges from 1 to 3% in the general population and 10–70% among TD patients [252, 253]. Other factors that play a role in the alloimmunization process include the immune competence of the recipient, the dose of the antigen to which the recipient is exposed, the frequency of exposure, antigen frequency in the population and the immunogenicity of the RBC antigen involved. Evidence-based best practice requires the implementation of a policy to carry out pre-transfusion alloantibody screen for all patients that require a red cell transfusion with the hope of detecting those that have atypical alloantibodies [252–254]. This implementation will facilitate the identification of the atypical antibodies and facilitate the indirect antiglobulin-based crossmatch of antigen negative red cells for the patient. Patients whose alloantibody screening test is positive should have a panel done to facilitate the identification of the alloantibody/ies present. This is to facilitate the crossmatch of units that have been phenotyped for the group specific antigen and found negative. The policy also recommends the provision of antigen negative units for patients in whom a clinically significant red cell alloantibodies was identified in the past but sub detectable in the current sample (alloantibody titre drops below detectable levels). The implementation of this policy is to ensure that the aim of giving the red cells transfusion is to optimize the haemoglobin level of the patients and by extension improve the oxygen carrying capacity or tissue perfusion in the recipient. It also reduces the risk of acute/delayed haemolytic transfusion reaction that can result when patients with a clinically significant alloantibody is transfused with donor unit positive for the group specific antigen. The national blood transfusion service should be able to test a percentage of all donations for Rh phenotype, K and other clinically significant red cell phenotypes such as Duffy (Fya) and Kidd (Jka) negative are generally in stock. Evidence-based best practice recommend that extended phenotyping be carried out for all transfusion-dependent patients (thalassemia, sickle cell disease and myelodysplastic syndrome) who are chronically transfused for Rh (C, c, E, e) and Kell antigens before the initial RBC transfusion [255]. This is to ensure that they are transfused at least ABO, Rh (C, c, E, e) and Kell compatible units as a minimum [256–258]. The use of uncrossmatched O red cells can have a lifesaving potential in haemorrhaging patient when there is no time to carry out a full pre-transfusion testing. Blood group O negative units used in emergency for a woman of childbearing age should be rr (C-, D- and E-), K, CMV and High titre negative [259]. In many settings across the West African region red cell phenotyped for clinically significant red cell antigens are not readily available. Donors are tested for only the ABO and Rhesus D group. Many hospitals in the sub region do not routinely test patients requiring a red cell transfusion for the presence of alloantibodies and facilities for panel testing to identify the alloantibodies present are often not available. Countries across the sub region must implement best practices to prevent RBC alloimmunization and haemolytic transfusion reactions (HTRs) including routine testing of all patients that require a transfusion for the presence of alloantibodies, provision of extended phenotyping for all transfusion dependent patients, optimization of the method and scope of RBC antigen typing as well as the selection of antigen negative blood for crossmatch to facilitate the provision of timely, most compatible and safe blood for transfusion to patients.

3.9 Gamma irradiated blood products

Transfusion-associated graft-*versus*-host disease (TA-GvHD) is a rare, usually fatal, complication of transfusion that occur when the viable and potent lymphocytes in the donor engraft and destroy the host lymphocytes and by extension the host immune system. TA-GvHD can either occur when immunocompromised recipients are transfused with cellular blood components containing viable lymphocytes or when a recipient receives blood components from a human leucocyte antigen (HLA)-haploidentical unrelated donor or from their family member. Transfusion of potent donor (related and non-related) lymphocytes to HLA haploidentical recipient is documented as the most potent risk factor for the development of TA-GvHD [260]. The transfusion of pre- storage leuco depleted blood products can reduce the risk of TA-GvHD. In the developed world all transfused units are universally leucocyte depleted. The implementation of this best practice has brought about a significant reduction in the residual cases of TA-GvHD. A previous report reported a TA-GvHD prevalence of 18·9% (66 out of the 348) between 2000 and 2013 [261]. Irradiation by exposing donor blood products to irradiation using Gamma rays and X-rays (a minimum of 25 Gy) is the principal of inactivating lymphocytes in the transfused component. Transfusion of washed red cells is not as effective in preventing TA-GvHD as irradiation. Gamma irradiated blood product is clinically indicated in the following patients groups; foetus and neonate who are immunological immature and whose lymphocytes are naive, patients needing intrauterine blood transfusion (IUT) including those requiring routine 'top-up' neonatal transfusions following IUT [262], recipients of allogeneic HSCT, adults and children with Hodgkin's Lymphoma (HL), patients treated with purine analogues (fludarabine, cladribine bendamustine and pentostatin) which are known to induce profound lymphopenia with associated low CD4 counts, CLL patients treated with alemtuzumab, aplastic anaemia patients undergoing treatment with ATG or alemtuzumab and patients receiving ATG or other T-lymphocyte-depleting serotherapy for rare types of immune dysfunction) [263–266]. The median time from transfusion to presentation among TA- GvHD patients is 11 days and commonly associated symptoms include rash (80·2%), fever (67·5%), elevated liver enzymes (66·4%), pancytopenia (65·2%), diarrhoea (43·1%), bone marrow aplasia (22·7%) and hypocellularity (17·2%) and hepatomegaly (13·5%). Laboratory information management systems (LIMS) should be updated with relevant information for patients in whom gamma irradiated blood products are clinically indicated. Evidence-based best practice in the management of patients in whom irradiated blood products are indicated requires the following; effective communication among those involved in the care of these patients (clinical areas and transfusion laboratories) as well as between transfusion laboratories particularly during patient transfers from one hospital to another and carrying of treatment information cards to facilitate the provision of appropriate components [267]. In emergency situations, where non-irradiated components are unavailable and where delay in sourcing gamma irradiated red cells or platelets can be life- threatening, leuco depleted blood or platelets can be sourced promptly as a minimum requirement. The justification for this must be included in the patient case note and such a patient should be observed for possible evidence of TA-GvHD for few weeks. Many of the above best practices are not readily available in blood centres in the sub-region. There is urgent need for the implementation of gamma irradiated products for patients in whom gamma irradiated red cell, platelet and granulocyte components is clinically indicated across the West African sub region as a way of optimizing the transfusion service delivery in the sub region and reduce the risk of TA-GvHD.

4. HLA and HPA matched platelets

Platelets are anucleate cellular elements that play a role in haemostasis. Platelet concentrate is used to manage thrombocytopenic patients with haematological oncological disorders including the management of haemorrhaging patients. Platelet can be transfused either as apheresis platelet concentrate (APC) or pooled platelet concentrate (RPC) [268]. The absolute clinical indications for apheresis platelets include patients who require HLA compatible and/or HPA matched platelets (platelet refractoriness due to the presence of HLA and/or HPA antibodies), patients with neonatal alloimmune thrombocytopenia (NAIT) and patients who require IgA deficient platelets. Apheresis derived platelets concentrate are associated with a lower risk of alloimmunization and subsequent development of platelet refractoriness, the risk of TTIs is less because the recipient is exposed to a single donor. Also, the platelet yield from apheresis is about 6 times more in pooled platelets [269–272]. The cost of producing platelet concentrate is higher with apheresis compared with pooled platelets. Also, the risk of allergic adverse reactions is about four times higher with apheresis derived platelet concentrate [273]. Other aspects may impact the decision: the fact that using APC in place of RPC reduces the total donor exposure of patients was considered critical in some countries to reduce the risk of transmission of blood transmissible disease. Finally, the cost of the components, much higher for APC, may be considered. Platelet refractoriness is a term used to describe the failure to achieve an adequate increase in platelet count of a recipient after two consecutive transfusions of random platelets. The common cause can either be immunologic (HLA - class I specific antibodies, HPA - antibodies or ABO - antibodies – mediated resulting from the transfusion of ABO incompatible platelets to a recipient who is positive for high titre anti-A or anti-B haemolysin) or non-immunologic (platelet sequestration and consumption) in nature resulting from non-immune destruction of transfused donor platelets [273]. Alloimmunization to human leukocyte antigens (HLA) class or human platelet antigens (HPA) can result in platelet refractoriness [274]. Patients with these anti-leucocyte or platelet antibodies will need to be provided HLA class I and HPA compatible/matched platelets [275, 276]. Refractoriness to platelet transfusion is usually caused by alloimmunization to either HLA/platelet antigens or as a result on non-immune destruction of platelets and is commonly seen in 14% of haematology patients receiving platelet transfusions with HLA alloimmunization as a major cause [277, 278]. Alloimmunization to HLA/platelet antigens and by extension platelet refractoriness can be reduced by transfusion of leucodepleted products, use of irradiation or transfusion of HLA/HPA matched platelet transfusions [279, 280]. Despite the importance of platelet concentrate in the management of thrombocytopenic haematology, oncology and haemorrhaging patients, the product is seldom available in most settings across the sub region. Government of West African states will need to show more commitment to the provision of a quality blood transfusion service by investing significantly in transfusion-related infrastructure with the hope of achieving improvement in transfusion service delivery.

4.1 Washed red cells

Washing of red cells is often carried out for three major clinically relevant reasons; to reduce the amount of cytokines [causes of febrile non-haemolytic transfusion reactions (FNHTRs), reduce the level of allergen proteins to reduce the risk of allergic reactions resulting from contaminating plasma proteins (including IgA) as well as to reduce the concentration of potassium that leaked from the intracellular during storage to reduce the detrimental effect of hyperkalaemia in the recipient [281]. Patients who are IgA deficient run the risk of developing allergic reaction if they are transfused with IgA- rich donor blood. Washing can potentially remove a significant 90–95% plasma resulting in a significant reduction of the IgA content to <0·05 mg/dl IgA –a level common seen in IgA deficient patients. Washed leucodepleted red cells reduce the risk of alloimmunization to HLA. Washing is often performed by normal saline (0.9% NaCl) in either an open or a closed system. RBCs washed in an open system should be used within 24 hours (prevent bacterial contamination) of washing while that washed in a closed system have a shelf life of 14 days post washing [282]. Red cell washing increases the RBC osmotic fragility and increased haemolysis post transfusion [283]. Washed red cells are associated with less systemic inflammation and lower levels of free plasma haemoglobin with its nitric oxide scavenging property which has been shown to be independent predictor of mortality in septic patients [284].

4.2 CMV negative unit

Cytomegalovirus (CMV) infection is endemic globally. In the USA the seroprevalence of the disease range from 30 to 97% [285]. Cytomegalovirus (CMV) is a significant contributor to increased morbidity, mortality and cost of management of immunocompromised patients [286]. CMV is a highly contagious viral infection that is transmitted through close contact with bodily fluids (blood, saliva, urine and breast milk). CMV can also be transmitted by organ transplantation and blood transfusion, when the donor is CMV positive, and the recipient is CMV negative [287]. Common signs and symptoms associated with the disease include; fever, malaise, leukopenia and neutropenia. Immune-deficient individuals can suffer severe or even fatal disseminated infections. Evidence-based best practice in the developed economies recommend that the following patient's groups should be transfused with CMV negative cellular blood products, congenital immunodeficiency and HIV-infected patients, haematopoietic progenitor cell transplant recipients, low birth-weight infants, pregnant women till delivery and their foetuses (to prevent congenital CMV), severely immunosuppressed patients and recipients of solid-organ transplant recipients [288]. The risk of CMV transmission through blood transfusion can be prevented by two major ways; by transfusing vulnerable CMV naïve and profoundly immunocompromised with blood and blood products that are negative for CMV and by ensuring that cellular blood products are universally leucodepleted (fewer than 5×10^6 leukocytes per unit) [289]. CMV negative blood and components is critical to reducing the risk of transfusion- transmitted symptomatic CMV infection in recipients who are themselves CMV naïve. Other potential measures that can reduce the risk of transfusing CMV infected blood products include washing red cell units and removing the buffy coat, freezing, thawing and subsequent deglycerolizing. The major drawback associated with these measures include the fact that they are not practicable large scale and are associated with a significant cost implication [288]. The implementation of TT- CMV reduction strategies in the late 1980s requiring that seronegative marrow recipients and other high-risk groups receive CMV seronegative blood products has brought about a significant reduction in the risk of CMV infection from 28% -57 to <5% [290, 291]. Government of West African countries have a duty of care to implement CMV prevention strategies by ensuring that evidence-based best practices requiring that all cellular blood products transfused across the sub region are universally leukocyte reduced and screened serologically for CMV.

4.3 Optimizing safe blood donation in the West African sub-region

The two major challenges associated with blood transfusion service delivery across the West African sub region are access to safe and adequate supply of blood and product products [2, 292]. World Health Assembly resolutions WHA28.72 [293] and WHA58.13 [294] urge member states to develop national blood transfusion services based on VNRDs. A VNRD-based NBTS is key to sustained supply of safe and adequate blood and blood products. It is the only realistic way to ensure long-term and consistent supply of blood and blood products to eliminate the chronic shortage of safe blood and blood products particularly in low- and medium-income countries. Not only is blood donation level low in the West African sub region, but it is also predominantly family replacement donor-based rather than benevolent, non-remunerated donors (VNRBDs) who give blood out of altruism. The blood donation rate in sub-Saharan Africa is significantly lower (4–5 per 1000 population) compared to the developed economies (30 donations per 1000 population). WHO recommends that blood transfusion from regular VNRBDs have the lowest risk of TTIs. There are several factors militating against the low VNRBD levels in most West African countries: lack of organization and financial resources, but also, to some extent, of socio-cultural barriers such as limited levels of education, religious and mystic beliefs and misconceptions about blood use [295]. Voluntary, non-remunerated blood donation is the cornerstone of a safe and adequate national blood supply that meets the transfusion requirements of all patients. VNRBDs represent less than 50% of whole blood donations in low-income countries compared with 76–100% in high-income countries [296]. The low VNRBD levels in the sub region can be attributable to several reasons: lack of organization and financial resources, socio-cultural barriers, low levels of education, religious and erroneous beliefs and misconceptions about blood donations [297]. Government across the West African sub region must implement innovative ways to recruit and retain voluntary donors; celebration of the gift of blood donation from voluntary blood donors; increasing public awareness of voluntary non-remunerated blood donation; educating the public on the importance of regular, voluntary, non-remunerated blood donation; educating the public on the benefits of voluntary non-remunerated blood donation to recipients; promoting healthy living (nutrition, exercise, lifestyle); and provision of noncash incentives to encourage people to donate blood.

4.4 Implementation of cell-free foetal DNA testing across the West African subregion

Haemolytic disease of the foetus and newborn (HDFN) is an alloimmune disease associated with alloantibody developed by the mum triggered by a previous incompatible blood transfusion or a transplacental haemorrhage during a previous pregnancy associated with foreign red cell antigen entering the maternal circulation and sensitizing her to produce alloantibody. These alloantibodies, being low molecular weight antibodies can pass through placenta in subsequent pregnancy involving a foetus with a red cell antigen to which the maternal alloantibody is specific. This maternal alloantibody usually will cross the placenta barrier into the foetal circulation and coat the foetal red cell containing the group specific antigen and induce haemolysis. The disease often results from maternal immunological incompatibility with foetal blood groups leading to the production of alloantibodies. The rate of antibody production depends on the red cell antigen dose that enters the maternal circulation, the immune competence of the mum and the immunogenicity of the foetal antigen [297]. Clinical presentation of the disease ranges from asymptomatic mild anaemia to hydrops foetalis or stillbirth resulting from severe anaemia and jaundice. Management options include; the use of amniocentesis (an invasive procedure to obtain amniotic fluid which is analysed for product of haemoglobin breakdown to identify the severity of the disease), serial Doppler ultrasonography measurements to diagnose foetal anaemia, in utero, intrauterine transfusion, titration and quantification of alloantibody level, controlled early delivery, top up transfusion and exchange transfusion in the management of severely alloimmunized foetuses [298, 299]. Anti-RhD is the most incriminated alloantibody responsible for the majority of HDFN. However, the availability and widespread implementation of antenatal and postpartum Rhesus immune globulin prophylaxis particularly in the West has resulted in a marked decrease in the prevalence of alloimmunization to the RhD antigen among pregnant women. Other commonly encountered antibodies include anti-c, anti-K, E, AB0, JK (Kidd), and FY (Duffy) [300]. The most important blood groups are D, c, E, and K with respect to antenatal foetal blood group determination using cell-free foetal DNA (cfDNA) [301]. cfDNA derived from the foetus circulates in maternal blood. cfDNA testing is a non-invasive prenatal screening carried out on maternal plasma of pregnant women to predict foetal blood groups with the aim of; assessing the risk of haemolytic disease of the foetus and newborn (HDFN) in previously alloimmunized women and also to determine the Rhesus D group of the baby in order to determine if a non-previously immunized mum will need to be recruited into the RAADP program and will require anti-D prophylaxis following a potentially sensitizing event during pregnancy [302]. The cfDNA test can help identify women who have red cell alloantibodies and may be affected by haemolytic disease of the foetus and newborn (HDFN). cfDNA testing is carried out on maternal blood and can predict the foetal RhD, RhC, Rhc, RhE and K status of the foetus and by extension the risk of HDFN [303]. Early in pregnancy, small amounts of foetally derived cfDNA exist, but the fraction of foetal cfDNA in the maternal circulation increases with advancing gestational age [304]. The clinical implementation of this technology should be encouraged across the West African sub region. There are many advantages associated with this implementation [305, 306]. The test is significantly sensitive and specific with diagnostic sensitivity ranging from 95 to 100% and specificities over 99% [307–309]. The prevalence of Rh D negative varies widely between Caucasians with a prevalence >14% [307–310] compared to ethnic groups of sub-Saharan Africa with a prevalence ranging between 2.4 and 4.5% [311]. Evidence has shown that 40% of Rhesus D negative women carry D Negative foetuses. It is evidence-based best practice that all Rhesus D negative pregnant women who are not previously immunized are universally offered anti-D prophylaxis at the 3rd trimester under the RAADP program. NICE guidance released in 2008 recommend that a single dose of anti-D (1500iu) given to Rhesus D negative not previously sensitized pregnant women between weeks 28 and 30 would also be cost-effective in potentially preventing anti-D HDFN in subsequent pregnancy [312]. The use of cfDNA testing for the determination of the predicted Rh D group of the foetus has several advantages; allow for the rational implementation of antenatal immuno-prophylaxis for women in whom it is not clinically indicated who are predicted to be carry Rh D negative foetus rather than providing the prophylaxis universally to all Rh D negative non-previous immunized women. cfDNA testing can potentially predict 40% of these women who are carrying D negative babies for which Rh D prophylaxis will be a waste of a scarce human resource [313–316]. Also, the feto-maternal haemorrhage testing carried out during a potentially sensitizing event during pregnancy and post-delivery will not be required (reagent and time to carry out the testing) if the baby is predicted to be Rhesus D negative. The prophylactic anti-D offered to these Rh D negative women is a human blood product with reduce potential to transmit hepatitis C and prion type diseases [317]. The women whose babies are predicted to be Rhesus D negative with will be spared the pain and associated cost of travel to hospital to receive the anti-D prophylaxis [318]. Government across the West African sub region will need to live to their responsibility by implementing evidence-based best practices; cell-free DNA testing, provision of anti-D prophylaxis for non-previously sensitized Rh D negative women, feto maternal haemorrhage testing, non-invasive serial sonograms with Doppler of the Median Cerebral Artery (MCA) to determine the peak systolic velocity (PSV) and by extension foetal anaemia, amniocentesis and provision of blood that meet the minimum requirement for intrauterine transfusion for foetus severely affected with HDFN in utero and facility for sonographic guided intrauterine transfusion through the umbilical vein should be implemented across the sub region to optimize the obstetric and neonatal care offered.

4.5 Quality management issues in blood transfusion service delivery in West Africa

Blood transfusion process comprises a series of steps ranging from ordering of blood or blood products, administration, monitoring of the transfused patient, managing of adverse reactions and events as well as documentation of transfusion adverse events and outcomes [319]. Quality management in blood transfusion is the sum of all the processes put in place to ensure that blood products and services are produced consistent, safe, efficacious service that meet the need of the customers [320]. There is increasing advocacy to ensure the efficacy, quality and safety of blood and blood products. The sum total of all the processes in place to ensure safety of blood and blood product from the point of collection of blood and blood products from blood donors to the point of administration to the recipients [321]. Quality management in blood transfusion encompasses the organization and her quality management system, personnel and organization, quality policy, organograms with responsibilities of staff, job description for staff members, change control of documents, continuous training based on SOPs (should be approved before distribution and the correct versions should be provided at the points of use), collection of blood and blood components, non-conformance, deviations, complaints, recall, corrective and preventive actions, self-inspection, audits, and improvements [322, 323]. The blood transfusion organization must ensure that they understand and meet the current and future requirements of the customers. The Blood Service must ensure that adequate resources are provided to implement and operate the quality management system, to continually improve its effectiveness and to satisfy customer requirements. The physical resources (equipment, consumables, work areas and utilities) to undertake the work must be suitable to attain the required standards.

4.6 Personnel and organization

It is a general requirement that all personnel responsible for blood transfusion service delivery should have the right skills, experience, education/training, certification, competence and regularly trained and retrained [324]. It is expected that appropriate staffing levels involvement should ensure the safe and effective delivery of all transfusion service activities and be subjected to annual review [325]. All personnel shall have up-to-date job descriptions that clearly set out their tasks and responsibilities. Blood transfusion organizations shall have separate persons as training officer and quality manager. Provision of training to the personnel on safe blood transfusion, hazards, and appropriate implementation of corrective and preventative measures, as well as abiding with standard safety guidelines are vital and must be implemented throughout the entire blood transfusion process [326]. In every step in the blood transfusion process there are potential risks, such as errors in patient identification, blood typing, cross-matching, administration and other human errors. Many errors which result in serious morbidity or mortality that occur in the blood transfusion process and by extension in healthcare delivery are related to human error with training and competency issues a major contributory factor [327, 328]. All personnel should be appropriately trained, and their competency assessed before being allowed to work unsupervised. The contents of training being implemented should be periodically assessed and the competence of personnel evaluated regularly. Employers must develop personal development plan (PDP) for all staff involved in the blood transfusion process that ensures that staff develop in a continual format to enable the delivery of a continually improving quality service tailored towards meeting the present and strategic future needs of the organization and her customers. Personnel are required to participate in a lifelong continuing professional development (CPD). There is also the need to ensure that transfusion staff are adequately remunerated. Efforts should be made to employ, motivate and retain the best staff, adequate number of staff and mix as well as ensuring that there are opportunities for professional growth and development and that staff are not working excess unsocial hours with inadequate recovery time. Previous report indicates that these issues can affect staff turnaround, result in burn out, low morale, high sickness absences, increased error rate, poor team spirit, diminished productivity, and suboptimal blood transfusion service delivery [329]. The healthcare delivery system in the West African sub region faces many challenges including human resource inadequacy. Migration of health workers (brain drain) defined as the movement of health personnel in search of a better standard of living and life quality, higher remuneration, better working condition, wellbeing, access to advanced technology and more stable political conditions has made the human resource challenge in the sub region even worse [330]. The best of West African human resources in healthcare who should be offering excellent care to citizens in their home nations have emigrated to developed countries. The physician-to-population ratio is estimated to be 13/100,000 in Africa, compared with 280/100,000 in the United States [331]. Although there is a hypothesis that brain drain could be beneficial and impart positively on medical education fostering international collaboration in healthcare research and development [332]. This argument will only be substantive if these health professionals return periodically or permanently after practicing abroad for a while. The economic effect of brain drain on the economy of developing countries is huge [333]. There are several reasons for the poor retention of healthcare workers in the West African sub region: poor remuneration, lack of opportunity, high unemployment in health labour markets and the deplorable state of healthcare infrastructure in the sub region. Leaders of West African countries must take realistic steps to ensure that all staff involved in blood transfusion service delivery across the sub region are adequately trained, remunerated, motivated, and retained to ensure high morale, increased productivity and to prevent the risk of brain drain. These have the potential to reduce the reduce the error rate, brain drain and suboptimal blood transfusion service delivery.

4.7 Premises and environment

The premises and environment where all processes involved in blood transfusion delivery is implemented must be enabling and must be conducive for activities being carried out. The work environment (processes, systems, structures and tools or conditions) in the blood transfusion workplace that can potentially impact the staff favourably and by extension their performance and productivity should be provided [334]. The work done must be process oriented, associated with effective cleaning and maintenance protocols, and arranged in such a way as to minimize the risk of errors, injury and to minimize the risk of contamination. There should be a separate area (Donation, testing and processing, storage and waste management) that is optimally endowed (human and materials). Donation area should be endowed with facilities to allow for confidential interviews and assessment of individuals to determine their eligibility to donate blood. Collection area should be appropriately equipped to facilitate the safe collection of blood and blood products as well as manage adverse reactions or injuries from events associated with donation. The safety of the transfusion staff and donors must be maintained. The environment where the blood transfusion process is implemented must be enabling in terms of space, safety and infrastructural endowment (equipment, availability of piped borne water, soap, appropriate sanitation facilities, handwashing facilities, availability of adequate infection control measures including personal protective equipment (PPE) and waste management as well as availability of uninterrupted power supplies) [335–337]. The blood transfusion organization should have a dedicated laboratory for donor testing and should be separated from the processing areas to prevent the risk of contamination. There should be restricted access (limited to authorized staff) to the testing and processing areas. There should also be a dedicated storage area for the blood components (red cells, plasma, and platelets). There should be an area set aside for the secure and segregated storage of different blood components including a separate area for quarantine (not fit to use) and released (fit to use) as well as blood products collected for dedicated use (autologous donation) [338]. The storage area must have access to uninterrupted power supply and back up fridges, freezers and alternative sources of power in the event of equipment or power failure. Provision of adequate and safe blood transfusion service delivery is associated with the generation of waste which is potentially hazardous and may carry a potential for infection and injury [339]. Suboptimal and inappropriate handling of healthcare-related waste can have serious public health consequences and a significant impact on the environment [340]. The blood transfusion organization should have a system for the effective management of waste. The waste generated during production of blood and blood component carries a higher potential for infection and injury. Waste generated should be segregated [domestic non-hazardous, hazardous healthcare waste including sharps (needles, hypodermic needles, scalpels, blades, lancet, infusion sets, broken glass and pipettes) and chemical and radioactive waste] and disposed appropriately. In most West African countries, unsustainable management of waste is common. Open dumping and open burning are commonly implemented as waste treatment and final disposal systems. Illegal dumping of waste onto sidewalks, open fields, storm water drains and rivers is commonplace with negative economic, social and environmental impacts. Also, waste management involves the activity of the informal sector including waste pickers and scavengers with a significant associated health risks from potentially hazardous waste [341]. There is need for the implementation of effective waste management across the West African sub region by taking realistic steps at waste reduction, reuse if safe, recycling, recovery and treatment to achieve sustainable and environmentally sound management of all wastes [342, 343].

4.8 Equipment and materials

All equipment for use in the blood transfusion organization must have Equipment Operating Procedure (EOPs), be validated prior to implementation, regularly calibrated, and maintained [343]. The acquisition of any equipment must be justified and constitute value for money and should be carefully chosen to minimize any hazard to the blood donors, the personnel, or the blood components itself [344]. The transfusion organization must carry out validation of equipment, certification and pre-acceptance testing of all reagents to establish that the performance characteristics of the method meet the requirements for the intended analytical application. Validation is a pre-defined exercise to confirm that equipment or a procedure (either current or proposed) is fit for its intended purpose and meets its pre-defined specification. The benefits of validation include assurance that critical aspects of a process are in control, increased probability of uniform product quality, reduced product waste and reduced customer complaints. Reagent certification of reagents ensures that reagents are performing to the quality standards of the manufacturers and fit for diagnostic work. Only reagents and materials from approved suppliers that meet the documented requirements, certification and specifications shall be used. The blood organization should have a robust computerized LIMS with back-up procedures. The LIMS should be validated before use [345]. All the associated hardware and software shall be protected against unauthorized use and changes. The back-up system must prevent loss of or damage to data [346]. The blood transfusion organization should implement a documented change control process that facilitate the suggestion of changes to the process by staff involved in the process that is beneficial, potentially save cost, remove bureaucratic aspects, and will optimize the safety of donors and personnel. The change control is planned and implemented in a controlled way, the possible re- training for staff involved in the process following the standard operating procedures (SOPs), shall ensure there is a record of the processes operated before and after the change, that the date of the change is known, and that material processed through the changed system can be identified. There should also be a system to ensure that the effectiveness of the newly implemented process is monitored and opportunities for further improvement are investigated and, where relevant, implemented. It shall support the organization in trying to learn from incidents, accidents, near misses, complaints, and other event information. The objective analysis of these and implementation of corrective and preventive measures in an action-planned format will facilitate the delivery of a continually improving quality blood transfusion service across the West African sub region [347, 348].

4.9 Recall and traceability

Effective blood transfusion service delivery requires that a system be in place to allow 100% accountability of donated blood and blood products [349]. The implementation of traceability facilitates the easy and prompt recall of products that is identified to be suboptimal or have potential to cause the recipient after release from the national blood transfusion service to hospital blood bank or from the hospital blood bank to the ward or satellite fridges can be recalled [350]. The recall system should be such that it is prompt and can be triggered at any time. All recalled products should be separated and kept away from other units that are fit for use to prevent its accidental release until a decision is made on the final fate (release to the pool or discarded). The recall process should be reviewed regularly to ensure its continued effectiveness. Most countries, particularly those in developing countries were poorly implementing sub-indicators of haemovigilance particularly in the area of legal provisions, arrangement for effective organization and human resources indicators [351]. There must be a system to ensure that materials can be traced through the entire process from procurement, testing, production, issue from the NBTS to the hospital blood bank and subsequently to the recipient. There must be 100% traceability for all donated units (who donated the unit, when the blood was released to hospital blood bank and when unit was transfused to the recipient or discarded). For all donated units, traceability must be maintained from vein to vein from donor to the patient. In Morocco for example, the traceability rates were around 51% in Casablanca [352] and 15.5% in Rabat [353].

5. Ensuing a continuous quality improvement-oriented blood transfusion service across the West African sub-region

The blood transfusion organization must strive for Continuous Quality Improvement (CQI) by the regular and objective evaluation of overall performance using indices such as incidents, errors, near misses, complaints, audit and accreditation (internal and external), litigation and customer satisfaction surveys to determine the quality of service delivered on a continual basis [354]. At the root of CQI is culture of root cause analysis as a problem-solving tool to identify nonconformities with the hope of identifying corrected and preventive actions (CAPA) that needs to be implemented in an action planned format (what is to be done, why, how, by whom and time frame to achieve the task) to nip the non-conformance in the bud. All complaints from the customer and other relevant information, including any serious adverse reactions and serious adverse events lined to a defective blood component should be reported, documented, and promptly investigated to identify the causative factor/s of the defect and promptly recall the affected unit if necessary [355]. All serious adverse reactions or serious adverse events should be reported to appropriate regulatory authorities.

5.1 Quality audit and accreditation

A Quality audit is a planned systematic, independent and documented process of evaluating elements of a quality management system. It assesses whether quality activities and related results comply with planned arrangements [356]. Audits can either be internal or external and ensure that process are being operated as stated in the SOP and that procedures and associated quality assurance comply with Good Manufacturing Practice (GMP) principles. Audits should be carried out by a competent and trained individual who is knowledgeable about the process. The results of all audits and all non-conformances identified should be documented to allow for the implementation of root causes and action-planned implementation of corrective and preventive actions in a timely manner [357]. Unlike their Western counterparts, many countries in the West African sub region do not have a fit for purpose, centralized and coordinated blood transfusion services and the safety, quality, efficacy and regulatory framework remain significantly poor. The implementation of quality management system in blood transfusion across the West African region is relatively naïve. The issues surrounding the safety of production, supply, distribution, administration, and clinical use is poorly developed. Blood transfusion service delivery across the

West African sub region can be optimized. Audits of practice and incident reporting to national haemovigilance schemes have shown that poor hospital transfusion practice is frequent and occasionally results in catastrophic consequences for patients [358]. There is the need for governments of countries in the sub region to take steps to ensure the implementation of a quality management system-oriented blood transfusion process across the sub-region. Quality efforts should be made to ensure that blood transfusion is efficacious by the objective implementation of a high level of quality and safety throughout the transfusion chain (blood collection, testing, processing, storage, distribution, matching, delivery and clinical use of the blood products.

5.2 Providing safe blood transfusion across the West African sub-region

Blood transfusion is an indispensable component of modern healthcare delivery and saves millions of lives annually. Blood transfusion is often required to manage anaemia, bleeding following trauma, intra and post- operative, obstetric haemorrhage (ante and post-partum) and to manage several medical diseases including haematological conditions [349]. For blood transfusion to have life- saving potential, it must be safe. Safe blood transfusion is the right blood collected from the right voluntary non remunerated donor and transfused to the right patient at the right quantity, at the right time, in the right place and based on the right clinical indication [359]. Safe blood transfusion is not wishful thinking. It is achieved by implementing evidence-based best practices in key areas including patient identification, documentation, communication, patient consent, request for transfusion, pre transfusion sampling, collection of blood and delivery in the clinical area, safe administration of blood and monitoring during a blood transfusion. A significant number of patients worldwide are administered with wrong blood annually with sometimes fatal consequences. Many of these incidents are preventable and predominantly due to human errors [360]. The common root causes of these errors are poor patient identification, misidentification of patient during pre-transfusion sampling, errors during laboratory testing, error during collection of blood from the blood bank and errors during blood administration. Previous report indicates that as many as 40% of mis transfusions are due to errors in the post-analytic phase: often failures in the final check of the right blood and the right patient at the bedside [361]. There is need for healthcare professionals involved in the blood transfusion process including biomedical scientist, medical doctors and nursing staff practice in environments that recognize the importance of reducing error and improving safety using non-punitive system approaches that encourages the reporting and objective investigation of incidents, accidents, near misses and errors [362, 363].

5.3 Patient identification

Positive patient identification is fundamental to safe blood transfusion. It is essential to ensure that the right blood is given to the right patient. Patient misidentification can have a potentially fatal consequence for patients [364]. Errors in the whole-blood transfusion chain - from initial recipient identification to final blood administration - occur with a frequency of approximately 1 in 1000 events [365]. Among pre-analytical errors, misidentification and mis transfusion are still regarded as a considerable problem, posing serious risks for patient health and carrying huge expenses for the healthcare system [366]. Patient identification errors in pre- transfusion blood sampling ('wrong blood in tube') are a persistent area of risk in blood transfusion errors [367]. Evidenced best practice in the West requires that all patient for which blood transfusion is intended wear an identification band containing the minimum patient identifiers (surname, forename, date of birth and hospital number) to facilitate an unmistakable patient identification during pre-transfusion sample collection and during blood administration. In accident and emergency units, patients presenting in coma who cannot be immediately identified must be given at least one unique identifier (A&E or trauma number and patient gender). Prior to collecting or administering blood to a patient, the patient, carer or parent in case of children should be requested to state their full name and date of birth and this information must be compared to what is on the patient wrist band. It is only when there is a match that a patient is said to have been positively identified for sample collection and administration purposes. All identification discrepancies at any stage of the transfusion process must be investigated and resolved before moving to the next stage to prevent transfusion errors.

5.4 Documentation

In blood transfusion the golden rule is that anything not written down was done. Blood transfusion documentation is critical to ensuring 100% traceability of all donated donor units. Documentation (hard copy or electronic) to capture events at every stage of the transfusion process (pre-transfusion, during transfusion and post transfusion) should be kept in a clear, legible, readable, auditable, and user-friendly format. Vital information including transfusion prescription sheet, crossmatch worksheet, temperature, monitoring records, reagent storage, equipment validation, reagent certification and monitoring charts must be kept providing a clear audit trail [350]. Previous report indicates that use of barcode reader and related electronic technology can be adapted to improve transfusion safety and reduce the risk of human errors at all steps of the blood transfusion process [368]. All transfusion documentation should include the minimum patient identifiers (name, date of birth and hospital number). Pre-transfusion related information including laboratory data and clinical indication for transfusion, information that the potential risks, benefits and alternatives have been discussed with the patient and that written informed consent was obtained, the dose/volume and rate of transfusion and information of any special transfusion requirement for the patient such as CMV negative, antigen negative blood, gamma irradiated components, etc.). Previous report indicates that bedside ABO-typing and checklist prior to blood transfusion can control the ABO-mismatched transfusion if done timely and correctly [369]. Intra transfusion documentation must contain vital information; medical staff who started the transfusion, date and time transfusion commenced and completed, details of blood component (component type, bag numbers and any special requirement) as well as information on observation prior, during and post transfusion (temperature, blood pressure, respiratory rate and pulse). Post-transfusion documentation must include information on clinical outcome of any transfusion, adverse reaction or events and evidence that transfusion was beneficial and accomplished the desired outcome (HB optimization and improvement in anaemia and related symptoms) [370]. Previous report indicates that training and education of health-care staff on transfusion-related documentation at the bedside is vital to reducing blood transfusion related errors, morbidities, and mortalities [371].

5.5 Communication

Communication (verbal and written) between clinical, laboratory staff and porters should be clear and unambiguous as it is critical to patient safety. Misunderstanding and transcription error are common communication- related issues associated with transfusion errors. Effective commination among the health-care care workers involved in the blood transfusion process is critical to limiting transfusion-related errors [372]. Written or electronic communication should be used wherever possible with request for urgent transfusion supplemented by telephone request with laboratory staff. Good communication is especially important at times of staff handover between shifts, both on the wards and in the laboratory, and can be enhanced by a standardized and documented process. Handovers should be built into transfusion laboratory routine practices, ensuring effective transfer of information and appropriate follow up actions are taken [373]. Hospital transfer of patients is common- place in healthcare delivery. Effective transfer of relevant transfusion information relating to patient care is vital in blood transfusion service delivery [374].

5.6 Patient consent

Under the principle of medical ethics, a competent patient's autonomy and right to determine his or her treatment is widely recognized in medical practice. Evidence-based best practice recommends that patients are informed about and understand the purpose, benefits and potential risks of transfusion as well as available alternatives. The Advisory Committee on the Safety of Blood, Tissues, and Organs (SaBTO) recommends that 'valid consent' for blood transfusion should be obtained and documented in the clinical record (signed consent) [375]. Blood transfusion is not an entirely safe form of treatment. It is sometimes associated with adverse effects and events. Blood transfusion must not be given lightly but rather it must be given only when there are no safer alternatives. Its use must not only be based on laboratory results alone but also on the clinical presentation and presence of symptoms. The potential risk, benefits and alternatives must be discussed with patients to enable them to make an informed decision. A survey of the use of blood in the UK indicates that 20% or more of transfusions are inappropriate and that many patients could benefit from safer alternatives [376]. However, in emergency situations the inability to obtain a consent must not prevent or delay the need for essential urgent lifesaving transfusion. The only exception is patients that have a valid Advance Decision Document declining transfusion. Most Jehovah's witnesses carry a written advance directive declaring their religious convictions not to take a blood transfusion [377]. The blood refusal card directs that no blood is to be given to the owner under any circumstance, even if physicians believe transfusion will be lifesaving [378]. The right of such patients not to be transfused should be respected [379]. However, in the emergency, in the absence of blood refusal card or if there is a reasonable doubt about the validity of a treatment refusal, the physician has a duty of care to take decision that they believe is in the best interest of the patients and render life-saving treatment [380]. The issue of informed consent to have a transfusion is critical because transfused patients potentially lose their ability to be blood donors. In many developed countries, transfusion dependent patients are offered a modified form of consent that requires them to go through an annual review and re-consent [381].

5.7 Prescribing and request for transfusion

The process of prescribing blood components is not necessarily legally restricted to registered medical practitioners. From a safety and efficiency and saving lives point of view, there are clear advantages in allowing non-medical practitioners to authorize transfusion in certain situations. Evidence-based best practice recommends that appropriately trained and competent practitioners including registered nurses and midwives can make clinical decisions and provide written instruction for blood component transfusion. This practice has the potential to deliver a more patient-centred quality service [382, 383]. It is vital that all transfusion prescriptions or written authorization to transfuse a patient blood must be permanent part of a patient clinical records and should contain vital information including patient's minimum identifiers, information on the blood component to be transfused, the dose, volume rate and any special requirements [384].

5.8 Pre transfusion sampling

Wrong blood in tube' (WBIT) errors and misidentification at blood sampling, where the blood in the tube is not that of the patient identified on the label is a major cause of ABO incompatible transfusion and fatal haemolytic transfusion reactions. The consequence of these errors can be catastrophic [385]. This type of error is difficult to identify particularly when there is no historic blood group documented in the patients records on the LIMS [386]. Sub optimally labelled samples carry a significantly increased risk of containing blood from the wrong patient. There are several steps that can potentially reduce the risk of this kind of errors; use of electronic systems, ensuring that phlebotomist responsible for sample collection are adequately trained and competent tested; patients must be positively identified and their details (name, date of birth and hospital number) on the sample, dated, timed, and must match those on the request form and patient wrist band [386]. It is generally expected that all inpatients must wear an identity band and the collection and labelling of the sample tubes must be performed at the patient bedside as one uninterrupted process involving one trained and competent staff and one patient. Other requirements include; sample tubes must not be pre-labelled prior to sample collection; sample tubes must be hand labelled legibly; addressograph or printed labels must not be used on the transfusion sample and the transfusion laboratory must maintain a zero-tolerance policy for rejecting samples that do not meet the above minimum requirements [387–389]. It is also evidence-based best practice to implement a two- specimen rule to allow for the verification of ABO/Rh for blood transfusion [390, 391]. This implementation of two concordant ABO typing results has the potential to detect wrong blood in the tube and prevent the risk of haemolytic transfusion reaction resulting from the transfusion of ABO incompatible blood particularly when there is a discrepancy in the blood group obtained from both sample [392]. Many countries in the West African sub region do not seem to have a LIMS nor a barcode-based identification. The 2-sample rule is also not being implemented and documentation tends to be hardcopy and paper-based [393]. Countries in the sub region will need to start implementing these best practices to the latter to enhance the safety of blood transfusion service delivery and to reduce the risk of incompatible blood transfusion.

5.9 Collection of blood and delivery in the clinical area

Errors during blood collection of blood from the blood bank have been reported as predominant root cause of wrong blood transfusion and associated haemolytic transfusion reaction [393]. All staff responsible for collecting blood from the blood bank or satellite refrigerators must be trained and competency tested. There is increasing advocacy for the replacement of the predominant manual documentation of blood collection using a transfusion register which is predominant in many settings in the West Africa sub region to the less error- prone electronic blood-tracking systems [394]. This manual documentation system in operation in most settings in the sub region is risky particularly because people bear similar names thus increasing the risk of potentially taking blood meant for a different patient [395]. Electronic blood-tracking systems has a number of advantages over the traditional hardcopy register system; improved quality of transfusion service delivery by reducing transfusion errors; it allows for timely collection and delivery to clinical area, enhances the productivity of nursing staff as well as reduced blood wastage, prevent the risk of taking blood for a wrong patient and unallocated or de-reserved units, provides audit trail as only staff who have been trained and competency tested are given barcode and password to identify themselves on the system. Staff collecting blood is expected to scan the patient barcode containing the minimum patient identifiers which must be checked against the details on the transfusion laboratory-generated crossmatch label attached to the blood pack. Normally if there is no blood allocated for the patient in the fridge the staff will be denied access to the fridge. The system only ensures that only blood that is within its expiry time and date and meant for the desired patient is released for collection. Other advantages of the computer-controlled, electronically-linked information management system is that; minimize the risk of transfusing units that have been out of temperature-controlled storage for too long (>30 minutes); provides a full audit trail of all activity and frees up nursing resources allowing them concentrate on other core nursing duties, prevents the transfusion of incorrectly stored units and out of date product or quarantined; facilitate inventory control management, delivery, tracking and documentation as well as audit trails. Access to electronic databases have greatly facilitated product traceability and biovigilance efforts and it can be linked to LIMS and other IT systems, providing robust documentation and data relevant to transfusion at all stages of the transfusion process (blood sample collection, laboratory testing, blood unit collection from the blood bank and transfusion of blood to the patient, ensuring full documentation and audit trail at every stage [396]. Electronic blood-tracking systems ensure that the right patient receives the right blood component at the right time [397].

6. Receiving blood in the clinical area and safe administration of blood

Transfusion of wrong blood or blood component is the most important error associated with serious morbidity or mortality. Provision of training and competency for healthcare workers involved in blood transfusion, developing standard safety guidelines, raising of hazards and implementation of appropriate preventative measures are critical during all steps of blood and blood component transfusion [397]. There are evidence-based practices that clinical staff involved in blood transfusion will have to implement to prevent transfusion errors. Before attempting to collect blood from the blood bank they must ensure that patient is wearing an identity band, has given consent for transfusion, the transfusion 'prescription' has been completed, there is venous access and staff are available to start the transfusion promptly and monitor it correctly. Also except in case of major haemorrhage requiring rapid transfusion of large quantities, only one unit should be collected at a time. Also, transfusion of not urgent blood at night should be avoided. Effective identity checks between patient and the blood unit including the component special requirements are key requirements as it constitutes the final opportunity to avoid potentially fatal mis transfusion (last chance/bus stop to prevent mis transfusion). The check must be performed by two clinical staff for every unit transfused. The unit must be inspected thoroughly for signs of leakage, discoloration or clumps. The prescription and other relevant paperwork should be signed by the person administering the component including the component donation number, date, time of starting and stopping the transfusion, dose/volume of component transfused, and name of the administering practitioner should be recorded in the clinical record. Correct patient identification is crucial in transfusion safety. Failure in patient identification can result in wrong blood typing or transfusion of the wrong blood component. Many of these kinds of incidents are preventable by carefully checking patient data at the bedside prior to commencing the transfusion [398]. Changes in vital signs are regularly seen during transfusion. There is need for clinical staff to be aware of common transfusion reaction signs and symptoms to enable them to differentiate between a normal patient response from a life-threatening reaction [399, 400].

6.1 Monitoring during a blood transfusion

Blood transfusion is associated with adverse reactions or events. Patients having a blood transfusion should be regularly monitored before, during and post transfusion. Patients must be encouraged to report new symptoms. By monitoring and recording vital signs such as temperature, pulse, respiratory rate, and blood pressure regularly we can tell if a patient is having a transfusion reaction. These parameters are determined at baseline (at least 60 minutes) before commencement of the transfusion, 15 minutes after the start and regularly during and after the transfusion. Patient monitoring during transfusion is of paramount importance for prompt detection of transfusion reactions [401]. Transfusion reaction associated with transfusion of ABO incompatibility or bacterial transmission present early after commencing the transfusion [402]. Sometimes patients can have delayed transfusion reaction that will become evident 24 hours post transfusion. It is vital that the transfusion recipient is monitored over the next 24 hours. Any reaction observed during and after the transfusion of a blood component must be reported promptly and investigated. The guidelines of the British Committee for Standards in Haematology recommends that when any of the associated signs and symptoms of transfusion reactions occur, the initial treatment should be based on signs and symptoms rather than on classification [403].

6.2 Enhancing blood transfusion safety across the West African sub-region

Safe blood is a crucial component in improving health care and in preventing the transmission of infections. The two major challenges associated with blood transfusion service delivery across the West African sub region is that adequacy and safety [2, 404]. Developing countries have continued to lag behind in contributing her own quota to the allogenic blood pool globally. Out of the 92 million blood units were donated worldwide in 2008, only an insignificant 4 million (4.3%) were donated in sub-Saharan Africa- a continent that is home to approximately 12% of the global population [405]. The rate of blood donation across the region has remained consistently lower than rates in developed economies (4–5 per 1000 compared to 30 donations per 1000) respectively [406]. The World Health Organization recommends blood transfusion from low risk and altruistic regular voluntary non-remunerated blood donors (VNRBDs). However, VNRBDs represent <50% of whole blood donations in low-income countries compared with 76–100% in developed economies. The sub-region will need to abolish the unsafe commercial remunerated blood donation. Efforts should be made to enlighten the sub-region that family replacement donors are unsafe, there is difficulty in replacing blood in quantity and type through family replacement donation and blood donated can put transfusion recipient who are females of childbearing age at risk of developing alloantibodies that can cause HTR and HDFN if they receive blood from their husbands and his relatives. The region will need to look for innovative ways to encourage community members to change their mentality from being family replacement donors to becoming voluntary non-remunerated donors. VNRBDs are key to the maintenance of a safe and adequate blood supply. Education and public enlightenment, innovation, and pragmatic approach in the aspect of recruitment, retention, non-cash motivation and renewal of an active volunteer and non-remunerated donor pool from the massive young population in the sub region is key to safe and sustainable blood transfusion service delivery [407]. Transfusion-transmissible infections, such as HIV, hepatitis B virus (HBV), hepatitis C virus (HCV), syphilis, and malaria are prevalent across the sub region and have remained a source of safety concern for transfusion recipients. Transfusion of sub- optimally screened blood is the cause of 5–10% of HIV infections in sub-Saharan Africa and about 12.5% of transfusion recipients in the region are at risk of post-transfusion hepatitis [408]. Unsafe blood transfusion has a significant effect (socio, economic and health) on the sub region, families, communities, and the wider society [409]. The various markers of infection for these infective agents appear at different times after infection. The window periods (period between infection and availability of screening marker in the blood of the donor) vary depending on the infective agent (range from few days to months), the infectious agent and the screening marker and the technology used. In the window period a screening marker may not be detectable in a recently infected donor even though the donor may be infectious. Nucleic acid (RNA/DNA of the infectious agent) is the first detectable target to appear in blood, followed by the antigen (produced by the infectious agent), and finally the antibody following an immune response in the donor. The sub region will need to implement a policy of universal/mandatory screening of blood donors for HIV-1 and HIV-2, Hepatitis B, Hepatitis C and Syphilis as a minimum requirement [410]. The infectious agent, the screening marker, and the minimum technology to be employed should be defined by way of policy. For HIV-1 and HIV-2 screening using a combination of HIV antigen-antibody or HIV antibodies as a minimum and where possible nucleic acid testing is advocated. Screening for hepatitis B using hepatitis B surface antigen (HBsAg). Hepatitis C screening for either a combination of HCV antigen-antibody or HCV antibodies and where possible nucleic acid testing while for syphilis (Treponema pallidum) screening for specific treponemal antibodies should be implemented across the sub region. The use of only antibody-based test for screening donors for HIV and HCV should be discouraged to prevent the risk of introducing donor blood in the window phase of infection into the blood donor pool [411]. All efforts and energy need to be invested by member countries of ECOWAS to minimize the risks of transfusion-transmitted infection particularly during the window phase of infectious agent to make blood safer [2]. Implementation of stringent donor selection criteria and deferral system is the first step in determining the suitability of a potential blood donor to donate blood [412]. It can determine eligibility and identify donors whose behaviours put them potentially at risk for blood donation warranting either temporal or permanent deferral. The implementation of a robust donor deferral strategy can have a positive impact on transfusion safety in the West African sub-region [413]. A better understanding of the reasons for deferral of potential blood donors across the sub region could assist in donor recruitment planning and gives insight into the general health of the population in terms of prevalence of TTIs and anaemia. The presence of anaemia and risk of TTIs are the predominant contributors to donor deferral among donors [414, 415]. Member countries in the sub region will need to improve on the donor screening and deferral procedures as well as serologic testing. The aim of deferral is to facilitate the exclusion of donors from potentially higher risk populations to enhance patient safety [416]. The sub region will need to develop an efficient donor screening and deferral system to ensure the safety of both prospective donors and recipients [417]. The need for allogenic blood in the West African sub region has continued to be on the increase for several reasons; increase in the number of elective surgeries, failure to match demand and supply, suboptimal functioning of the national blood transfusion services, lack of relevant policies, trained personnel, funding and appropriate infrastructure in member states, dominance of unsafe family replacement and commercial remunerated blood transfusion rather than safe and altruistic voluntary non-remunerated blood donors, old and emerging threats of transfusion-transmitted infection, poor management of coagulopathy, major haemorrhage and bleeding disposition in surgical patients and pregnant women, prevalent insurgencies and communal clashes, increase in road traffic accidents due to poor road infrastructure in some member states, armed conflicts, insurgency and banditry, high prevalence of sickle cell disease, nutritional and malaria associated anaemia and pregnancy-related complications. All these factors have made allogenic blood a vital but limited commodity across the sub region. The region will need to think strategically out of the box to identify innovative ways to recruit and retain voluntary low-risk blood donors. Education, public enlightenment, and collaboration with stakeholders are key to changing the erroneous belief of the people towards donation of blood [418]. Countries in the West African sub region need to be smart, flexible and do things differently to ensure the adequacy and safety of blood transfusion service delivery in the sub region. Efforts should be made to make transfusion safer by implementing best practices in donor selection and screening. The use of other alternatives to allogenic blood (autologous transfusion, use of pharmacologic agents like oral, IV iron and erythropoietin to optimize haemoglobin of patients particularly those going for elective surgery, optimal management of trauma and associated major haemorrhage (trauma, surgical, ante and post-partum) by using haemorrhage limiting medication like antifibrinolytic, prothrombin complex concentrate, Novo7 and vitamin K [419]. The implementation of component therapy and universal leucodepletion of blood products will go a long way in ensuring the optimal management and safety of our limited allogenic blood stock. The need for the National blood transfusion services across the sub region to work synergistically under the umbrella of ECOWAS cannot be over emphasized to drive the organization and management, blood donor recruitment, collection, testing of donor blood and appropriate clinical use of blood. The sub region will need to invest significantly on human and infrastructural capital development by increasing the budget for training aimed at an increasing the number of transfusions service-related skilled workforce, providing an enabling working environment and proper renumeration of health workers. These implementations have the potential to improve the access to adequate and safe blood transfusion across the sub region.

7. Conclusion and recommendations

Blood transfusion service delivery across the west African sub region faces daunting but surmountable challenges bordering around adequacy and safety. The challenge of providing adequate and safe blood and blood product across the sub region is multi-dimensional and include; lack of transfusion policies and a fit for purpose National blood transfusion service in some ECOWAS countries, reliance on unsafe family replacement and commercial remunerated donors rather than safe benevolent voluntary non-remunerated donors who donate blood for altruistic purpose, suboptimal funding required to fund a quality blood transfusion service, inadequate number of skilled manpower, lack of political will to implement the haemovigilance system, reliance on suboptimal antibody-based screening method for donor screening for HIV, transfusion of leucocyte rich whole blood rather than leuco-depleted component therapy, suboptimal pre-transfusion screening of patients that require a red cell transfusion, poor cold chain management of blood and blood products, absence of specialized blood products like gamma irradiated blood CMV negative and antigen negative blood etc. required by certain patients group, poor management of Rh negative pregnancy and absence of universal access to anti-D prophylaxis, absence of a quality management system-based blood transfusion service, absence of indication coding tool to facilitate the effective clinical use of blood, lack of alloantibody prevention measures, poor management of haemolytic disease of the foetus and newborn, suboptimal use of laboratory testing to determine the coagulopathic status of patients billed for surgery to facilitate the effective management of the coagulopathy prior to surgery to reduce the risk of haemorrhage, poor management of major haemorrhage, suboptimal use of pharmacologic and non-pharmacologic alternatives to allogenic blood in anaemic and bleeding patients. These factors affect the adequacy and safety of blood transfusion across the sub-region.

8. Recommendations

We recommend the implementation of the following evidence-based best practices to ensure the safety, adequacy and timely provision of blood and blood products across the West African sub-region.

1. Countries in the sub region should implement a blood component to facilitate the optimum utilization of donated blood.

2. Implementation of a policy on universal leucodepletion of blood products transfused across the sub region to prevent the challenges associated with the transfusion of leucocyte- rich blood products.

3. There is need for government across the sub region to invest significantly in funding the national blood transfusion services to facilitate the safety and adequacy of blood transfusion.

4. Governments across the ECOWAS region need to invest in critical infrastructure including the utilization of the readily available green solar energy resource to manage the cold chain management of blood and blood products.

5. There should be the implementation of evidence-based best practices in alloimmunization prevention to prevent the incidence of haemolytic disease of the foetus and newborn across the sub-region.

6. Implementation of best practices in pre-transfusion testing including alloantibody screening and panel testing for patients whose alloantibody screening is positive to facilitate the provision of antigen negative donor blood for transfusion to the recipient.

7. There is need for a paradigm shift from the use of the less sensitive conventional tube method to the more sensitive column agglutination technique for blood transfusion testing including blood group, alloantibody testing and crossmatching.

8. There is need to develop a major haemorrhage protocol for use across the region to facilitate the effective management of patients with major haemorrhage.

9. Implementation of a donor screening algorithm for use across the sub region that reduces the risk of introducing donor blood in the window phase of transfusion -transmissible viral infection into the subregional blood pool.

10. There is need to develop a sub-regional protocol for the management of transfusion dependent patients to implement best practices like the implementation of extended phenotyping and universal access to use of chelating agents in these patients.

11. Implementation of a sub-regional indication coding tool to facilitate the effective clinical use of blood and blood products.

12. Provision of specialized products that is clinically indicated in several patients' groups like gamma irradiated blood, CMV negative blood, antigen negative blood, etc.

13. Implementation of a quality management-oriented blood transfusion service across the sub region that facilitates the delivery of a continually improving quality transfusion service.

14. There is need for the optimum remuneration, motivation and retention of healthcare workers involved in the entire blood transfusion process to prevent the brain drain of the sub-region human resource assets.

15. There is need for countries across the sub region to provide adequate budgetary allocation for the running of National Blood Transfusion services to facilitate the adequacy and safety of blood transfusion service delivery.

16. The is need for implementation of best practices, in patient identification, informed consent, prescription, pre- transfusion sampling, collection of blood from storage area, receipt of blood in clinical area, administration and monitoring during blood of transfusion.

17. There is need for the implementation of a sub-regional policy that promote the use of pharmacologic and non-pharmacologic alternatives in anaemic and bleeding patients to facilitate the optimum utilization of our limited allogenic blood stock on patients in whom these alternatives are contraindicated.

18. The implementation of a policy on universal access to anti-D prophylaxis in non-previously sensitized pregnant Rhesus D negative women as well as the introduction of cell-free foetal DNA testing for all Rh D negative pregnant women across the sub region to identify those carrying Rh D negative foetuses for which the use of the prophylaxis can be spared.

19. Facilities for non-invasive foetal maternal haemorrhage testing (Kleihauer or flow cytometry) should be provided to facilitate the optimum management of Rhesus D negative non-previously sensitized pregnant women following a potential sensitizing event to facilitate the administration of optimum dose of anti-D prophylaxis to prevent the women from being sensitized.

20. There is urgent need for the implementation of a unified haemovigilance system across the sub region that facilitates the reporting of all near misses, adverse events and reaction associated with donation and transfusion of blood allowing for the provision of a continually improving transfusion service delivery across the sub region.

21. There is need for the implementation of a policy that promotes safe and altruistic voluntary non- remunerated donor run national blood transfusion service rather than the unsafe family replacement donor system.

22. There should be a sub-regional policy to outlaw unsafe commercial remunerated donation of blood.

Author details

Osaro Erhabor[1,2]*, Josephine O. Akpotuzor[3], Edward Yaw Afriyie[4], Godswill Chikwendu Okara[5], Tosan Erhabor[6], Donald Ibe Ofili[6], Teddy Charles Adias[7], Idris Ateiza Saliu[8], Evarista Osime[9], Alhaji Bukar[10], Oyetunde B. Akinloye[11], Zakiya Abdul-Mumin[12], John Ocquaye-Mensah Tetteh[13], Edwin G. Narter-Olaga[14], Andrews Yashim-Nuhu[15], Folashade Aturamu[15], Ayodeji Olusola Olayan[16], Adeyinka Babatunde Adedire[17], Oyeronke Suebat Izobo[18], Kolawole A. Fasakin[19], Onyeka Paul[20], Collins Ohwonigho Adjekuko[21], Elliot Eli Dogbe[22] and Uloma Theodora Ezeh[23]

1 Blood Transfusion Faculty, West African Postgraduate College of Medical Laboratory Science, Wupa, Nigeria

2 Department of Haematology and Blood Transfusion Science, Usmau Danfodiyo University Sokoto, Sokoto, Nigeria

3 Department of Haematology and Blood Transfusion Science, University of Calabar, Nigeria

4 KNUST/KATH, Kumasi, Ghana

5 West African Postgraduate College of Medical Laboratory Science, Nigeria

6 Medical Laboratory Science Council of Nigeria, Abuja Nigeria

7 Federal University Utuoke Bayelsa State, Nigeria

8 Safe Blood for Africa Foundation, South Africa

9 University of Benin, Benin City Edo State, Nigeria

10 Medical Laboratory Science Department, University of Maiduguri/Blood Bank, University of Maiduguri Teaching Hospital, Nigeria

11 Association of Medical Laboratory Scientists of Nigeria (AMLSN), Nigeria

12 Tamale Teaching Hospital, Ghana

13 National Blood Service, Ghana

14 Department of Blood Bank and Serology, Ghana Association of Medical Laboratory Scientists –GAMLS, Ghana

15 National Hospital, Abuja, Nigeria

16 Department of Medical Laboratory Science Afe Babalola University, Nigeria

17 Federal Medical Center, Owo, Nigeria

18 Lagos State College of Health Technology Yaba, Nigeria

19 Federal Teaching Hospital, Ido Ekiti, Nigeria/ ELIZADE University, Ilaramokin, Nigeria

20 University of Abuja Teaching Hospital Gwagwalada, Abuja, Nigeria

21 University of Delta, Agbor, Nigeria

22 Komfo Anokye Teaching Hospital, Ghana

23 Department of Haematology and blood transfusion, Nnamdi Azikiwe University Teaching Hospital Nnewi, Nigeria

*Address all correspondence to: n_osaro@yahoo.com

References

[1] Barro L, Drew VJ, Poda GG, Tagny CT, El-Ekiaby M, Ofori SO, et al. Blood transfusion in sub-Saharan Africa: Understanding the missing gap and responding to present and future challenges. Vox Sanguinis. 2018;**113**(8):726-736

[2] Erhabor O, Adias TC. The challenges of meeting the blood transfusion requirements in sub-Saharan Africa: The need for the development of alternatives to allogenic blood. Journal of Blood Medicine. 2011;**2**:7-21

[3] Pape A, Stein P, Horn O, Habler O. Clinical evidence of blood transfusion effectiveness. Blood Transfusion. 2009;**7**(4):250-258

[4] Letowska M. Patient-specific component requirements: 'Right blood, right patient, right time, right place. ISBT Science Series. 2009;**4**:52-55

[5] World Health Organization. Global Status Report on Blood Safety and Availability. Geneva, Switzerland: World Health Organization; 2016

[6] Evans R, Ferguson E. Defining and measuring blood donor altruism: A theoretical approach from biology, economics, and psychology. Vox Sanguinis. 2014;**106**(2):118-126

[7] Tagny CT, Laperche S, Murphy EL. Francophone Africa network for transfusion medicine research. Updated characteristics of blood services, donors and blood products in 11 French-speaking African countries. Vox Sanguinis. 2018;**113**(7):647-656

[8] Kanagasabai U, Michelle S, Chevalier BD, Mili FD, Qualls ML, Bock N, et al. Trends and gaps in National Blood Transfusion Services — 14 sub-Saharan African countries, 2014-2016. Morbidity and Mortality Weekly Report (MMWR). 2018;**67**(50):1392-1396

[9] Hensher M, Jefferys E. Financing blood transfusion services in sub-Saharan Africa: A role for user fees. Health Policies and Planning. 2000;**15**(30):287-295

[10] Asamoah-Akuoko L, Hassall OW, Bates I, Ullum H. Blood donors' perceptions, motivators and deterrents in sub-Saharan Africa – A scoping review of evidence. British Journal of Haematology. 2017;**177**(6):864-877

[11] Roman L, Armstrong B, Smart E. Donation testing and transfusion transmissible infections. ISBT Science Series. 2020;**15**:192-206

[12] Pruett CR, Vermeulen M, Zacharias P, Ingram C, Tagny CT, Bloch EM. The use of rapid diagnostic tests for transfusion infectious screening in Africa: A literature review. Transfusion Medicine Reviews. 2015;**29**:35-44

[13] Vamvakas EC, Blajchman MA. Universal WBC reduction: The case for and against. Transfusion. 2001;**41**:691-712

[14] Erhabor O, Adias TC. From whole blood to component therapy: The economic, supply/demand need for implementation of component therapy in sub-Saharan Africa. Transfusion Clinique et Biologique. 2011;**18**(5-6):516-526

[15] Samukange WT, Kluempers V, Porwal M, et al. Implementation and performance of haemovigilance systems in 10 sub-Saharan African countries

is sub-optimal. BMC Health Services Research. 2021;**21**:1258. DOI: 10.1186/s12913-021-07235-0

[16] Patidar GK, Kaur D. Audit and education: Role in safe transfusion practice. Asian Journal of Transfusion Science. 2018;**12**(2):141-145

[17] Stanworth SJ, Walwyn R, Grant-Casey J, et al. Effectiveness of enhanced performance feedback on appropriate use of blood transfusions: A comparison of 2 cluster randomized trials. JAMA Network Open. 2022;**5**(2):e220364

[18] Zomorrodi A, Picciola EA, Hotwagner DT. Determining the need for blood transfusion. [updated 2021 Oct 21]. In: StatPearls. Treasure Island (FL): StatPearls Publishing; 2022. [Internet] Available from: https://www.ncbi.nlm.nih.gov/books/NBK564300/

[19] Basu D, Kulkarni R. Overview of blood components and their preparation. Indian Journal of Anaesthesia. 2014;**58**(5):529-537

[20] Erhabor O, Adias TC. From whole blood to component therapy: The economic, supply/demand need for implementation of component therapy in sub-Saharan Africa. Transfusion Clinique et Biologique. 2011;**18**(5-6, 526):516

[21] Kumar H, Gupta PK, Mishra DK, Sarkar RS, Jaiprakash M. Leucodepletion and blood products. Medical Journal, Armed Forces India. 2006;**62**(2):174-177

[22] Pruss A, Kalus U, Radtke H, Koscielny J, Bsumsnn-Zbaretti B. Balzer universal leukodepletion of blood components results in a significant reduction of febrile non-hemolytic but not allergic transfusion reactions. Transfusion and Apheresis Science. 2004;**30**:41-46

[23] Tagny CT, Diarra A, Yahaya R, et al. Characteristics of blood donors and donated blood in sub-Saharan Francophone Africa. Transfusion. 2009;**49**:1592-1599

[24] Stacy A, Gurevitz MD. Update and utilization of component therapy in blood transfusions. Laboratory Medicine. 2010;**41**(2):739-744

[25] Benedict N, Aigberadion U, Nwannadi IA, Aigbe I. Knowledge, attitude, and practice of voluntary blood donation among physicians in a tertiary health facility of a developing country. International Journal of Blood Transfusion and Immunohematology. 2012;**2**(2):4-10

[26] Aliyu I, Michael G, Ibrahim H, Ibrahim ZF, Aliyu G, Isaiah AT. Blood transfusion request pattern in a medical Centre in North-western Nigeria. Global Journal of Transfusion Medicine. 2017;**2**(1):52-55

[27] Arewa OP. One-year clinical audit of the use of blood and blood components at a tertiary hospital in Nigeria. Nigerian Journal of Clinical Practice. 2009;**12**(4):429-433

[28] Obi E, Diette-Spiff C, Omunakwe H. Knowledge and practices of physicians on blood component therapy: A cross-sectional study from two tertiary hospitals in Nigeria. African Health Sciences. 2021;**21**(3):1230-1236

[29] Tapko JB, Toure B, Sambo LG. Status of Blood Safety in the Who African Region. Report of the 2010 Survey. Regional Office for Africa: World Health Organization. 2014;**2014**:14-16

[30] Sawadogo S, Nébié K, Kafando E, et al. Preparation of red cell concentrates

in low-income countries: Efficacy of whole blood settling method by simple gravity in Burkina Faso. International Journal of Blood transfusion and Immunohematology. 2016;**6**:20-29

[31] Ala F, Allain JP, Bates I, et al. External financial aid to blood transfusion services in sub-Saharan Africa: A need for reflection. PLoS Medicine. 2012;**9**:e1001309

[32] Manning, R. and Grabowski, H. Key economic and value considerations in the U.S. market for plasma protein therapies. 2018. Available from: https://www.bateswhite.com/newsroom-insight-197.html. [Accessed on January 4, 2020].

[33] Burnouf T. Current status and new developments in the production of plasma derivatives. ISBT Science Series. 2016;**11**(2):18-25

[34] Aalaei S, Amini S, Keramati MR, Shahraki H, Eslami S. Monitoring of storage and transportation temperature conditions in red blood cell units: A cross-sectional study. Indian Journal of Hematology & Blood Transfusion. 2019;**35**(2):304-312

[35] Shabihkhani M, Lucey GM, Wei B, Mareninov S, Lou JJ, Vinters HV, et al. The procurement, storage, and quality assurance of frozen blood and tissue biospecimens in pathology, biorepository, and biobank settings. Clinical Biochemistry. 2014;**47**(4-5):258-266

[36] Ramirez-Arcos S, Mastronardi C, Perkins H, Kou Y, Turner T, Mastronardi E, et al. Evaluating the 4-hour and 30-minute rules: Effects of room temperature exposure on red blood cell quality and bacterial growth. Transfusion. 2013;**53**(4):851-859

[37] Norfolk D. UK blood transfusion services. In: Handbook of Transfusion Medicine. 5. London: Stationery Office; 2013

[38] Groth S. Manual on the Management, Maintenance and Use of Blood Cold Chain Equipment. Geneva: World Health Organization; 2005

[39] James V, McClelland B. Guidelines for the Blood Transfusion Services in the United Kingdom. London: The Stationery Office; 2005

[40] Sigle JP, Holbro A, Lehmann T, Infanti L, Gerull S, Stern M, et al. Temperature-sensitive indicators for monitoring RBC concentrates out of controlled temperature storage. American Journal of Clinical Pathology. 2015;**144**(1):145-150

[41] Ramirez-Arcos S, Mastronardi C, Perkins H, Kou Y, Turner T, Mastronardi E, et al. Evaluating the 4-hour and 30-minute rules: Effects of room temperature exposure on red blood cell quality and bacterial growth. Transfusion. 2013;**53**(4):851-859

[42] Dumani D, Goldfinger D, Ziman A. Is the 30-minute rule still applicable in the 21st century? Transfusion. 2013;**53**(6):1150-1152

[43] Thomas S, Wiltshire M, Hancock V, Fletcher S, McDonald C, Cardigan R. Core temperature changes in red blood cells. Transfusion. 2011;**51**(2):442-443

[44] Yu YB, Briggs KT, Taraban MB, et al. Grand challenges in pharmaceutical research series: Ridding the cold chain for biologics. Pharmaceutical Research. 2021;**38**:3-7

[45] Mitra R, Mishra N, Rath GP. Blood groups systems. Indian Journal of Anaesthesia. 2014;**58**(5):524-528

[46] Avent ND, Reid ME. The Rhesus blood group system. Journal of

American Society of Hematology. 2000;**95**(2):375-387

[47] Jeremiah ZA. An assessment of the clinical utility of routine antenatal screening of pregnant women at first clinic attendance for haemoglobin genotypes, haematocrit, ABO and Rh blood groups in Port Harcourt, Nigeria. African Journal of Reproductive Health. 2005;**9**:112-117

[48] Loua A, Lamah MR, Haba NY, Camara M. Frequency of blood groups ABO and rhesus D in the Guinean population. Transfusion Clinique et Biologique. 2007;**14**:435-439

[49] Tagny CT, Fongué VF, Mbanya D. The erythrocyte phenotype in ABO and Rh blood groups in blood donors and blood recipients in a hospital setting of Cameroon: Adapting supply to demand. Revue Médicale de Bruxelles. 2009;**30**:159-162

[50] Bergstrom S, Pereira C, Hagstrom U, Safwenberg J. Obstetric implications of rhesus antigen distribution in Mozambican and Swedish women. Gynecologic and Obstetric Investigation. 1994;**38**:82-86

[51] Weinstein L. Irregular antibodies causing haemolytic disease of the newborn: A continuing problem. Clinical Obstetrics and Gynecology. 1982;**25**:321-332

[52] Bowman J. Hemolytic disease (erythroblastosis fetalis). In: Creasy R, Resnik R, editors. Prevention of Rh Alloimmunization. Philadelphia, PA: WB Saunders Co; 1999. pp. 736-738

[53] Catrina FR. Hemolytic disease of the newborn. REX Lab Bulletin. 2007;**126**:1-4

[54] Belinga S, Ngo SF, Bilong C, Manga J, Mengue MA, Tchendjou P. High prevalence of anti-D antibodies among women of childbearing age at Centre Pasteur of Cameroon. African Journal of Reproductive Health. 2009;**13**:47-52

[55] Gajjar K, Spencer C. Diagnosis and management of non-anti-D red cell antibodies in pregnancy. The Obstetrician and Gynaecologist. 2009;**11**:89-95

[56] Kumar S, Regan F. Management of pregnancies with RhD alloimmunisation. British Medical Journal. 2005;**330**:1255-1258

[57] Erhabor O, Isaac Z, Yakubu A, Adias T. Abortion, ectopic pregnancy, and miscarriage in sub Saharan Africa: Challenges of rhesus isoimmunization in rhesus negative women. Open Journal of Obstetrics and Gynecology. 2013;**3**:15-26

[58] Avent ND. RHD genotyping from maternal plasma: Guidelines and technical challenges. Methods in Molecular Biology. 2008;**444**:185-201

[59] Harkness M, Freer Y, Prescott RJ, Warner P. Implementation of NICE recommendation for a policy of routine antenatal anti-D prophylaxis: A survey of UK maternity units. Transfusion Medicine. 2008;**18**:292-295

[60] McBain RD, Crowther CA, Middleton P. Anti-D administration in pregnancy for preventing rhesus alloimmunisation. Cochrane Database of Systematic Reviews. 2015;**2015**(9):CD000020

[61] Carroli G, Rooney C, Villar J. How effective is antenatal care in preventing maternal mortality and serious morbidity? An overview of the evidence. Paediatric and Perinatal Epidemiology. 2001;**15**:1-42

[62] Correa P, Linhard J, Diebolt G, Diadhiou F. Study of bilirubin in

amniotic fluid associated with fetomaternal isoimmunization at Dakar. Bulletin de la Société Médicale d'Afrique Noire de Langue Française. 1969;**14**:262-266

[63] Verkuyl DA. Economics of anti-rhesus prophylaxis in an African population. The Central African Journal of Medicine. 1987;**33**:32-37

[64] Ahman E, Shah I. Unsafe abortion: Worldwide estimates for 2000. Reproductive Health Matters. 2002;**10**:13-17

[65] Osaro E, Charles AT. Rh isoimmunization in sub-Saharan Africa indicates need for universal access to anti-RhD immunoglobulin and effective management of D-negative pregnancies. International Journal of Women's Health. 2010;**2**:429-437

[66] Cakana AZ, Ngwenya L. Is antenatal antibody screen worthwhile in the Zimbabwean population? The Central African Journal of Medicine. 2001;**47**:26-28

[67] Toure Ecre A, Horo FM, Konan SK, Ble R, Kone M. Management of rhesus alloimmunisation by spectrophotometry: About one case at the Yopougon teaching hospital, Côte- d'Ivoire. Bulletin de la Société de Pathologie Exotique. 2006;**99**:245-249

[68] Darmstadt GL, Lee AC, Cousens S, et al. 60 million non-facility births: Who can deliver in community settings to reduce intrapartum-related deaths? International Journal of Gynaecology and Obstetrics. 2009;**107**(1):S89-S112

[69] Kotila TR, Odukogbe AA, Okunlola MA, Olayemi O, Obisesan KA. The pregnant rhesus negative Nigerian woman. The Nigerian Postgraduate Medical Journal. 2005;**12**:305-307

[70] Lapierre Y, Riga D, Adam J, Josef D, Meyer F, Greber S, et al. The gel test: A new way t~ detect red cell antigen-antibody reactions. Transfusion. 1990;**30**:109-113

[71] Dara RC, Tiwari AK, Mitra S, Acharya D, Aggarwal G, Arora D, et al. Comparison of a column agglutination technology-based automated immunohematology analyzer and a semiautomated system in pretransfusion testing. Asian Journal of Transfusion Science. 2019;**13**(2):115-119

[72] Duguid KM. (1997) uses of column technology in blood transfusion. Hematology. 1997;**2**(6):485-489

[73] Varshney L, Gupta S. Comparison between conventional tube technique and column agglutination technique for antibody screening and identification at Mgm blood Bank, Navi Mumbai. Journal of Evolution of Medical and Dental Sciences. 2017;**6**(92):6551

[74] Das SS, Chaudhary R, Khetan D. A comparison of conventional tube test and gel technique in evaluation of direct antiglobulin test. Hematology. 2007;**12**(2):175-178

[75] Raos M. Evaluation of antibody screening and identification pre-transfusion tests using DG gel cards. Journal of Applied Health Sciences. 2018;**4**(2):179-186

[76] Finck R, Lui-Deguzman C, Teng SM, et al. Comparison of a gel microcolumn assay with the conventional tube test for red blood cell alloantibody titration. Transfusion. 2013;**53**(4):811-815

[77] Winters JL, Richa EM, Bryant SC, et al. Polyethylene glycol antiglobulin tube versus gel microcolumn: Influence on the incidence of delayed haemolytic transfusion reactions and delayed

serologic reactions. Transfusion. 2010;**50**(7):1444-1452

[78] Patil V, Shetmahajan M. Massive transfusion and massive transfusion protocol. Indian Journal of Anaesthesia. 2014;**58**(5):590-955

[79] Calvert C, Thomas SL, Ronsmans C, Wagner KS, Adler AJ, Filippi V. Identifying regional variation in the prevalence of postpartum haemorrhage: A systematic review and meta-analysis. PLoS One. 2012;7(7):e41114

[80] GBD 2015 Maternal Mortality Collaborators. Global, regional, and national levels of maternal mortality,1990-2015: A systematic analysis for the global burden of disease study 2015. Lancet. 2016;**388**:1775-1812

[81] Lancaster L, Barnes RFW, Correia M, Luis E, Boaventura I, Silva P, et al. Maternal death and postpartum hemorrhage in sub-Saharan Africa - a pilot study in metropolitan Mozambique. Research and Practice in THROMBOSIS AND Haemostasis. 2020;**4**(3):402-412

[82] Kavle JA, Stoltzfus RJ, Witter F, Tielsch JM, Khalfan SS, Caulfield LE. Association between anaemia during pregnancy and blood loss at and after delivery among women with vaginal births in Pemba Island, Zanzibar, Tanzania. Journal of Health, Population, and Nutrition. 2008;**26**:232-240

[83] WOMAN Trial Collaborators. Effect of early tranexamic acid administration on mortality, hysterectomy, and other morbidities in women with post-partum haemorrhage (WOMAN): An international, randomised, double-blind, placebo-controlled trial. Lancet. 2017;**389**:2105-2116

[84] Li B, Miners A, Shakur H, Roberts I. Tranexamic acid for treatment of women with post-partum haemorrhage in Nigeria and Pakistan: A cost-effectiveness analysis of data from the WOMAN trial. The Lancet Global Health. 2018;**6**:e222-e228

[85] Black RE, Levin C, Walker N, Chou D, Liu L, Temmerman M. Reproductive, maternal, newborn, and child health: Key messages from disease control priorities 3rd edition. Lancet. 2016;**388**:2811-2824

[86] Bazirete O, Nzayirambaho M, Umubyeyi A, Karangwa I, Evans M. Risk factors for postpartum haemorrhage in the Northern Province of Rwanda: A case control study. PLoS One. 2022;**17**(2):e0263731

[87] Asamoah-Akuoko L, Hassall OW, Bates I, Ullum H. Blood donors' perceptions, motivators and deterrents in sub-Saharan Africa- a scoping review of evidence. British Journal of Haematology. 2017;**177**:864-877

[88] Nyflot LT, Sandven I, Stray-Pedersen B, Pettersen S, Al-Zirqi I, Rosenberg M, et al. Riskfactors for severe postpartum haemorrhage: A case-control study. BMC Pregnancy and Childbirth. 2017;**17**:17

[89] Knight M, Callaghan WM, Berg C, Alexander S, Bouvier-Colle MH, Ford JB, et al. Trends in postpartum hemorrhage in high resource countries: A review and recommendations from the international postpartum hemorrhage collaborative group. BMC Pregnancy and Childbirth. 2009;**9**:55

[90] Kyei-Nimakoh M, Carolan-Olah M, McCann TV. Access barriers to obstetric care at health facilities in sub-Saharan Africa-a systematic review. Systematic Reviews. 2017;**6**(1):110

[91] Heitkamp A, Aronson SL, van den Akker T, et al. Major obstetric

haemorrhage in metro east, Cape Town, South Africa: A population-based cohort study using the maternal near-miss approach. BMC Pregnancy and Childbirth. 2020;**20**:14. DOI: 10.1186/s12884-019-2668-x

[92] Ejekam CS, Okafor IP, Anyakora C, Ozomata EA, Okunade K, Oridota SE, et al. Clinical experiences with the use of oxytocin injection by healthcare providers in a southwestern state of Nigeria: A cross-sectional study. PLoS One. 2019;**14**(10):e0208367

[93] Lalonde A, Davis BA, Acosta A, Herschderefer K. Postpartum haemorrhage today: ICM/FIGO initiative 2004-2006. IJGO. 2006;**94**:243-253

[94] Hill K, Thomas K, AbouZahar C, et al. Estimates of maternal mortality worldwide between 1990 and 2005: An estimate of available data. Lancet. 2007;**370**:1311-1319

[95] Obaid T. No woman should die giving life. Lancet. 2007;**370**:1287-1288

[96] International Federation of Gynecology & Obstetrics. Prevention and treatment of postpartum haemorrhage. New Advances for Low Resource Settings. ICM/FIGO Joint Statement. FIGO Safe Motherhood and Newborn Health (SMNH) Committee / International Journal of Gynecology and Obstetrics. 2012;**70**:108-118

[97] Ronsmans C, Graham W. Maternal mortality: Who, when where and why. Lancet. 2006;**368**:1189-1200

[98] Say L, Chou D, Gemmill A, Tunçalp Ö, Moller AB, Daniels J, et al. Global causes of maternal death: A WHO systematic analysis. The Lancet. Global Health. 2014;**2**:323-333

[99] Cantwell R, Clutton-Brock T, Cooper G, Dawson A, Drife D, Garrod D, et al. Saving mothers' lives: Reviewing maternal deaths to make motherhood safer: 2006-2008. An Int J Obstet Gynaecol. 2011;**118**:1-203

[100] Booth C, Allard S. Major haemorrhage protocols. ISBT Science Series. 2018;**13**:219-228

[101] Zehtabchi S, Nishijima DK. Impact of transfusion of fresh-frozen plasma and packed red blood cells in a 1:1 ratio on survival of emergency department patients with severe trauma. Academic Emergency Medicine. 2009;**16**:371-378

[102] Murad, M.H., Stubbs, J.R., Gandhi,M.J., Wang, A.T., Paul, A., Erwin, P.J., Montori, V.M. & Roback, J.D. The effect of plasma transfusion on morbidity and mortality: A systematic review and meta- analysis. Transfusion2010; 50:1370– 1383.

[103] Cardenas JC, Rahbar E, Pommerening MJ, Baer LA, Matijevic N, Cotton BA, et al. Measuring thrombin generation as a tool for predicting haemostatic potential and transfusion requirements following trauma. Journal of Trauma and Acute Care Surgery. 2014;**7**:839-845

[104] Davenport RA, Guerreiro M, Rourke C, Platton S, Cohen M, Pearse R, et al. Activated protein C drives the hyperfibrinolysis of acute traumatic coagulopathy. Anesthesiology. 2017;**126**:115-127

[105] Schochl H, Cotton B, Inaba K, Nienaber U, Fischer H, Voelckel W, et al. FIBTEM provides early prediction of massive transfusion in trauma. Critical Care. 2011a;**15**:R265

[106] Hiippala ST, Myllyla GJ, Vahtera EM. Hemostatic factors and replacement of major blood loss with plasma-poor red cell concentrates.

Anesthesia and Analgesia. 1995;**81**:360-365

[107] Spahn DR, Bouillon B, Cerny V, et al. The European guideline on management of major bleeding and coagulopathy following trauma: Fifth edition. Critical Care. 27 Mar 2019;**23**(1):98. DOI: 10.1186/s13054-019-2347-3

[108] Schöchl H, Maegele M, Solomon C, Görlinger K, Voelckel W. Early and individualized goal- directed therapy for trauma-induced coagulopathy. Scand J trauma Resusc. Emergency Medicine. 2012;**20**:15. DOI: 10.1186/1757-7241-20-15

[109] Joint United Kingdom (UK). Blood transfusion and tissue transplantation services professional advisory committee. Transfusion management of major haemorrhage. Last updated01/04/2020

[110] Ghadimi K, Levy JH, Welsby IJ. Prothrombin complex concentrates for bleeding in the perioperative setting. Anesthesia and Analgesia. 2016;**122**(5):1287-1300

[111] Lau P, Ong V, Tan WT, Koh PL, Hartman M. Use of activated recombinant factor VII in severe bleeding - evidence for efficacy and safety in trauma, postpartum Hemorrhage, cardiac surgery, and gastrointestinal bleeding. Transfusion Medicine and Hemotherapy. 2012;**39**(2):139-150

[112] Wikkelsø A, Wetterslev J, Møller AM, Afshari A. Thromboelastography (TEG) or thromboelastometry (ROTEM) to monitor haemostatic treatment versus usual care in adults or children with bleeding. Cochrane Database of Systematic Reviews. 2016;**2016**(8):CD007871

[113] Curry NS, Davenport R. Transfusion strategies for major haemorrhage in trauma. British Journal of Haematology. 2019;**184**(4):508-523

[114] Cotton BA, Reddy N, Hatch QM, LeFebyre E, Wade CE, Kozar RA, et al. Damage control resuscitation is associated with a reduction in resuscitation volumes and improvement in survival in 390 damage control laparotomy patients. Annals of Surgery. 2011a;**254**:598-605

[115] Hunt BJ, Allard S, Keeling D, et al. A practical guideline for the haematological management of major haemorrhage. British Journal of Haematology. 2015;**170**:788-803

[116] Bates I, Owusu-Ofori S. Blood transfusion. Manson's Tropical Diseases. 2009:229-234. DOI: 10.1016/B978-1-4160-4470-3.50018-5

[117] World Health Organization (WHO). Screening donated blood for transfusion-transmissible infections: Recommendations. In: 4, Screening for Transfusion-Transmissible Infections. Geneva: World Health Organization; 2009. Available from: https://www.ncbi.nlm.nih.gov/books/NBK142989/

[118] Scott SR, Zunyou W. Risks and challenges of HIV infection transmitted via blood transfusion. Biosafety and Health. 2019;**1**(3):124-128

[119] Bianco C, Kessler D. Donor notification and counselling management of blood donors with positive test results. Vox Sanguinis. 1994;**67**(3):255-259

[120] World Health Organization (WHO). Screening Donated Blood for Transfusion-Transmissible Infections. Geneva: World Health Organization; 2010. [17 August 2012] Available from: http://www.who.int/bloodsafety/publications/bts_screendondbloodtransf/en/index.html

[121] Polizzotto MN, Wood EM, Ingham H, Keller AJ. Australian red cross blood service donor and product safety team. Reducing the risk of transfusion-transmissible viral infection through blood donor selection: The Australian experience 2000 through 2006. Transfusion. 2008;**48**(1):55-63

[122] Dwyre DM, Fernando LP, Holland PV. Hepatitis B, hepatitis C and HIV transfusion-transmitted infections in the 21st century. Vox Sanguinis. 2011;**100**:92-98

[123] Chaurasia R, Zaman S, Das B, Chatterjee K. Screening donated blood for transfusion transmitted infections by serology along with NAT and response rate to notification of reactive results: An Indian experience. Journal of Blood Transfusion. 2014;**2014**:412105. DOI: 10.1155/2014/412105

[124] Nübling CM, Heiden M, Chudy M, Kress J, Seitz R, Keller-Stanislawski B, et al. Experience of mandatory nucleic acid test (NAT) screening across all blood organizations in Germany: NAT yield versus breakthrough transmissions. Transfusion. 2009;**49**(9):1850-1858

[125] Hans R, Marwaha N. Nucleic acid testing-benefits and constraints. Asian Journal of Transfusion Science. 2014;**8**(1):2-3

[126] Aneke JC, Okocha CE. Blood transfusion safety; current status and challenges in Nigeria. Asian Journal of Transfusion Science. 2017;**11**(1):1-5. DOI: 10.4103/0973-6247.200781

[127] World Health Organization. Modern list of essential medicines for 2019. Available from: https://apps.who.int/iris/bitstream/handle/10665/325771/WHO-MVP-EMPIAU-2019.06-eng.pdf. [Last accessed on May 20, 2021]

[128] WHO. Universal Access to Safe Blood. 2010. Feb 11, [Last accessed on 2013 Dec 06]. Available from: http://www.who.int/bloodsafety/universalbts/en/index.html

[129] Jeremiah ZA, Koate B, Buseri F, Emelike F. Prevalence of antibodies to hepatitis C virus in apparently healthy Port Harcourt blood donors and association with blood groups and other risk indicators. Blood Transfusion. 2008;**6**:150-155

[130] Buseri FI, Muhibi MA, Jeremiah ZA. Sero-epidemiology of transfusion-transmissible infectious diseases among blood donors in Osogbo, South-West Nigeria. Blood Transfusion. 2009;7:293-299

[131] Okocha EC, Aneke JC, Ezeh TU, Ibeh NC, Nwosu GA, Okorie IO, et al. The epidemiology of transfusion-transmissible infections among blood donors in Nnewi, South-East Nigeria. African Journal of Medical and Health Sciences. 2015;**14**:125-129

[132] Ahmed SG, Ibrahim UA, Hassan AW. Adequacy and pattern of blood donations in north-eastern Nigeria: The implications for blood safety. Annals of Tropical Medicine and Parasitology. 2007;**101**:725-731

[133] Emeribe AO, Ejele AO, Attai EE, Usanga EA. Blood donation and patterns of use in Southeastern Nigeria. Transfusion. 1993;**33**:330-332

[134] Okocha EC, Aneke JC, Ezeh TU, Ibeh NC, Nwosu GA, Okorie IO, et al. The epidemiology of transfusion-transmissible infections among blood donors in Nnewi, south-East Nigeria. African Journal of Medical and Health Sciences. 2015;**14**:125-129

[135] Bolarinwa RA, Aneke JC, Olowookere SA, Salawu L. Seroprevalence

of transfusion transmissible viral markers in sickle cell disease patients and healthy controls in Ile-Ife, southwestern Nigeria: A case-control study. Journal of Applied Hematology. 2015;**6**:162-167

[136] Kassim OD, Oyekale TO, Aneke JC, Durosinmi MA. Prevalence of seropositive blood donors for hepatitis B, C and HIV viruses at the Federal Medical Centre, Ido-Ekiti, Nigeria. Annals of Tropical Pathology. 2012;**3**:47-55

[137] Ugwu A, Madu A, Efobi C, et al. Pattern of blood donation and characteristics of blood donors in Enugu, Southeast Nigeria. Nigerian Journal of Clinical Practice. 2018;**21**:1438-1444

[138] Loua A, Sonoo J, Musango L, et al. Blood safety status in WHO African region countries: Lessons learnt from Mauritius. Journal of Blood Transfusion. 2017;**2017**:e1970479

[139] Klein HG, Spahn DR, Carson JL. Red blood cell transfusions in clinical practice. Lancet. 2007;**370**:415-436

[140] Tayler VV. Blood Bank Technical Manual, 13th Ed. Maryland, USA: AABB; 1999. pp. 175-176

[141] Kientz D, Laforet M, Isola H, Cazenave JP. Leukodepletion of platelet concentrates and plasma collected with haemonetics MCS+ apheresis system. Experience of EFS-Alsace. Transfusion and Apheresis Science. 2001;**25**:55-59

[142] Pruss A, Kalus U, Radtke H, KoscielnyJ, Bsumsnn-ZbarettiBB. Universal Luekodepletion of blood components results in a significant reduction of febrile non-hemolytic but not allergic transfusion reactions. Transfusion and Apheresis Science. 2004;**30**:41-46

[143] Begue S. Leukocyte depletion. Transfusion Clinique et Biologique. 1998;**5**:411-414

[144] Hitzler WE. Apherese- und Pool-Thrombozytenkonzentrat--Wertigkeit und Bewertung beider Blutkomponenten [single-donor (apheresis) platelets and pooled whole-blood-derived platelets--significance and assessment of both blood products]. Clinical Laboratory. 2014;**60**(4):S1-S39

[145] Cazzola M, Borgna-Pignatti C, Locatelli F, et al. A moderate transfusion regimen may reduce iron loading in beta-thalassemia major without producing excessive expansion of erythropoiesis. Transfusion. 1997;**37**:135-140

[146] Schiffer CA. Diagnosis, and management of refractoriness to platelet transfusion. Blood Reviews. 2001;**15**(4):175-180

[147] Cheng CK, Lee CK, Lin CK. Clinically significant red blood cell antibodies in chronically transfused patients: A survey of Chinese thalassemia major patients and literature review. Transfusion. 2010;**52**:2220-2224

[148] Rios M, Hue-Roye K, Storry JR, Reiss RF. Cell typing the sensitized transfusion-dependent patient. Annals of Clinical and Laboratory Science. 2000;**30**(4):379-386

[149] Joint United Kingdom (UK). Blood transfusion and tissue transplantation services professional advisory committee. Transfusion in Surgery. Last updated01/04/2020. 5th edition, Handbook for Transfusion Medicine; Jan 2014

[150] Liumbruno GM, Bennardello F, Lattanzio A, Piccoli P, Rossetti G. Italian Society of Transfusion Medicine and Immunohaematology Working Party. Recommendations for the transfusion management of patients in the peri-operative period. III. The post-operative period. Blood Transfusion. 2011;**9**(3):320-335

[151] Elmistekawy E, Rubens F, Hudson C, McDonald B, Ruel M, Lam K, et al. Preoperative anaemia is a risk factor for mortality and morbidity following aortic valve surgery. European Journal of Cardio-Thoracic Surgery. 2013;**44**(6):1051-1056

[152] Thachil J, Gatt A, Martlew V. Management of surgical patients receiving anticoagulation and antiplatelet agents. The British Journal of Surgery. 2008;**95**(12):1437-1448

[153] Polania Gutierrez JJ, Rocuts KR. Perioperative anticoagulation management. In: StatPearls [Internet]. Treasure Island (FL): StatPearls Publishing; 2022. [Updated 2022 Jan 26] Available from: https://www.ncbi.nlm.nih.gov/books/NBK557590/

[154] Kay LA, Noble RS. Systematic pre-deposit autologous blood provision for elective surgery: An important contribution to hospital blood supply. Vox Sanguinis. 1990;**59**(1):23-25

[155] Kawahara Y, Ohtsuka K, Tanaka K, et al. Use of laboratory testing for prediction of postoperative bleeding volume in cardiovascular surgery. Thrombosis. 2021:70. DOI: 10.1186/s12959-021-00324-4

[156] Jakoi A, Kumar N, Vaccaro A, et al. Perioperative coagulopathy monitoring. Musculoskeletal Surgery. 2014;**98**:1-8

[157] Themistoklis T, Theodosia V, KonstantinosK, GeorgiosDI. Perioperative blood management strategies for patients undergoing total knee replacement: Where do we stand now? World Journal of Orthopedics. 2017;**8**(6):441-454

[158] Pei Z, Szallasi A. Prevention of surgical delays by pre-admission type and screen in patients with scheduled surgical procedures: Improved efficiency. Blood Transfusion. 2015;**13**(2):310-312

[159] Spahn DR, Spahn GH, Stein P. Evidence base for restrictive transfusion triggers in high-risk patients. Transfusion Medicine and Hemotherapy. 2015;**42**(2):110-114

[160] Loor G, Rajeswaran J, Li L, et al. The least of 3 evils: Exposure to red blood cell transfusion, anemia, or both? The Journal of Thoracic and Cardiovascular Surgery. 2013;**146**:1480-1487

[161] Vaglio S, Prisco D, Biancofiore G, Rafanelli D, Antonioli P, Lisanti M, et al. Recommendations for the implementation of a patient blood management programme. Application to elective major orthopaedic surgery in adults. Blood Transfusion. 2016;**14**(1):23-65

[162] Lawson T. Ralph, C, Perioperative Jehovah's witnesses: A review. BJA: British Journal of Anaesthesia. 2015;**115**(5):676-687

[163] Mundy GM, Birtwistle SJ, Power RA. The effect of iron supplementation on the level of Hb after lower limb arthroplasty. Journal of Bone and Joint Surgery. British Volume (London). 2005;**87-B**:213-217

[164] Muñoz M, Naveira E, Seara J, Cordero J. Effects of postoperative intravenous iron on transfusion requirements after lower limb arthroplasty. British Journal of Anaesthesia. 2012;**108**:532-534

[165] Hofmann A, Farmer S, Shander A. Five drivers shifting the paradigm from product-focused transfusion practice to patient blood management. The Oncologist. 2011;**16**(3):3-11

[166] Steuber TD, Howard ML, Nisly SA. Strategies for the Management of Postoperative Anemia in elective Orthopedic surgery. The Annals of Pharmacotherapy. 2016;**50**(7):578-585

[167] Thavarajah S, Choi MJ. The use of erythropoiesis-stimulating agents in patients with CKD and cancer: A clinical approach. American Journal of Kidney Diseases. 2019;**74**(5):667-674

[168] Singer ST, Wu V, Mignacca R, Kuypers FA, et al. Alloimmunization and erythrocyte autoimmunization in transfusion-dependent thalassemia patients of predominantly Asian descent. Blood. 2000;**96**:3369-3373

[169] Thompson AA, Cunningham MJ, Singer ST, et al. Red cell alloimmunization in a diverse population of patients with thalassaemia. British Journal of Haematology. 2011;**153**:121-128

[170] Ugwu NI, Awodu OA, Bazuaye GN, Okoye AE. Red cell alloimmunization in multi-transfused patients with sickle cell anemia in Benin City, Nigeria. Nigerian Journal of Clinical Practice. 2015;**18**:522-526

[171] Ugwu A, O, Madu AJ, Anigbogu IO. Blood transfusion in sub-Saharan Africa: Historical perspective, clinical drivers of demand and strategies for increasing availability. African Sanguine. 2021;**23**(1):14-20

[172] Ugwu NI, Awodu OA, Bazuaye GN, Okoye AE. Red cell alloimmunization in multi-transfused patients with sickle cell anemia in Benin City, Nigeria. Nigerian Journal of Clinical Practice. 2015;**18**:522-526

[173] Kangiwa U, Ibegbulam O, Ocheni S, Madu A, Mohammed N. Pattern and prevelence of alloimmunization in multiply transfused patients with sickle cell disease in Nigeria. Biomarker Research. 2015;**3**:26

[174] Jeremiah ZA, Mordi A, Buseri FI, Adias TC. Frequencies of maternal red blood cell alloantibodies in Port Harcourt, Nigeria. Asian J Transfus Sci. 2011;**5**:39-41

[175] Nadarajan SN, Hlaing AA, Maung TH, Jeyajoti I, Kyu TN, Ranjana KJ, et al. Incidence of red cell alloantibodies in a multi-ethnic hospital patient population. Vox Sanguinis. 2007;**93**:63-64

[176] Schonewille H, van de Watering LMG, Loomans DSE, Brand A. Red blood cell alloantibodies after transfusion: Factors influencing incidence and specificity. Transfusion. 2006;**46**:250-256

[177] Yousuf R, Abdul Aziz S, Yusof N, Leong CF. Incidence of red cell alloantibody among the transfusion recipients of Universiti Kebangsaan Malaysia medical Centre. Indian Journal of Hematology and Blood Transfusion. 2013;**29**(2):65-70

[178] Qureshi H, Massey E, Kirwan D, Davies T, Robson S, White J, et al. BCSH guideline for the use of anti-D immunoglobulin for the prevention of haemolytic disease of the foetus and newborn. Transfusion Medicine. 2014;**24**(1):8-20

[179] Clausen FB, Christiansen M, Steffensen R, et al. Report of the first nationally implemented clinical routine screening for fetal RHD in D– pregnant women to ascertain the requirement for antenatal RhD prophylaxis. Transfusion. 2012;**52**:752-758

[180] Lindemburg ITM, van Kamp IL, van Zwet EW, et al. Increased perinatal

loss after intrauterine transfusion for alloimmune anaemia before 20 weeks of gestation. BJOG: An International Journal of Obstetrics andGynaecology. 2013;**120**:847-852

[181] Smith HM, Shirey RS, Thoman SK, Jackson JB. Prevalence of clinically significant red blood cell alloantibodies in pregnant women at a large tertiary care facility. Immunohematology. 2013;**29**:127-130

[182] Wassie GT, Belete MB, Tesfu AA, Bantie SA, Ayenew AA, Endeshaw BA, et al. Association between antenatal care utilization pattern and timely initiation of postnatal care checkup: Analysis of 2016 Ethiopian demographic and health survey. PLoS One. 2021;**16**(10):e0258468

[183] Okeke TC, Ocheni S, Nwagha UI, Ibegbulam OG. The prevalence of rhesus negativity among pregnant women in Enugu, Southeast Nigeria. Nigerian Journal of Clinical Practice. 2012;**15**(4):400-402

[184] Smith HM, Shirey RS, Thoman SK, Jackson JB. Prevalence of clinically significant red blood cell alloantibodies in pregnant women at a large tertiary care facility. Immunohematology. 2013;**29**:127-130

[185] Pegoraro V, Urbinati D, Visser GHA, Di Renzo GC, Zipursky A, Stotler BA, et al. Hemolytic disease of the fetus and newborn due to Rh(D) incompatibility: A preventable disease that still produces significant morbidity and mortality in children. PLoS One. 2020;**15**(7):e0235807

[186] Krywko DM, Yarrarapu SNS, Shunkwiler SM. Kleihauer Betke test. In: StatPearls [Internet]. Treasure Island (FL): StatPearls Publishing; 2022. [Updated 2021 Aug 11] Available from: https://www.ncbi.nlm.nih.gov/books/NBK430876/

[187] Kim YA, Makar RS. Detection of fetomaternal hemorrhage. American Journalof Hematology. 2012;**87**(4):417-423

[188] Tiblad E, Taune Wikman A, Ajne G, Blanck A, Jansson Y, Karlsson A, et al. Targeted routine antenatal anti-D prophylaxis in the prevention of RhD immunisation--outcome of a new antenatal screening and prevention program. PLoS One. 2013;**8**(8):e70984

[189] Urgessa F, Tsegaye A, Gebrehiwot Y, Birhanu A. Assessment of feto-maternal haemorrhage among rhesus D negative pregnant mothers using the Kleihauer-betke test (KBT) and flow cytometry (FCM) in Addis Ababa, Ethiopia. BMC Pregnancy and Childbirth. 2014;**14**(1):358

[190] Golassa L, Tsegaye A, Erko B, Mamo H. High rhesus (Rh(D)) negative frequency and ethnic- group based ABO blood group distribution in Ethiopia. BMC Research Notes. 2017;**10**(1):330

[191] McBain RD, Crowther CA, Middleton P. Anti-D administration in pregnancy for preventing rhesus alloimmunisation. Cochrane Database of Systematic Reviews. 2015;**2015**(9):CD000020

[192] Ayenew AA. Prevalence of rhesus D-negative blood type and the challenges of rhesus D immunoprophylaxis among obstetric population in Ethiopia: A systematic review and meta-analysis. Maternal Health, Neonatology and Perinatology. 2021;**7**(1):8

[193] National Institute for Health and Clinical Excellence (NICE G156). 2008 WHO Reproductive Health Library. WHO Recommendation on Antenatal Anti-D Immunoglobulin Prophylaxis. December 2016

[194] Chanko KP. Frequency of ABO blood group and Rh (D) negative mothers among pregnant women attending at antenatal Care Clinic of Sodo Health Center, SNNPR, Ethiopia. American Journal of Clinical and Experimental Medicine. 2020;**8**:10-14

[195] Chilcott J, Lloyd JM, Wight J, Forman K, Wray J, Beverley C, et al. A Review of the Clinical Effectiveness and Cost-Effectiveness of Routine Anti-D Prophylaxis for Pregnant Women Who Are Rhesus-Negative. United Kingdom: NICE Technology Appraisal Guidance; 2022. p. 41

[196] Nadarajan SN, Hlaing AA, Maung TH, Jeyajoti I, Kyu TN, Ranjana KJ, et al. Incidence of red cell alloantibodies in a multi-ethnic hospital patient population. Vox Sanguinis. 2007;**93**:63-64

[197] Schonewille H, van de Watering LMG, Loomans DSE, Brand A. Red blood cell alloantibodies after transfusion: Factors influencing incidence and specificity. Transfusion. 2006;**46**:250-256

[198] Yousuf R, Abdul Aziz S, Yusof N, Leong CF. Incidence of red cell alloantibody among the transfusion recipients of Universiti Kebangsaan Malaysia medical Centre. Indian Journal of Hematology and Blood Transfusion. 2013;**29**(2):65-70

[199] Xie XFQ, Bao Z, Zhang Y, Zhou D. Clinical value of different anti-D immunoglobulin strategies for preventing Rh haemolytic disease of the foetus and newborn: A network meta-analysis. PLoS One. 2020;**15**(3):e0230073

[200] American College of Obstetricians and Gynaecologists. ACOG practice bulletin No. 181: Prevention of Rh D alloimmunization. Clinical management guidelines for obstetrician-gynaecologists. Obstetrics & Gynaecology. 2017;**130**(2):e57-e70

[201] De Vries RR, Faber JC, Strengers PF. Haemovigilance: An effective tool for improving transfusion practice. Vox Sanguinis. 2011;**100**:60-67

[202] Wood EM, Ang AL, Bisht A, Bolton-MaggsPH,BokhorstAG,FleslandO, et al. International haemovigilance: What have we learned and what do we need to do next? Transfusion Medicine. 2019;**29**:221-230

[203] Diekamp U, Gneißl J, Rabe A, Kießig ST. Donor Hemovigilance with blood donation. Transfusion Medicine and Hemotherapy. 2015;**42**(3):181-192

[204] Stainsby D, Faber JC, Jorgensen J. Overview of hemovigilance. In: Simon TL, Solheim BG, Straus RG, Snyder EL, Stowell CP, editors. Rossi's Principles of Transfusion Medicine. 4th ed. West Sussex: Blackwell Publishing; 2009. p. 694

[205] Jean-Claude F. Hemovigilance: Definition and overview of current Hemovigilance systems. Transfusion Alternatives in Transfusion Medicine. 2008;**5**(1):237-245

[206] Ministry of Health and Family Welfare, Government of India. National Blood Policy. New Delhi: National AIDS Control Organisation; 2003

[207] Faber JC. The European blood directive: A new era of blood regulation has begun. Transfusion Medicine. 2004;**14**:257-273

[208] Watson R. EU tightens rules on blood safety. BMJ. 2005;**331**:800

[209] Proposed standard definitions for surveillance of noninfectious

adverse transfusion rections [Internet] International Haemovigilance Network. 2011. [Last Accessed on 2012 Jun 25]. Available from: http://www.isbtweb.org/fileadmin/user_upload/WP_on_Haemovigilance/ISBT_definitions_final_2011_.pdf

[210] Samukange WT, Kluempers V, Porwal M, Mudyiwenyama L, Mutoti K, Aineplan N, et al. Implementation and performance of haemovigilance systems in 10 sub-saharan African countries is sub-optimal. BMC Health Services Research. 2021;**21**(1):1258

[211] Lemssahli I, Hajjout K, Benajiba M, Belmekki A. Haemovigilance recipients at the Rabat regional blood transfusion Center 2015-2019. Acta Scientific Paediatrics. 2021;**4**(3):56-62

[212] Dahourou H, Tapko JB, Nébié Y. et al, Implementation of hemovigilance in sub-Saharan Africa. Transfusion clinique et biologique : journal de la Société française de transfusion sanguine. 2012;**19**:39-45

[213] Ogunbanjo G. Are there alternatives to the shortage of blood in South Africa? South African Family Practice. 2014;**56**:5. DOI: 10.1080/20786190.2014.1002985

[214] Kleinman S, Chan P, Robillard P. Risks associated with transfusion of cellular blood components in Canada. Transfusion Medicine Reviews. 2003;**17**:120-162

[215] Jimenez K, Kulnigg-Dabsch S, Gasche C. Management of iron deficiency anemia. Gastroenterología y Hepatología. 2015;**11**(4):241-250

[216] Muñoz M. Editorial: Iron therapy in clinical practice: An overview. Transfusion Alternatives in Transfusion Medicine. 2012;**12**(3-4):41-43. DOI: 10.1111/j.1778-428X.2012.01179.x

[217] Mpoya A, Kiguli S, Olupot-Olupot P, et al. Transfusion and treatment of severe anaemia in African children (TRACT): A study protocol for a randomised controlled trial. Trials. 2015;**6**:593. DOI: 10.1186/s13063-015-1112-4

[218] Khalafallah A, Dennis A, Bates J, Bates G, Robertson IK, Smith L, et al. A prospective randomized, controlled trial of intravenous versus oral iron for moderate iron deficiency anaemia of pregnancy. J intern med. 2010 Sep;268(3):286-95Marik PE, Corwin HL. Efficacy of red blood cell transfusion in the critically ill: A systematic review of the literature. Critical Care Medicine. 2008;**36**:2667-2674

[219] Villanueva C, Alan C, Alba B, et al. Transfusion strategies for acute upper gastrointestinal bleeding. The New England Journal of Medicine. 2013;**368**(1):11-21

[220] Goodnough LT. Iron deficiency syndromes and iron-restricted erythropoeisis. Transfusion. 2012;**52**:1584-1592

[221] KDOQI, National Kidney Foundation. II. Clinical practice guidelines and clinical practice recommendations for anaemia in chronic kidney disease in adults. American Journal of Kidney Diseases. 2006;**47**(5):S16-S85

[222] Hofmann A, Farmer S, Towler SC. Strategies to preempt and reduce the use of blood products: An Australian perspective. Current Opinion in Anaesthesiology. 2012;**25**:66-73

[223] Munoz M, Gomez-Ramirez S, Bhandari S. The safety of available treatment options for iron- deficiency anemia. Expert Opinion on Drug Safety. 2018;**17**(2):149-159

[224] Shin HW, Park JJ, Kim HJ, You HS, Choi SU, Lee MJ. Efficacy of perioperative intravenous iron therapy for transfusion in orthopedic surgery: A systematic review and meta-analysis. PLoS One. 2019;**14**(5):e0215427

[225] Lyseng-Williamson KA, Keating GM. Ferric carboxymaltose: A review of its use in iron-deficiency anaemia. Drugs. 2009;**69**:739-756

[226] Fishbane S. Review of issues relating to iron and infection. American Journal of Kidney Diseases. 1999;**34**(4):S47-S52

[227] Litton E, Xiao J, Ho KM. Safety and efficacy of intravenous iron therapy in reducing requirement for allogeneic blood transfusion: Systematic review and meta-analysis of randomized clinical trials. BMJ. 2015;**347**:f4822.

[228] Ionescu A, Sharma A, Kundnani NR, et al. Intravenous iron infusion as an alternative to minimize blood transfusion in peri-operative patients. Scientific Reports. 2020;**10**:18403. DOI: 10.1038/s41598-020-75535-2

[229] Jelkmann, W. Physiology and Pharmacology of Erythropoietin. Transfusion Medicine Hemotherapy (Switzerland). 2013;**40**(5):302-309

[230] Jelkmann W. Erythropoietin. Frontiers of Hormone Research. 2016;**47**:115-127

[231] Zarychanski R, Turgeon AF, McIntyre L, et al. Erythropoietin-receptor agonists in critically ill patients: A meta-analysis of randomized controlled trials. CMAJ. 2007;**177**:725-734

[232] Corwin HL, Gettinger A, Fabian TC, et al. Efficacy and safety of epoetin alfa in critically ill patients. The New England Journal of Medicine. 2007;**357**:965-976

[233] Shin HJ, Ko E, Jun I, Kim HJ, Lim CH. Effects of perioperative erythropoietin administration on acute kidney injury and red blood cell transfusion in patients undergoing cardiac surgery: A systematic review and meta-analysis. Medicine (Baltimore). 2022;**101**(9):e28920

[234] Alghamdi AA, Albanna MJ, Guru V, Brister SJ. Does the use of erythropoietin reduce the risk of exposure to allogeneic blood transfusion in cardiac surgery? A systematic review and meta-analysis. Journal of Cardiac Surgery. 2006;**21**(3):320-326

[235] Jelkmann W. Physiology and pharmacology of erythropoietin. Transfusion Medicine and Hemotherapy. 2013 Oct;**40**(5):302-309

[236] McCullough PA, Barnhart HX, Inrig JK, Reddan D, Sapp S, Patel UD, et al. Cardiovascular toxicity of epoetin-alfa in patients with chronic kidney disease. American Journal of Nephrology. 2013;**37**(6):549-558

[237] Gershanik J, Boecler B, Ensley H, McCloskey S, George W. The gasping syndrome and benzyl alcohol poisoning. The New England Journal of Medicine. 1982;**307**(22):1384-1388

[238] Adias TC, Jeremiah Z, Uko E, Osaro E. Autologous blood transfusion – A review. SAJS. 2006;**44**(3):114-118

[239] Blumberg N, Vanderlinde ES, Heal JM. Autologous transfusion. BMJ. 2002;**324**:772-775

[240] Parker-Williams EJ. Autologous blood transfusion. Postgraduate Doctor: Africa. 1989;**11**:52-56

[241] Goodnough LT, Brecher ME, Kanter MH, et al. Transfusion medicine. Second of two parts — Blood conservation. The New England Journal of Medicine. 1999;**340**:525-533

[242] Huet C, Salmi LR, Fergusson D, et al. A meta-analysis of the effectiveness of cell salvage to minimize perioperative allogeneic blood transfusion in cardiac and orthopedic surgery. International Study of Perioperative Transfusion (ISPOT) Investigators Anesth Analg. 1999;**89**:861-869

[243] Hayden SJ, Albert TJ, Watkins TR, Swenson ER. Anemia in critical illness: Insights into etiology, consequences, and management. American Journal of Respiratory and Critical Care Medicine. 2012;**185**(10):1049-1057

[244] Hébert PC, Wells G, Blajchman MA, et al. A multicenter, randomized, controlled clinical trial of transfusion requirements in critical care. Transfusion requirements in critical care investigators, Canadian critical care trials group. The New England Journal of Medicine. 1999;**340**:409-417

[245] Lacroix J, Hébert PC, Hutchison JS, et al. Transfusion strategies for patients in paediatric intensive care units. The New England Journal of Medicine. 2007;**356**:1609-1619

[246] Tinmouth AT, McIntyre LA, Fowler RA. Blood conservation strategies to reduce the need for red blood cell transfusion in critically ill patients. CMAJ. 2008;**178**(1):49-57

[247] Kirpalani H, Whyte RK, Andersen C, et al. The premature infants in need of transfusion (PINT) study: A randomized, controlled trial of a restrictive (low) versus liberal (high) transfusion threshold for extremely low birth weight infants. The Journal of Pediatrics. 2006;**149**:301-307

[248] Wu WC, Rathore SS, Wang Y, et al. Blood transfusion in elderly patients with acute myocardial infarction. The New England Journal of Medicine. 2001;**345**:1230-1236

[249] Hardy JF, de Moerloose P, Samama CM. The coagulopathy of massive transfusion. Vox Sanguinis. 2005;**89**:123-127

[250] Snyder EL. Component therapy to cellular therapy and beyond—A Darwinian approach to transfusion medicine. Transfusion. 2008;**48**(9):2000-2007

[251] Makarovska-Bojadzieva T, Blagoevska M, Kolevski P, Kostovska S. Optimal blood grouping and antibody screening for safe transfusion. Contributions / Macedonian Academy of Sciences and Arts, Section of Biological and Medical Sciences. 2009;**30**(1):119-128

[252] Hoeltge GA, Domen RE, Rybicki LA, Schaffer PA. Multiple red cell transfusions and alloimmunization. Experiences with 6996 antibodies detected in a total of 159,262 patients from 1985-1993. Archives of Pathology & Laboratory Medicine. 1995;**119**:42-45

[253] Boisen ML, Collins RA, Yazer MH, Waters JH. Pretransfusion testing and transfusion of uncrossmatched erythrocytes. Anesthesiology. 2015;**122**:191-195

[254] Makarovska-Bojadzieva T, Velkova E, Blagoevska M. The impact of extended typing on red blood cell Alloimmunization in transfused patients. Open Access Macedonian Journal of Medical Sciences. 2017;**5**(2):107-111

[255] Azarkeivan A, Ansari S, Ahmadi MH, Hajibeigy B, Maghsudlu M, Nasizadeh S, et al. Blood transfusion

and alloimmunization in patients with thalassemia: Multicenter study. Pediatric Hematology and Oncology. 2011;**28**(6):479-485

[256] Sanz C, Nomdedeu M, Belkaid M, Martinez I, Nomdedeu B, Pereira A. Red blood cell alloimmunization in transfused patients with myelodysplastic syndrome or chronic myelomonocytic leukemia. Transfusion. 2013;**53**(4):710-715

[257] Vichinsky EP, Luban NL, Wright E, Olivieri N, Driscoll C, Pegelow CH, et al. Prospective RBC phenotype matching in a stroke-prevention trial in sickle cell anaemia: A multicenter transfusion trial. Transfusion. 2001;**41**(9):1086-1092

[258] Mark HY, Jonathan HW, Philip C. Spinella on behalf of the AABB (formerly known as the American Association of Blood Banks)/trauma, Hemostasis, oxygenation resuscitation network (THOR) working party; use of Uncrossmatched erythrocytes in emergency bleeding situations. Anesthesiology. 2018;**128**:650-656

[259] Anderson KC, Weinstein HJ. Transfusion-associated graft-versus-host disease. The New England Journal of Medicine. 1990;**323**:315-321

[260] Kopolovic I, Ostro J, Tsubota H, Lin Y, Cserti-Gazdewich CM, Messner HA, et al. A systematic review of transfusion-associated graft-versus-host disease. Blood. 2015;**126**:406-414

[261] Manduzio P. Transfusion-associated graft-versus-host disease: A concise review. Hematology Reports. 2018;**10**(4):7724

[262] Hutchinson K, Kopko PM, Muto KN, Tuscano J, O'Donnell RT, Holland PV, et al. Early diagnosis and successful treatment of a patient with transfusion associated GVHD with autologous peripheral blood progenitor cell transplantation. Transfusion. 2002;**42**:1567-1572

[263] Leitman SF, Tisdale JF, Bolan CD, Popovsky MA, Klippel JH, Balow JE, et al. Transfusion-associated GVHD after fludarabine therapy in a patient with systemic lupus erythematosus. Transfusion. 2003;**43**:1667-1671

[264] Slivnick DJ, Ellis TM, Nawrocki JF, Fisher RI. The impact of Hodgkin's disease on the immune system. Seminars in Oncology. 1990;**17**:673-682

[265] Treleaven J, Gennery A, Marsh J, Norfolk D, Page L, Parker A, et al. Guidelines on the use of irradiated blood components prepared by the British Committee for Standards in haematology blood transfusion task force. British Journal of Haematology. 2011;**152**:35-51

[266] Robinson S, Harris A, Atkinson S, Atterbury C, Bolton-Maggs P, Elliott C, et al. The administration of blood components: A British Society for Haematology guideline. Transfusion Medicine. 2018;**28**(1):3-21

[267] Vassallo RR, Murphy S. A critical comparison of platelet preparation methods. Current Opinion in Hematology [Review]. 2006;**13**(5):323-330

[268] Gurkan E, Patah PA, Saliba RM, Ramos CA, Anderson BS, Champlin R, et al. Efficacy of prophylactic transfusions using single donor apheresis platelets versus pooled platelet concentrates in AML/MDS patients receiving allogeneic hematopoietic stem cell transplantation. Bone Marrow Transplant. [Comparative Study Evaluation Studies]. 2007;**40**(5):461-464

[269] Schrezenmeier H, Seifried E. Buffy-coat-derived pooled platelet concentrates and apheres is platelet concentrates: Which product type should be preferred? Vox Sanguinis [Review]. 2010;**99**(1):1-15

[270] Heddle NM, Arnold DM, Boye D, et al. Comparing the efficacy and safety of apheresis and whole blood-derived platelet transfusions: A systematic review. 2008. In: Database of Abstracts of Reviews of Effects (DARE): Quality-Assessed Reviews [Internet]. York (UK): Centre for Reviews and Dissemination (UK); 1995. Available from: https://www.ncbi.nlm.nih.gov/books/NBK75900/

[271] Andreu G, Vasse J, Sandid I, Tardivel R, Semana G. Use of random versus apheresis platelet concentrates. Transfusion Clinique et Biologique. 2007;**14**(6):514-521

[272] Hod E, Schwartz J. Platelet transfusion refractoriness. British Journal of Haematology. 2008;**142**(3):348-360

[273] Belizaire R, Makar RS. Non-Alloimmune mechanisms of thrombocytopenia and refractoriness to platelet transfusion. Transfusion Medicine Reviews. 2020;**34**(4):242-249

[274] Kekomäki R. Use of HLA- and HPA—Matched platelets in alloimmunized patients. Vox Sanguinis. 1998;**74**(2):359-363

[275] Saris A, Pavenski K. Human leukocyte antigen Alloimmunization and Alloimmune platelet refractoriness. Transfusion Medicine Reviews. 2020;**34**(4):250-257

[276] Rebulla P. A mini review on platelet refractoriness. Haematologica. 2005;**90**(2):247-253

[277] Marktel S, Napolitano S, Zino E, et al. Platelet transfusion refractoriness in highly immunized beta thalassemia children undergoing stem cell transplantation. Pediatric Transplantation. 2010;**14**(3):393-401

[278] Cohn CS. Platelet transfusion refractoriness: How do I diagnose and manage? Hematology. American Society of Hematology. Education Program. 2020;**2020**(1):527-532

[279] Amemiya Y. Platelet transfusion refractoriness and effective management of platelet alloimmunization. Nihon Rinsho. 1997;**55**(9):2392-2398

[280] Cardigan R, New HV, Tinegate H, Thomas S. Washed red cells: Theory and practice. Vox Sanguinis. 2020;**115**(8):606-616

[281] Acker JP, Hansen AL, Yi QL, et al. Introduction of a closed-system cell processor for red blood cell washing post implementation monitoring of safety and efficacy. Transfusion. 2016;**56**(1):49-57

[282] Masalunga C, Cruz M, Porter B, Roseff S, Chui B, Mainali E. Increased hemolysis from saline pre-washing RBCs or centrifugal pumps in neonatal ECMO. Journal of Perinatology. 2007;**27**(6):380-384

[283] Liu C, Liu X, Janes J, et al. Mechanism of faster NO scavenging by older stored red blood cells. Redox Biology. 2014;**2**:211-219

[284] Razonable RR, Humar A. AST infectious diseases Community of Practice. Cytomegalovirus in solid organ transplantation. American Journal of Transplantation. 2013;**13**(4):93-106

[285] Kotton CN. CMV: Prevention, diagnosis and therapy. American Journal of Transplantation. 2013;**13**(3):24-40

[286] Azevedo LS, Pierrotti LC, Abdala E, Costa SF, Strabelli TM, Campos SV, et al.

Cytomegalovirus infection in transplant recipients. Clinics (São Paulo, Brazil). 2015;**70**(7):515-523

[287] Jebakumar D, Bryant P, Linz W. Risk of cytomegalovirus transmission by blood products after solid organ transplantation. Proceedings (Baylor University. Medical Center). 2019;**32**(2):222-226

[288] Sharma RR, Marwaha N. Leukoreduced blood components: Advantages and strategies for its implementation in developing countries. Asian Journal of Transfusion Science. 2010;**4**:3-8

[289] Myers JD, Flournoy N, Thomas ED. Risk factors for cytomegalovirus infection after human marrow transplantation. The Journal of Infectious Diseases. 1986;**153**:478-488

[290] Kotton CN, Kumar D, Caliendo AM, et al. Transplantation society international CMV consensus group. The third international consensus guidelines on the management of cytomegalovirus in solid-organ transplantation. Transplantation. 2018;**102**:900-931

[291] Tagny CT, Mbanya D, Tapko JB, Lefrère JJ. Blood safety in sub-Saharan Africa: A multi- factorial problem. Transfusion. 2008;**48**(6):1256-1261

[292] World Health Assembly resolution WHA28.72 Utilization and Supply of Human Blood and Blood Products. 1975

[293] World Health Assembly resolution WHA58.13 (Blood Safety) Proposal to Establish World Blood Donor Day. 2005WHA58/2005/REC/1. 2005

[294] World Health Organization Global database on blood safety: report 2001-2002. Available from: http://www.who.int/bloodsafety/GDBS_Report_2001-2002.pdf. [Accessed Nov 8 2010]

[295] Murphy E, Sanchez-Guerrero SA, Valiente-Banuet L, et al. Demographic characteristics, and infectious disease markers in blood donors in the Mexico-US border region (abstract). Vox Sanguinis. 2010;**99**:2

[296] Urbaniak SJ, Greiss MA. RhD haemolytic disease of the foetus and the newborn. Blood Reviews. 2000;**14**:44-461

[297] Liu KL, Li N, Li BJ, Peng JY, Shu XW, Yu YY. Clinical significance of anti-D IgG screening and titer detection in 286 RhD negative pregnant women. Zhongguo Dang Dai Er Ke Za Zhi. 2009;**11**(3):185-187

[298] Mari G, Deter RL, Carpenter RL, Rahman F, Zimmerman R, Moise KJ Jr, et al. Non-invasive diagnosis by Doppler ultrasonography of foetal anaemia due to maternal red cell alloimmunization. Collaborative Group for Doppler Assessment of the blood velocity in anaemic foetuses. The New England Journal of Medicine. 2000;**342**:9-14

[299] Moise KJ. Fetal anemia due to non-Rhesus-D red-cell alloimmunization. Seminars in Fetal & Neonatal Medicine. 2008;**13**:207-214

[300] Nordvall M, Dziegiel M, Hegaard HK, Bidstrup M, Jonsbo F, Christensen B, et al. Red blood cell antibodies in pregnancy and their clinical consequences: Synergistic effects of multiple specificities. Transfusion. 2009;**49**:2070-2075

[301] Eryilmaz M, Müller D, Rink G, Klüter H, Bugert P. Introduction of non-invasive prenatal testing for blood group and platelet antigens from

cell-free plasma DNA using digital PCR. Transfusion Medicine and Hemotherapy. 2020;**47**(4):292-301

[302] Armstrong-Fisher S, Koushki K, Mashayekhi K, Urbaniak SJ, Schoot E, Varzi AM. Confirmed non-invasive prenatal testing for foetal Rh blood group genotyping along with bi-allelic short insertion/deletion polymorphisms as a positive internal control. Transfusion Medicine. 2022;**32**(2):141-152. DOI: 10.1111/tme.12858

[303] Rieneck K, Clausen FB, Dziegiel MH. Non-invasive antenatal determination of foetal blood group using next-generation sequencing. Cold Spring Harbor Perspectives in Medicine. 2015;**6**(1):a023093

[304] Clausen FB, Jakobsen TR, Rieneck K, Krog GR, Nielsen LK, Tabor A, et al. Pre-analytical conditions in non-invasive prenatal testing of cell-free fetal RHD. PLoS One. 2013;**8**:e76990

[305] Rieneck K, Bak M, Jønson L, Clausen FB, Krog GR, Tommerup N, et al. Next-generation sequencing: Proof of concept for antenatal prediction of the fetal Kell blood group phenotype from cell-free foetal DNA in maternal plasma. Transfusion. 2013;**53**:2892-2898

[306] Condero D, Stampalija T, Bolzicco D, Castro Silva E, Candolini M, Cortivo C, et al. Fetal RHD detection from circulating cell-free fetal DNA in maternal plasma: Validation of a diagnostic kit using automatic extraction and frozen DNA. Transfusion Medicine. 2019;**29**(6):408-414

[307] Finning KM, Martin PG, Soothill PW, Avent ND. Prediction of fetal D status from maternal plasma: Introduction of a new non-invasive foetal RHD genotyping service. Transfusion. 2002;**42**:1079-1085

[308] Van der Schoot CE, Hayn S, Chitty LS. Non-invasive prenatal diagnosis and determinism of fetal Rh status. Seminars in Fetal & Neonatal Medicine. 2008;**13**(2):63-68

[309] Zipursky A, Paul VK. The global burden of Rh disease. Archives of Disease in Childhood. Fetal and Neonatal Edition. 2011;**96**:84-85

[310] Tagny CT, Fongué VF, Mbanya D. Erythrocyte phenotype in ABO and Rh blood groups in blood donors and blood recipients in a hospital setting of Cameroon: Adapting supply to demand. Revue Médicale de Bruxelles. 2009;**30**:159-162

[311] Mwangi J. Blood group distribution in an urban population of patient targeted blood donors. East African Medical Journal. 1999;**76**:615-618

[312] Loua A, Lamah MR, Haba NY, Camara M. Frequency of blood groups ABO and rhesus D in the Guinean population. Transfusion Clinique et Biologique. 2007;**14**:435-439

[313] NICE. The clinical effectiveness and cost effectiveness of routine anti-D prophylaxis for RhD-negative women in pregnancy. Technology appraisals TA41. 2002

[314] Ford J, Soothill P. Cell-free DNA foetal blood group testing for RhD-negative pregnant women: Implications for midwifery. Clinical Practice. British Journal of Midwifery. 2016;**2**(2)

[315] Finning K, Martin P, Summers J, et al. Effect of high throughput RHD typing of fetal DNA in maternal plasma on use of anti-RhD immunoglobulin in RhD negative pregnant women: Prospective feasibility study. BMJ. 2008;**336**(7648):816-818

[316] Kenny-Walsh E. Clinical outcomes after hepatitis C infection from contaminated anti-D immune globulin. Irish hepatology research group. The New England Journal of Medicine. 1999;**340**(16):1228-1233

[317] van der Schoot CE, Soussan AA, Koelewijn J, Bonsel G, Paget-Christiaens LG, de Haas M. Non-invasive antenatal RHD typing. Transfusion Clinique et Biologique. 2006;**13**(1-2):53-57

[318] Natukunda B, Schonewille H, Smit Sibinga CT. Assessment of the clinical transfusion practice at a regional referral hospital in Uganda. Transfusion Medicine. 2010;**20**(3):134-139

[319] Smit-Sibinga CT. Total quality management in blood transfusion. Vox Sanguinis. 2000;**78**(2):281-286

[320] Berte LM. Tools for improving quality in the transfusion service. American Journal of Clinical Pathology. 1997;**107**(4 Suppl 1):S36-S42

[321] Commission directive 2005/61/EC of 30 September 2005 implementing directive 2002/98/EC of the European Parliament and of the council as regards traceability requirements and notifications of serious adverse reactions and events. Official Journal of the European Union. 2005;**L256**:32

[322] Strengers P. Key elements of a blood transfusion quality management system, the tools and objectives. Special Issue: State of the Art Presentations. 21st Regional Congress of the ISBT. Europe-Lisbon, Portugal, Vox Sanguine. 2011;**101**(1):1-370

[323] Chaffe B, Glencross H, Jones J, Staves J, Capps-Jenner A, Mistry H, et al. UK transfusion laboratory collaborative: Minimum standards for staff qualifications, training, competency and the use of information technology in hospital transfusion laboratories 2014. Transfusion Medicine. 2014;**24**(6):335-340

[324] NHS England. 2014. Pathology quality assurance review. Available from: http://www.england.nhs.uk/publications/ind-rev/ [Accessed 21/10/14]

[325] Najafpour Z, Hasoumi M, Behzadi F, Mohamadi E, Jafary M, Saeedi M. Preventing blood transfusion failures: FMEA, an effective assessment method. BMC Health Services Research. 2017;**17**(1):453

[326] Sazama K. Reports of 355 transfusion-associated deaths:1976 through 1985. Transfusion. 1990;**30**:583-590

[327] Kohn LT, Corrigan JM, Donaldson MS. To err is human: Building a safer health system. In: Committee on Health Care in America. Institute of Medicine. Washington (DC): National Academy Press; 1999

[328] Osaro E, Chima N. Challenges of a negative workload and implications on morale, productivity and quality of service delivered in NHS laboratories in England. Asian Pacific Journal of Tropical Biomedicine. 2014;**4**(6):421-429

[329] Misau YA, Al-Sadat N, Gerei AB. Brain-drain and health care delivery in developing countries. Journal of Public Health in Africa. 2010;**1**(1):e6

[330] Hagopian A, Thompson MJ, Fordyce M, et al. The migration of physicians from sub-Saharan Africa to the United States of America: Measures of the African brain drain. Human Resources for Health. 2004;**2**:17

[331] Astor A, Akhtar T, Matallana MA, et al. Physician migration: Views from professionals in Colombia, Nigeria, India, Pakistan and the Philippines. Social Science & Medicine. 2005;**61**:2492-2500

[332] Kirigia JM, Gbary AR, Muthuri LK, et al. The cost of health professionals' brain drain in Kenya. BMC Health Services Research. 2006;**6**:89

[333] Haynes BP. An evaluation of the impact of the office environment on productivity. Facilities. 2008;**26**(5/6):178-195

[334] Cronk R, Bartram J. Environmental conditions in health care facilities in low- and middle- income countries: Coverage and inequalities. International Journal of Hygiene and Environmental Health. 2018;**221**(3):409-422

[335] World Health Organization. Essential Environmental Health Standards in Health Care WHO. Geneva: Switzerland; 2008

[336] Erasmus V, Daha TJ, Brug H, Richardus JH, Behrendt MD, Vos MC, et al. Systematic review of studies on compliance with hand hygiene guidelines in hospital care. Infection Control and Hospital Epidemiology. 2010;**31**(3):283-294

[337] Basu D, Kulkarni R. Overview of blood components and their preparation. Indian Journal of Anaesthesia. 2014;**58**(5):529-537

[338] Altin S, Altin A, Elevli B, Cerit O. Determination of hospital waste composition and disposal methods: A case study. Polish Journal of Environmental Studies. 2003;**12**(2):251-255

[339] Diaz LF, Eggerth LL, Enkhtsetseg SH, Savage GM. Characteristics of health carewaste. Waste Management. 2008;**28**(7):1219-1226

[340] Imam A, Mohammed B, Wilson DC, Cheeseman CR. Solid waste management in Abuja, Nigeria. Waste Management. 2008;**28**:468-472

[341] Wilson DC, Velis CA. Waste management—Still a global challenge in the 21st century: An evidence-based call for action. Waste Management & Research. 2015;**33**(12):1049-1051

[342] Godfrey L, Ahmed MT, Gebremedhin KG, Katima JH, Oelofse S, Osibanjo O, et al. Solid waste Management in Africa: Governance failure or development opportunity? In: Edomah N, editor. Regional Development in Africa [Internet]. London: IntechOpen; 2019. DOI: 10.5772/intechopen.86974

[343] Wilkinson R. Equipment and materials management. Introduction to Blood Transfusion Technology. 2006;**3**(2):248-253

[344] Guide to the preparation, use and quality assurance of blood components. In: European Committee (Partial Agreement) on Blood Transfusion (CD-P-TS). 19th Edition. 2007:45-49

[345] Jones RG, Johnson OA, Batstone G. Informatics and the clinical laboratory. Clinical Biochemist Reviews. 2014;**35**(3):177-192

[346] Nevalainen DE. Documentation and record keeping: The key to compliance. In: Sibinga CTS, Das PC, Heiniger HJ, editors. Good Manufacturing Practice in Transfusion Medicine. Developments in Hematology and Immunology. Vol. 29. Boston, MA: Springer; 1994. DOI: 10.1007/978-1-4615-2608-7_16

[347] Ardenghi D, Martinengo M, Bocciardo L, Nardi P, Tripodi G. Near miss errors in transfusion medicine: The experience of the G. Gaslini transfusion medicine service. Blood Transfusion. 2007;**5**(4):210-216

[348] Jersild C, Hafner V. Blood transfusion services. International Encyclopedia of. Public Health. 2017:247-253. DOI: 10.1016/B978-0-12-803678-5.00037-0

[349] Uríz MJ, Antelo ML, Zalba S, Ugalde N, Pena E, Corcoz A. Improved traceability and transfusion safety with a new portable computerised system in a hospital with intermediate transfusion activity. Blood Transfusion. 2011;**9**(2):172-181

[350] Samukange WT, Kluempers V, Porwal M, Mudyiwenyama L, Mutoti K, Aineplan N, et al. Implementation and performance of haemovigilance systems in 10 sub-Saharan African countries is sub-optimal. BMC Health Services Research. 2021;**21**(1):1258

[351] Tazi I, Loukhmas L, Benchemsi N. Hémovigilance: bilan 1995-2003 Casablanca. Transfusion Clinique et Biologique. 2005;**12**(3):257-274

[352] Ouadghiri S, Atouf O, Brick C, Benseffaj N, Essakalli M. Traçabilité des produits sanguins labiles au Maroc: expérience de l'hôpital Ibn-Sina de Rabat entre 1999 et 2010. Transfusion Clinique et Biologique. 2012;**19**(1):1-4

[353] Hughes RG. Tools and strategies for quality improvement and patient safety. In: Hughes RG, editor. Patient Safety and Quality: An Evidence-Based Handbook for Nurses. Rockville (MD): Agency for Healthcare Research and Quality (US); 2008. Chapter 44 Available from: https://www.ncbi.nlm.nih.gov/books/NBK2682/

[354] Rodziewicz TL, Houseman B, Hipskind JE. Medical error reduction and prevention. In: StatPearls [Internet]. Treasure Island (FL): Stat Pearls Publishing; 2022. [Updated 2022May1] Available from: https://www.ncbi.nlm.nih.gov/books/NBK499956/

[355] Hergon E. L'audit qualité dans l'établissement de transfusion sanguine [The quality audit in a blood transfusion center]. Transfusion Clinique et Biologique. 1998;**5**(6):422-430

[356] John DC. Quality assurance in the blood transfusion services. Proceedings of the Royal Society of Edinburgh, Section B: Biological Sciences. 1993;**101**:241-249

[357] Murphy MF, Stanworth SJ, Yazer M. Transfusion practice and safety: Current status and possibilities for improvement. Vox Sanguinis. 2011;**100**(1):46-59

[358] World Health Organization (WHO). Towards 100% voluntary blood donation: A global framework for action. In: 2, Voluntary Blood Donation: Foundation of a Safe and Sufficient Blood Supply. Geneva: World Health Organization; 2010. Available from: https://www.ncbi.nlm.nih.gov/books/NBK305666/

[359] Stainsby D, Russell J, Cohen H, Lilleyman J. Reducing adverse events in blood transfusion. British Journal of Haematology. 2005;**131**:8-12

[360] Fastman BR, Kaplan HS. Errors in transfusion medicine: Have we learned our lesson? Mount Sinai Journal of Medicine. 2011;**78**(6):854-864

[361] Mancini ME. Performance improvement in transfusion medicine. What do nurses need and want? Archives of Pathology & Laboratory Medicine. 1999;**123**(6):496-502

[362] Lau FY, Cheng G. To err is human nature. Can transfusion errors due to human factors ever be eliminated? Clinica Chimica Acta. 2001;**313**:59-67

[363] Stout L, Joseph S. Blood transfusion: Patient identification and empowerment. The British Journal of Nursing. 2016;**25**(3):138-143

[364] Pagliaro P, Rebulla P. Transfusion recipient identification. Vox Sanguinis. 2006;**91**(2):97-101

[365] Lippi G, Plebani M. Identification errors in the blood transfusion laboratory: A still relevant issue for patient safety. Transfusion and Apheresis Science. 2011;**44**(2):231-233

[366] Oldham J. Blood transfusion sampling and a greater role for error recovery. The British Journal of Nursing. 2014;**23**(8):S28, S30-S28, S34

[367] Marconi M, Langeberg AF, Sirchia G, Sandler SG. Improving transfusion safety by electronic identification of patients, blood samples, and blood units. Immunohematology. 2000;**16**(2):82-85

[368] Moiza B, Siddiquib AK, Sanac N, Sadiqb MW, Karimd F, Alia N. Documentation errors in transfusion chain: Challenges and interventions. Transfusion and Apheresis Science. 2020;**59**:102812

[369] Robinson S, Harris A, Atkinson S, Atterbury C, Bolton-Maggs P, Elliott C, et al. The administration of blood components: a British Society for Haematology Guideline. Transfusion Medicine. 2018;**28**(1):3-21

[370] Fatima N, Anwar N, Ul Mujtaba H, Shamsi T. Compliance of documentation by health-care professionals: Evaluation of transfusion practices at bedside. Glob J Transfus Med. 2021;**6**:183-188

[371] O'Leary KJ, Buck R, Fligiel HM, et al. Structured interdisciplinary rounds in a medical teaching unit: Improving patient safety. Archives of Internal Medicine. 2011;**171**(7):678-784

[372] Tuckley V, Davies J, Poles D, Robbie C, Narayan S. Safe handovers: Safe patients-why good quality structured hand overs in the transfusion laboratory are important. Transfusion Medicine. 2022;**32**(2):135-140

[373] Zakrison TL, Rosenbloom B, McFarlan A, et al. Lost information during the handover of critically injured trauma patients: A mixed-methods study. BMJ Quality and Safety. 2016;**25**(12):929-936

[374] Murphy MF, Harris A, Neuberger J. SaBTO consent for transfusion working group. Consent for blood transfusion: Summary of recommendations from the advisory Committee for the Safety of blood, tissues, and organs (SaBTO). Clinical Medicine (London, England). 2021;**21**(3):201-203

[375] Serious Hazards of Transfusion. Annual SHOT Report 2019. SHOT. 2020. Available from: www.shotuk.org/wp-content/uploads/myimages/SHOT-REPORT-2019-Final-Bookmarked-v2.pdf

[376] Watson SB. Jehovah's witnesses and blood transfusion. Clinical Ethics Report. 1991;**5**(1):1-16

[377] Migden DR, Braen GR. The Jehovah's witness blood refusal card: Ethical and medicolegal considerations for emergency physicians. Academic Emergency Medicine. 1998;**5**(8):815-824

[378] Kleinman I. Written advance directives refusing blood transfusion: Ethical and legal considerations. The American Journal of Medicine. 1994;**96**(6):563-567

[379] Adams J. Respecting the right to be wrong. Academic Emergency Medicine. 1998;**5**(8):753-755

[380] Murphy MF, Harris A, Neuberger J. SaBTO consent for transfusion working group. Consent for blood transfusion: Summary of recommendations from the advisory Committee for the Safety of blood, tissues and organs (SaBTO). Clinical Medicine (London, England). 2021;**21**(3):201-203

[381] Pirie E, Green J. Should nurses prescribe blood components? Nursing Standard. 2007;**21**(39):35-41

[382] Latter S, Courtenay M. Effectiveness of nurse prescribing: A review of the literature. Journal of Clinical Nursing. 2004;**13**(1):26-32

[383] Klein AA, Arnold P, Bingham RM, Brohi K, Clark R, Collis R, et al. AAGBI guidelines: The use of blood components and their alternatives. Anaesthesia. 2016;**71**(7):829-842

[384] Bolton-Maggs PHB, Wood EM, Wiersum-Osselton JC. Wrong blood in tube – Potential for serious outcomes: Can it be prevented? British Journal of Haematology. 2015;**168**(1):3-13

[385] Askeland RW, McGrane SP, Reifert DR, Kemp JD. Enhancing transfusion safety with an innovative bar-code-based tracking system. Healthcare Quarterly. 2009;**12**:85-89

[386] BCSH, Milkins C, Berryman J, Cantwell C, Elliott C, Haggas R, et al. Guidelines for pre-transfusion compatibility procedures in blood transfusion laboratories. Transfusion Medicine. 2013;**23**:3-35

[387] Lumadue JA, Boyd JS, Ness PM. Adherence to a strict specimen-labeling policy decreases the incidence of erroneous blood grouping of blood bank specimens. Transfusion. 1997;**37**:1169-1172

[388] Gonzalez-Porras JR, Graciani IF, Alvarez M, Pinto J, Conde MP, Nieto MJ, et al. Tubes for pretransfusion testing should be collected by blood bank staff and hand labelled until the implementation of new technology for improved sample labelling. Results of a prospective study. Vox Sanguinis. 2008;**95**:52-56

[389] Thomas W, Davies J, Asamoah A, Scott-Molloy C, Sansom V, Kerr J. Two samples for blood transfusion: Single Centre experience. Transfusion Medicine. 2014;**24**:209-212

[390] Ashford P, Gozzard D, Jones J, Revill J, Wallis J, Bruce M. Guidelines for blood bank computing. Transfusion Medicine. 2000;**10**:307-314

[391] Davies A, Staves J, Kay J, Casbard A, Murphy MF. End-to-end electronic control of the hospital transfusion process to increase the safety of blood transfusion: Strengths and weaknesses. Transfusion. 2006;**46**:352-364

[392] Strobel E. Hemolytic transfusion reactions. Transfusion Medicine and Hemotherapy. 2008;**35**(5):346-353

[393] Dubin CH. Technology, vigilance, and blood transfusions: How U.S. hospitals and the federal government are working to reduce adverse events. P T. 2010;**35**(7):374-376

[394] Olaniyi JA. Blood transfusion reactions. In: Tombak A, editor. Blood Groups. London, UK, London: Intech Open; 2019. DOI: 10.5772/intechopen.85347

[395] Sharma G, Parwani AV, Raval JS, Triulzi DJ, Benjamin RJ, Pantanowitz L.

Contemporary issues in transfusion medicine informatics. Journal of Pathology Informatics. 2011;7(2):3

[396] Wong KF. Virtual blood bank. Journal of Pathology Informatics. 2011;**2**:6. DOI: 10.4103/2153-3539.76155

[397] Najafpour Z, Hasoumi M, Behzadi F, Mohamadi E, Jafary M, Saeedi M. Preventing blood transfusion. Failures: FMEA, an effective assessment method. BMC Health Services Research. 2017;**17**(1):453

[398] Bolton-Maggs P. Blood transfusion safety: Patients at risk from human errors. British Journal of Hospital Medicine (London, England). 2013;**74**(10):544-545

[399] Crookston KP, Koenig SC, Reyes MD. Transfusion reaction identification and management at the bedside. Journal of Infusion Nursing. 2015;**38**(2):104-113

[400] Cottrell S, Davidson V. National audit of bedside transfusion practice. Nursing Standard. 2013;**27**(43):41-48

[401] Todd O, Sikwewa K, Kamp J, et al. Inadequate monitoring risks safety of blood transfusion in rural Zambia. Critical Care. 2015;**19**:P338. DOI: 10.1186/cc14418

[402] Tinegate H, Birchall J, Gray A, et al. Guideline on the investigation and management of acute transfusion reactions. Prepared by the BCSH blood transfusion task force. British Journal of Haematology. 2012;**159**:143-153

[403] Bloch EM, Vermeulen M, Murphy E. Blood transfusion safety in Africa: A literature review of infectious disease and organizational challenges. Transfusion Medicine Reviews. 2012;**26**(2):164-180

[404] World Health Organisation (WHO). Blood Safety and Availability: Facts and Figures from the 2007 Blood Safety Survey. Geneva, Switzerland: World Health Organisation (WHO); 2007

[405] Diane MK, Dembele B, Konate S. Blood collection to cover national needs in sub-Saharan Africa: The reality of the Ivory Coast. Blood Transfusion. 2014;**12**(4):624-625

[406] Godin G, Sheeran P, Conner M, et al. Factors explaining the intention to give blood among the general population. Vox Sanguinis. 2005;**89**:140-149

[407] Nagalo MB, Sanou M, Bisseye C, Kaboré MI, Nebie YK, Kienou K. Seroprevalence of human immunodefi ciency virus, hepatitis B and C viruses and syphilis among blood donors in Koudougou (Burkina Faso) in 2009. Blood Transfusion. 2011;**9**:419-424

[408] Shiferaw E, Tadilo W, Melkie I, Shiferaw M. Sero-prevalence and trends of transfusion-transmissible infections among blood donors at Bahir Dar district blood bank, Northwest Ethiopia: A four-year retrospective study. PLoS One. 2019;**14**(4):e0214755

[409] World Health Organization (WHO). Screening donated blood for transfusion-transmissible infections: Recommendations. In: 4, Screening for Transfusion-Transmissible Infections. Geneva: World Health Organization; 2009. Available from: https://www.ncbi.nlm.nih.gov/books/NBK142989/

[410] Song Y, Bian Y, Petzold M, Ung COL. Prevalence, and trend of major transfusion-transmissible infections among blood donors in Western China, 2005 through 2010. PLoS One. 2018;**9**(4):e94528

[411] World Health Organization. Blood Donor Selection and Counselling. Available from: http:www.who.int/bloodsafety/voluntary_donation/blood_donor_selection/en/. [Last assessed on 2016 Mar 03].

[412] Schutz R, Savarit D, Kadjo JC, Batter V, Kone N, La Ruche G, et al. Excluding blood donors at high risk of HIV infection in a west African city. BMJ. 1993;**307**:1517-1519

[413] Ekwere T, Ino-Ekanem M, Motilewa O, Ibanga I. Pattern of blood donor deferral in a tertiary hospital, south-south, Nigeria: A three-year study review. International Journal of Blood Transfusion and Immunohematology. 2014;**4**:7-13

[414] McFarland W, Kahn JG, Katzenstein DA, Mvere D, Shamu R. Deferral of blood donors with risk factors for HIV infection saves lives and money in Zimbabwe. Journal of Acquired Immune Deficiency Syndromes and Human Retrovirology. 1995;**9**:183-192

[415] Beattie RH, Sturrock SM. What is the evidence for the change in the blood donation deferral period for high-risk groups and does it go far enough? Clinical Medicine. 2018;**18**(4):304-307

[416] Aneke CJ, Ezeh UT, Nwosu AG, Anumba EC. Retrospective evaluation of prospective blood donor deferral in a tertiary hospital-based blood bank in south-East Nigeria. Journal of Medicine in the Tropics. 2016;**18**:103-107

[417] Allain JP, Sarkodie F, Boateng P, et al. A pool of repeat blood donors can be generated with little expense to the blood center in sub-Saharan Africa. Transfusion. 2008;**48**:735-741

[418] Bates I, Chapotera GK, McKew S, et al. Maternal mortality in sub-Saharan Africa: The contribution of ineffective blood transfusion services. BJOG : An International Journal of Obstetrics and Gynaecology. 2008;**115**:1331-1339

[419] Tapko JP, Toure B, Sambo LG, et al. Status of Blood Safety in the WHO African Region: Report of the 2006 Survey. Available from: http://www.afro.who.int/en/divisions-a-programmes/dsd/health-technologies-a-laboratories.html

Chapter 8

Clinical Effects and Possible Mechanisms of Transfusion-Related Immunomodulation

Yavuz Memis Bilgin

Abstract

Allogeneic blood components are commonly transfused in trauma, surgery, and intensive care units and are related with adverse effects, such as postoperative infections, multi-organ failure, and mortality. The adverse effects of blood transfusions on the immune system are called as transfusion-related immunomodulation (TRIM). Many clinical trials are conducted to show the clinical effects of TRIM. They found in different clinical settings controversial results. There are many possible mechanisms of TRIM. Although until now, the exact mechanisms are not elucidated resulting in a challenge to unravel this complex interaction between immunomodulation and clinical events leading to morbidity and mortality. It has been postulated that allogeneic leukocytes are associated with the clinical adverse effects of TRIM that predominantly is observed in high-risk patients as cardiovascular surgery. Allogeneic leukocytes could activate inflammation cascade leading to adverse events in high-risk patients. Also other blood components as red cells, plasma, and platelets can play a role in the development of inflammatory complications after blood transfusions. In this review, we will discuss the clinical effects and the possible mechanisms of TRIM in relation with allogeneic leukocytes and mediators derived from allogeneic blood transfusions.

Keywords: transfusion-related immunomodulation, red cells, leukocytes, plasma, platelets, infections, multi-organ dysfunction syndrome, mortality, inflammatory response, coagulation system

1. Introduction

Until the discovery of the ***ABO blood groups*** in the early 1900s blood transfusions were a high-risk procedure: more than 50% of the recipients of blood did not survive. The discovery of the ABO blood groups followed by the development of citrate as anticoagulant to prevent clotting of blood enabled the start of a long history of transfusion medicine. Since blood component transfusion of red blood cells (RBCs), platelet concentrates, and plasma became possible over time, blood transfusions became gradually considered as safe for the treatment of blood loss and other causes of anemia [1]. Allogeneic blood components are commonly transfused in trauma, surgery, and intensive care units (ICUs); up to 60% of these patients receives a blood transfusion [2, 3]. It is known that allogeneic blood transfusions have adverse effects which can lead to deleterious outcome in recipients. These effects of allogeneic blood transfusions are called transfusion-related ***immunomodulation*** (TRIM). The clinical effects of TRIM are most seen in high-risk patients as to cardiac surgery [4]. In this review, we will focus on the clinical effects and possible mechanisms of TRIM, especially in patients at high risk.

2. Transfusion-related immunomodulation (TRIM) in different clinical settings

The existence and possible mechanisms of TRIM are not yet fully ***dis***covered. Many factors might contribute to TRIM. Allogeneic leukocytes and (leukocyte-derived) soluble mediators in blood products were considered as most important [4]. Through filtration, the number of allogeneic leukocytes in donated blood can be reduced by more than 99.9% with a residual leukocyte count of less than $1x10^6$/L. Leukocyte-depleted blood transfusions were applied since the 1980s to reduce nonhemolytic febrile transfusion reactions, human leukocyte ***antigen (HLA)*** allo-immuni***za***tion, and ***Cytomegalovirus (CMV) transmission*** in patients at risk. In early 2000s, in ***many Western*** countries, universal leukocyte depletion of allogeneic blood transfusion was implemented.

In the 1970s, it was ***dis***covered that pre***transplantation*** allogeneic blood transfusions improved a subsequent renal allograft survival [5]. It was hypothesized that allogeneic leukocytes present in the blood components could lead to an ***immunosuppressive*** transfusion effect resulting in impaired cancer surveillance and to su***scep-t***ibility for postoperative infections [4, 6, 7]. ***Although, two*** randomized controlled ***trials (RCT***s) compared ***buffy-coat-poor red*** blood ***cells (RBC***) with filtered RBC on cancer recurrence after colorectal surgery. Both studies found no difference in recurrence after 5 years [8, 9]. Therefore, a possible immu***nosup***pressive effect of allogeneic blood transfusion on cancer recurrence is not found.

On the other hand, many observational studies showed an association between postoperative infections ***and allogeneic*** blood transfusions. The presumption was that the immunosuppressive effect of ***leuko***cyte-containing RBC transfusions was responsible for postoperative infections. ***Many RCTs*** were conducted in various clinical settings, evaluated postoperative after ***leukoreduced (LR) RBC transfusions***. These studies varied as to ***single- or multiple-center*** design, clinical ***diagnosis, methods*** to document infections and proportion of transfused patients ranging between 14 and 95% and revealed different outcomes.

Several meta-analyses were performed investigating the effects of, allogeneic leukocyte-containing, buffy-coat-depleted (BCD) RBC transfusions, but these came also to controversial conclusions. Meta-analyses using intention-to-treat analyses seldom found an association between LR transfusions and postoperative infections [10]. A meta-analysis, restricted to transfused patients only, thereby excluding 36% of the study population, reported up to almost 60% reduction in postoperative infection after transfusion of LR RBC [11]. The effect of LR RBC was mainly observed in patients undergoing cardiac surgery. On the other hand, mortality was also investigated in different clinical settings. Overall, no adverse effect of leukocyte-containing transfusions on short-term mortality has been found. Only in cardiac surgery, the mortality rate was significantly decreased in patients who received LR RBC [10].

3. Cardiac surgery and allogeneic blood transfusions

Coronary artery bypass graft (CABG) surgery is a frequently performed intervention to re-vascularize the myocardium. Worldwide, approximately 1 million patients are undergoing cardiac surgery annually. The current mortality rate after cardiac surgery is low, and cardiac surgery has become a routine procedure. Although the number of patients who receive blood transfusions and the numbers of transfused blood products became lower in time, patients undergoing cardiac surgery still receive more blood transfusions compared to other surgical settings. Due to hemodilution and consumption of coagulation factors and platelets in the extracorporeal circuit, patients undergoing cardiac surgery can develop severe bleeding complications. In cardiac surgery, transfusion rate varies between 27 and 92% and estimated approximately 10% of the total blood supply worldwide [12]. Also platelets and plasma are frequently transfused to patients undergoing cardiac surgery.

After cardiac surgery, patients generally stay at an intensive care unit (ICU) for as long as mechanical ventilation and cardiac inotropic drug support is needed. Anemia is often encountered in the ICU in surgical patients and is of multifactorial origin. Besides, hemodilution by abundant intravenous infusions, decreased RBC production due to iron deficiency and inappropriate erythropoietin response due to inflammatory mediators in critically ill patients, reduced RBC survival, and increased (drug-induced) hemolysis may contribute further to postoperative anemia in ICU patients [13–15]. A prospective observational study in several ICUs found that approximately 29% of the patients reached a hemoglobin value of less than 6.2 mmol/l (10.0 gr/dl) with a transfusion rate of 37%. Of the patients with an ICU stay >7 days, 73% had received allogeneic RBC transfusions. Overall mortality was almost twice as high in patients who received RBC transfusions compared to patients who were not transfused. In critically ill patients, blood transfusions have been associated with mortality, ventilator-associated pneumonia, acute respiratory distress syndrome (ARDS), and bloodstream infections [16–20]. Also transfusion of platelets and plasma were reported to contribute to the development of these complications [21, 22].

The effect of allogeneic blood transfusions containing leukocytes was predominantly present in cardiac surgery. This was observed in two RCTs. One randomized controlled trial, aimed to investigate the development of HLA antibodies and postoperative infections after RBC transfusions in cardiac surgery (CABG +/− valve surgery), found surprisingly a higher mortality rate in patients receiving leukocyte-containing RBC transfusions [23]. Mortality due to multi-organ dysfunction syndrome (MODS) was the major cause of excess deaths after non-LR transfusions. In this study, patients were randomized to three different blood products; BCD RBCs were compared with two filtered RBCs: either fresh filtered RBCs before storage (FF) or stored filtered RBCs (SF). Between the two types of filtered RBCs, the mortality rate was not different. A subsequent RCT conducted in high-risk cardiac surgery (anticipating higher transfusion needs) investigated the effect of leukoreduction on the incidence of MODS but found no difference after BCD or LR RBCs [24]. However, MODS (with the presence of postoperative infections) as a cause of death occurred more often in patients who received BCD RBC [25]. Recently, in 150 patients undergoing cardiac surgery, it was found that patients receiving leukocyte-containing blood transfusions had longer ICU stay and hospital stay, and the duration of mechanical ventilation was longer. These patients had more risk for developing postoperative kidney injury [26]. A meta-analysis in patients undergoing cardiovascular surgery concluded that leukocyte-depleted blood transfusions resulted in significant reduction in postoperative infections (OR = 0.77, 95% CI = 0.66–0.91) and all-cause mortality (OR = 0.69, 95% CI = 0.53–0.90) [27]. Further, a large analysis enrolling >14.000 patients undergoing cardiac surgery and hip surgery or admitted to ICU after surgery or trauma observed after universal leukoreduction significant lower in-hospital mortality and decreased incidence of fever and antibiotic use in patients receiving blood transfusions [28]. The available findings support the standard use of LR in cardiac surgery, if universal leukoreduction is not implemented [29].

As possible explanation for these differences in cardiac surgery, it was postulated that patients undergoing cardiopulmonary bypass develop a systemic inflammatory response syndrome (SIRS), where allogeneic blood transfusions could have a complementary role. Generation of inflammatory mediators may be associated with more complex and longer surgery, whereas these patients receive also larger amounts of blood transfusions. During cardiac surgery, blood is exposed to the extracorporeal circuit, hypothermia, and ischemia/reperfusion injury. These insults are potent inducers of a stress response. SIRS usually resolves with adequate supportive therapy, and most of the patients recover. However, overwhelming SIRS can dominate and progress to MODS, which may lead to mortality [30]. Transfusion of leukocyte-containing RBCs to a patient with an already existing inflammatory cascade can contribute to an increased morbidity and mortality (second hit). It has been hypothesized that leukocyte-containing RBC transfusions can further imbalance SIRS leading to aggravation of MODS and could finally result in death [31].

4. Possible mechanisms of TRIM

Many factors present in allogeneic blood products have been proposed to induce TRIM. These can due to factors derived from leukocytes, red blood cells, platelets, and plasma [32, 33].

4.1 Leukocyte-derived factors

Clinical studies suggested that allogeneic leukocytes are responsible for the deleterious effects of (leukocyte-containing) blood transfusions. In blood products up to $5x10^6$/L, residual leukocytes can present. Probably by apoptosis, these residual leukocytes and leukocyte-derived mediators or residual leukocytes may induce immunomodulation [34]. Also after transfusion, microchimerism may be present 2 years after transfusion in 25% of trauma survivors, which can contribute to the development of immune suppression [35]. Further, interaction between residual leukocytes from allogeneic blood transfusion and recipient's lymphocytes may result in allo-immunization [36]. Also leukocytes became apoptotic during the storage of blood products. These factors can lead to immunomodulation [37, 38]. One study in cardiac surgery showed as a marker for apoptosis an increase in Fas ligand in patients receiving leukocyte-containing blood [26]. Although a direct causal interaction between residual leukocytes and postoperative complications related with allogeneic blood transfusions remains uncertain.

Soluble leukocyte-derived factors, like cytokines and HLA molecules, can modulate recipient's immune system. It has been suggested that pro-inflammatory and anti-inflammatory cytokines can accumulate during the storage of allogeneic blood transfusions [39]. Also degranulation products of remaining leukocytes like histamine, serotonin, elastase, and acid phosphatase can contribute to an immunomodulatory effect [40]. In a multivariate analysis, the number of contaminating leukocytes and the storage duration of RBCs were the most significant factors associated with febrile nonhemolytic transfusion reactions [41]. Further, it has been suggested that interleukin-8 may be the cause of transient posttransfusion leukocytosis in critically ill patients [42]. Few studies investigated the effect of allogeneic (leukocyte-containing) blood products on the cytokine balance. These studies compared cytokine profiles in patients receiving leukocyte-containing RBC transfusions with patients who did not receive any transfusions. In one study in cardiac surgery, an association was found between allogeneic RBC transfusions and postoperative increase of bactericidal/permeability-increasing protein (BPI), a marker of neutrophil activation, and the pro-inflammatory mediator IL-6 [43]. However, the interaction between blood products and the concentrations of inflammatory mediators in relation with the outcome of the patients is unknown. Although, in one RCT between stored and then filtered and fresh filtered (lacking soluble mediators) RBCs, no association was found in postoperative mortality. This finding suggests that there is not a causal role for soluble mediators [23].

It has been observed that allogeneic leukocytes can increase a T-helper-2 (Th-2) response and suppress Th-1 response [44]. This was supported by one RCT that measured the profiles of some inflammatory mediators investigating the differences between LD and BCD RBCs [45]. The IL-6 levels were significantly higher at arrival at ICU in patients after transfusion of >3 units BCD RBCs compared with LD. The IL-10 levels were not associated with number and type of transfusions in patients with or without complications, although higher IL-10 concentrations were associated with hospital mortality in both randomization arms. These results suggested that leukocyte-containing blood transfusions can aggravate the pro-inflammatory response after surgery.

4.2 Red blood cell-derived factors

During the storage of blood products, red blood cells alter and undergo rheologic changes, as impaired deformability, shape, and rigidity. Further, biochemical changes can occur as depletion of 2,3-diphosphoglycerate and nitric oxide scavenging, which result in impaired oxygen delivery [46, 47].

Hemolysis of red blood cells occurs during storage that can lead to accumulation of iron and heme, which can cause the formation of reactive oxygen species (ROS) and expression leading to tissue damage. Iron released during storage can lead to increased levels of non-transferrin-bound iron (NTBI) that can result in changes in leukocyte activation resulting in immunomodulation and production and release of pro-inflammatory cytokines [48]. Although, no difference in pro-inflammatory cytokine release was found in healthy individuals and prematures receiving old versus fresh red blood cell transfusions, while NTBI levels were significantly higher in patients receiving older RBCs [49, 50]. Also, phagocytosis of stored red blood cells in monocytes and macrophages can induce immunomodulation that results in production and release of pro-inflammatory cytokines [51]. Further, it was observed that microparticles from red blood cells accumulated during storage have also an inflammatory effect [52].

Several observational trials investigated the effect of storage time of red blood cells. These studies found controversial conclusions in different clinical settings [53–55]. Retrospective analysis suggested an association between transfusion of RBCs older than 14 days and postoperative infections after cardiac surgery. However, other studies could not confirm this and found also no association between mortality, infections, and hospital-stay [56]. However, others found no effect of storage of red blood cells on mortality in critically ill patients [57]. Meta-analysis concluded that the heterogeneity among available studies could not the question whether the storage of red blood cells can influence prognosis [58]. Until now, RCTs could not find any deleterious effects of transfusion of older RBCs compared with younger RBCs.

4.3 Platelet-derived factors

There are few data suggesting that platelets in stored blood products play a role in the development of TRIM. Platelets and platelet-derived particles can induce immune suppression and activation of an inflammatory response [59]. Also, platelets interact with leukocytes which results in the formation of aggregates and can involve in apoptosis and can thereby play a role in immunomodulation [60]. Leukocyte-containing RBCs contain prothrombotic soluble mediators, such as CD40L, which induce the synthesis of pro-inflammatory mediators that can further activate the coagulation system. Soluble CD40L and other cytokines released by platelets may play a key role in endothelial activation and can in turn activate the immune system leading to inflammation [61]. Whether platelets present in allogeneic red blood cell bags are involved in the development of TRIM is so far not known.

4.4 Plasma-derived factors

Plasma-derived products and all plasma-containing products can contribute to the development of transfusion-related acute lung injury (TRALI). Bioactive lipids which accumulate during the storage of plasma are involved in an immunomodulatory effect. In combination with neutrophil activation in plasma, bioactive lipids can induce TRALI [62]. TRALI is a life-threatening transfusion reaction with an estimated incidence of 1:1000 to 5000 plasma-containing blood transfusions. TRALI is defined as non-cardiogenic lung edema presenting within 6 hours after the completion of transfusion [63]. Endogenous neutrophil priming associated with the patient's underlying illness, combined with bioactive lipids and modifiers in blood products, can result in neutrophil-induced pulmonary endothelial damage leading to capillary leakage. It has been hypothesized that the presence of leukocytes contributes to the generation of bioactive lipids during storage, enhancing the accumulation of lipid-priming agents and neutrophil-priming factors [64]. Besides leukocyte-reactive antibodies present in donor plasma, soluble factors accumulating during the storage of red cells and platelet products have been associated with TRALI [65].

5. Effect of platelet and plasma transfusions on TRIM

A substantial proportion of patients undergoing major surgery and trauma receive, besides red blood cells, also platelet transfusions. In cardiac surgery, approximately 20% of patients suffer from bleeding and receive platelet transfusion. Studies in cardiac surgery showed that platelet transfusion was associated with threefold increase in stroke and fivefold increase in mortality [66]. In another study in cardiac surgery, platelet transfusions were associated with mortality in patients with post-operative infections [67]. However, other studies found not an association between platelet transfusions and postoperative complications [68–70]. Patients who receive platelet transfusions could be more sicker and have more complex course, so transfusion of platelets could be a surrogate marker.

Plasma transfusions are predominantly transfused to patients who also receive large numbers of RBC transfusions. It has been suggested that plasma transfusions are associated with adverse outcome after cardiac surgery. A predominant role of plasma transfusions in cardiac surgery outcome was reported in one study in cardiac surgery [71]. Other studies that focused on plasma transfusions reported inconsistent findings [68, 72]. In another study, plasma transfusions were associated with mortality (with the presence of infections) [67]. This suggests that plasma transfusions (with the presence of soluble mediators) can contribute to postoperative inflammation in cardiac surgery. Because patients who need plasma transfusions often receive red blood cell and platelet transfusions, it is difficult to determine whether plasma transfusions are independent risk factors or are only confounders. Also one study found in >10,000 patients that the storage time of plasma transfusions was associated with early mortality, although late mortality was not [73].

The presented findings underscore the need for further studies to investigate the effects of all the various blood components transfused in cardiac surgery, as well as differentiate between adverse effects possibly associated with a specific blood component(s).

6. Allogeneic transfusion and thrombosis

Patients undergoing surgery or who suffer from cancer have a higher risk for the development of venous thromboembolism (VTE). Most observational studies investigating VTE ignored the role of allogeneic blood transfusion as a causal factor. Few studies found in cancer and after surgery that blood transfusions were dose-dependently associated with VTE [74–76]. One study in 1070 patients undergoing cardiac surgery found a dose-dependent association with transfusion of blood products and VTE [77]. In patients receiving red blood cells, the incidence of VTE was 16.7% and patients who received also plasma transfusions, this was almost doubled. The hypercoagulability and immobility after surgery could result in the activation of coagulation system, and in combination with blood transfusions this could result in higher risk in VTE.

It has been shown that platelets contain prothrombotic soluble mediators, which interact with leukocytes preceding apoptosis subsequently producing microparticles with procoagulant activity [60]. Leukocyte-containing RBCs contain soluble mediators, such as CD40L, which induce the synthesis of pro-inflammatory mediators that can further activate the coagulation system [58]. Recently, one study found in the bronchoalveolar lavage fluid, besides an increase in pro-inflammatory mediators IL-8 and TNF-alpha and also an increase in trombine-antithrombin complex (TATc), indicating the activation of the coagulation system in the lung [78]. Another study found an increase in levels of von-Willebrand-factor antigen in critically ill patients receiving a RBC transfusion. The von Willebrand factor antigen has a causal role in the activation of endothelium and also in the development of thrombi formation [79]. After cardiovascular surgery, the levels of plasma tissue factor are persistent high for 30 days, which can increase the risk of VTE [80]. In combination with plasma-derived products in stored blood products, this can result in an increased activation of the coagulation system.

7. Interaction between inflammation and coagulation associated with blood transfusions

Patients undergoing major surgery or after trauma have a higher risk for the development of both inflammation and thrombo-embolic complications. In these patients, both the inflammatory response and the release of pro-inflammatory mediators lead to an activation of the coagulation system and downregulate the anticoagulant system [81]. Activation of the coagulation factors can in turn activate inflammation. This may enhance the development of infections and microvascular thrombi [82]. Both thrombi and infections can be involved in the development and aggravation of MODS [83]. Further, by increasing the circulating red blood cell mass and vascular rheologic deformations by red blood cell transfusions, this process can be more pronounced. Also plasma and platelet transfusions can aggravate the activation of coagulation and inflammatory response.

There is a possible association between allogeneic blood transfusions and the formation of thrombosis, as a factor aggravating VTE and having a role in the development of MODS which can lead to increased mortality in patients at high risk as in

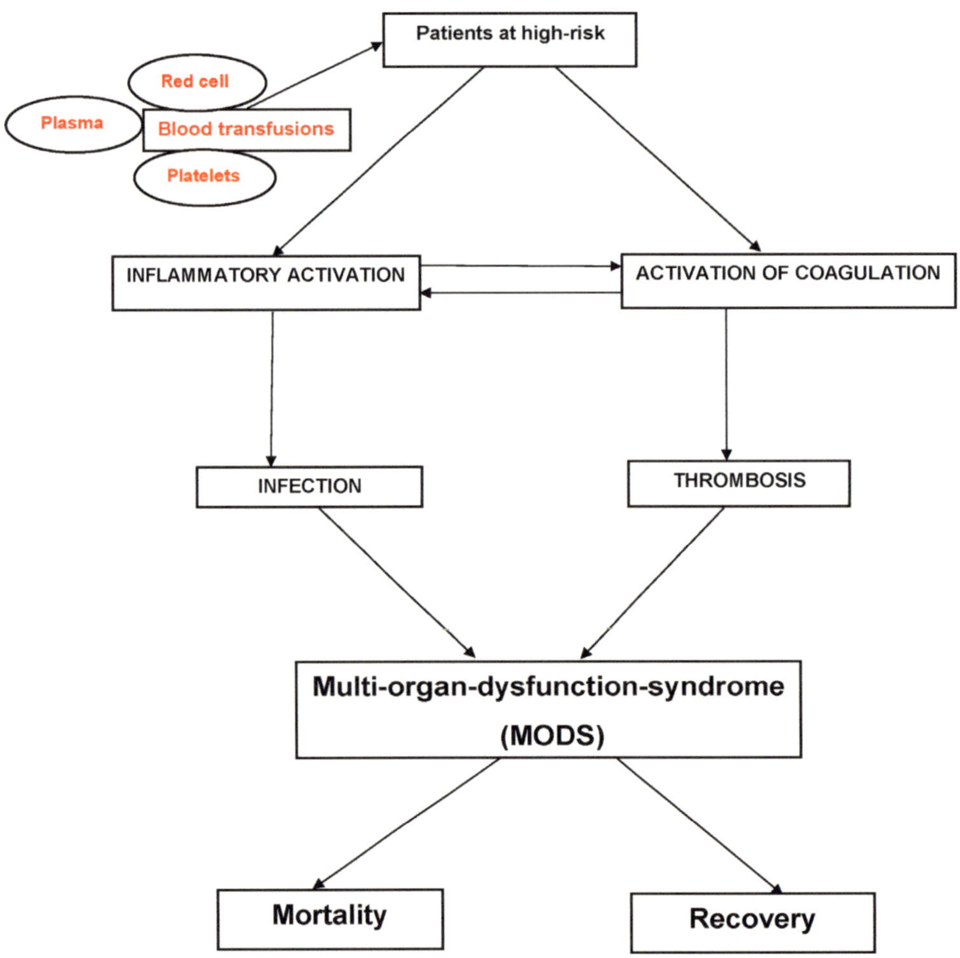

Figure 1.
Association between blood transfusions inflammation, coagulation and MODS.

cardiac surgery (**Figure 1**). This complex interaction and the role of allogeneic blood transfusions should be investigated in detail.

8. Conclusions

Nowadays, allogeneic blood transfusions are unavoidable. Although blood transfusions are safe today, there are still concerns about transfusion-related complications. The immune-mediated complications of blood transfusions are referred as transfusion-related immunomodulation. The effects of transfusion-related immunomodulation are mainly observed in major cardiovascular surgery. Patients undergoing cardiovascular surgery are transfused with large numbers of red cells, plasma, and platelets. Although, the exact mechanisms of these immune-mediated complications are still not elucidated. The past studies showed that allogeneic leukocytes in blood transfusions play a pivotal role in the development of transfusion-related immunomodulation. Nowadays, in many countries, leukocytes are removed from transfused blood components, although the discussion about the immunologic effects of blood transfusions is continuing. In addition, by the activation of inflammatory system and release of mediators, the storage of blood components and transfusion of plasma and platelets can contribute to the development of transfusion-related immunomodulation. Further, it has been suggested that allogeneic blood transfusions are associated with the development of thrombo-embolic events in high-risk patients as cancer and surgery. It has been suggested that allogeneic blood transfusions can activate an inflammatory response and a coagulation response. Both cascades can result in worse outcome in a high-risk patient. Probably, the term transfusion-related immunomodulation is not sufficient for both inflammation and coagulation activation after blood transfusion. The term transfusion-related inflammation and coagulation (TRIC) could be more comprehensive and includes the activation of both cascades. More research (clinical and laboratory) are needed to unravel the effects of allogeneic blood transfusions in the activation of the inflammatory and coagulation cascades.

Conflict of interest

The author declares no conflict of interest.

Author details

Yavuz Memis Bilgin
Department of Internal Medicine, Adrz, Goes, the Netherlands

*Address all correspondence to: y.bilgin@adrz.nl

References

[1] Ness P. Introduction: Recent evolution of transfusion medicine. In: Murphy MF, Pamphilon DH, Heddle NM, editors. Practical Transfusion Medicine. 4th ed. Chichester: Wiley-Blackwell; 2013. pp. 1-8

[2] Klein HG, Spahn DR, Carson JL. Red blood cell transfusion in clinical practice. Lancet. 2007;**370**:415-426

[3] Corwin HL. Anemia and red blood cell transfusion in the critically ill. Seminars in Dialysis. 2006;**19**:513-516

[4] Blumberg N, Heal JM. Effects of transfusion on immune function: Cancer recurrence and infection. Archives of Pathology & Laboratory Medicine. 1994;**118**:371-379

[5] Opelz G, Sengar DDS, Mickey MR, Terasaki PI. Effect of blood transfusions on subsequent kidney transplants. Transplantation Proceedings. 1973;**5**:253-259

[6] Gantt CL. Red blood cells for cancer patients. Lancet. 1981;**2**:363

[7] Burrows L, Tartter PI. Effect of blood transfusions on colonic malignancy recurrence rate. Lancet. 1982;**2**:662

[8] Skanberg J, Lundholm K, Haglind H. Effects of blood transfusion with leucocyte depletion on length of hospital stay, respiratory assistance and survival after curative surgery for colorectal cancer. Acta Oncologica. 2007;**46**:1123-1130

[9] van de Watering LMG, Brand A, Houbiers JGA, et al. Perioperative blood transfusions, with or without allogeneic leukocytes, relate to survival, not to cancer recurrence. The British Journal of Surgery. 2001;**88**:267-272

[10] Vamvakas EC. White-blood-cell-containing alloegenic blood transfusions and postoperative infection and mortality: An updated meta-analysis. Vox Sanguinis. 2007;**92**:224-232

[11] Blumberg N, Zhao H, Wang H, et al. The intention-to-treat principle in clinical trials and meta-analysis of leukoreduced blood transfusions in surgical patients. Transfusion. 2007;**47**:573-581

[12] Snyder-Ramos SA, Mohnle P, Weng YS, et al. The ongoing variability in blood transfusion practices in cardiac surgery. Transfusion. 2008;**48**:1284-1299

[13] Jelkman WE, Hellwig-Buergel T. Inhibition of erythropoetin production by cytokines. Implications for the anemia involved in inflammatory states. Annals of the New York Academy of Sciences. 1994;**718**:300-309

[14] Shander A. Anemia in the critically ill. Critical Care Clinics. 2004;**20**:159-178

[15] Rodriguez RM, Corwin HL, Gettinger A, et al. Nutritional deficiencies and blunted erythropoietin response as causes of the anemia of critical illness. Journal of Critical Care. 2001;**16**:36-41

[16] Shorr AF, Duh MS, Kelly KM, et al. Red blood cell transfusion and ventilator-associated pneumonia: A potential link? Critical Care Medicine. 2004;**32**:666-674

[17] Shorr AF, Jackson WL, Kelly KM, et al. Transfusion practice and blood stream infections in critically ill patients. Chest. 2005;**127**:1722-1728

[18] Zilberberg MD, Carter C, Lefebre P, et al. RBC transfusions and the risk of

ARDS among the critically ill: A cohort study. Critical Care. 2007;**11**:R63

[19] Taylor RW, Manganaro L, O'Brien J, et al. Impact of allogenic packed red blood cell transfusion on nosocomial infection rates in critically ill patient. Critical Care Medicine. 2002;**30**:2249-2254

[20] Gong MN, Thompson BT, Williams P, et al. Clinical predictors of and mortality in acute respiratory distress syndrome: Potential role of red cell transfusion. Critical Care Medicine. 2005;**33**:1191-1198

[21] Khan H, Belsher J, Yilmaz M, et al. Fresh-frozen plasma and platelet transfusions are associated with development of acute lung injury in critically ill medical patients. Chest. 2007;**131**:1308-1314

[22] Sarani B, Dunkman WJ, Dean L, et al. Transfusion of fresh frozen plasma in critically ill surgical patients is associated with an increased risk of infection. Critical Care Medicine. 2008;**36**:1114-1118

[23] van de Watering LM, Hermans J, Houbiers JG, et al. Beneficial effects of leukocyte depletion of transfused blood on postoperative complications in patients undergoing cardiac surgery: A randomized clinical trial. Circulation. 1998;**97**:562-568

[24] Bilgin YM, van de Watering LM, Eijsman L, et al. Double-blind, randomized controlled trial on the effect of leukocyte-depleted erythrocyte transfusions in cardiac valve surgery. Circulation. 2004;**109**:2755-2760

[25] Bilgin YM, van de Watering LM, Eijsman L, et al. Is increased mortality associated with post-operative infections after leukocytes containing red blood cell transfusions in cardiac surgery? An extended analysis. Transfusion Medicine. 2007;**17**:304-311

[26] Khan AI, Patidar GK, Lakshmy R, et al. Effect of leukoreduction on transfusion-related immunomodulation in patients undergoing cardiac surgery. Transf Med. 2020;**30**:497-504

[27] Simancas-Racines D, Arevalo-Rodriguez I, Urrutia G, et al. Leukodepleted packed red blood cells transfusion in patients undergoing major cardiovascular surgical procedure: Systemic review and meta-analysis. Cardiology Research and Practice. 2019;**2019**:7543917

[28] Hebert PC, Fergusson D, Blachjman MA, et al. Clinical outcomes following institution of the Canadian universal leukoreduction program for red blood cell transfusions. JAMA. 2003;**289**:1941-1949

[29] Boer C, Meesters MI, Milojevic M, et al. 2017 EACTS/EACTA guidelines on patient blood management for adult cardiac surgery. Journal of Cardiothoracic and Vascular Anesthesia. 2018;**32**:88-120

[30] Guidet B, Aegerter P, Gauzit R, et al. Incidence and impact of organ dysfunctions associated with sepsis. Chest. 2005;**127**:942-951

[31] Bilgin YM, van de Watering LM. Complications after cardiac surgery due to allogeneic blood transfusions. Journal of Clinical and Experimental Cardiology. 2013;**S7**:5

[32] Remy KE, Hall MW, Cholette J, et al. Mechanisms of red blood cell transfusion-related immunomodulation. Transfusion. 2018;**58**:804-815

[33] Maitta RW. Transfusion-related immunomodulation. In: Maitta RW,

editor. Immunologic Concepts in Transfusion Medicine. St.Louis: Elsevier; 2020. pp. 81-95

[34] Sut C, Tariker S, Chou ML, et al. Duraton of red blood cell storage and inflammatory marker generation. Blood Transfusion. 2017;**15**:145-152

[35] Lee TH, Paglieroni T, Ohto H, et al. Survival of donor leukocyte subpopulations in immunocompetent transfusion recipients: Frequent long-term microchimerism in severe trauma patients. Blood. 1999;**93**:3127-3139

[36] Saas P, Angelot F, Bardiaux L, et al. Phosphatidylserine-expressing cell by-products in transfusion: A pro-inflammatory or an anti-inflammatory effect? Transfusion Clinique et Biologique. 2012;**19**:90-97

[37] Frabetti F, Musiani D, Marini M, et al. White cell apoptosis in packed red cells. Transfusion. 1998;**38**:1082-1089

[38] Hod EA, Zhang N, Sokal SA, et al. Transfusion of red blood cells after prolonged storage produces harmful effects that are mediated by iron and inflammation. Blood. 2010;**115**:4284-4292

[39] Nagura Y, Tsuno NH, Tanaka M, et al. The effect of pre-storage whole-blood leukocyte reduction on cytokines/chemokines levels in autologous CPDA-1 whole blood. Transfusion and Apheresis Science. 2013;**49**:223-230

[40] Nielsen HJ, Reinert CM, Pedersen AN, et al. Time-dependent spontaneous release of white cell-and platelet-derived bioactive substances from stored human blood. Transfusion. 1996;**36**:960-965

[41] Heddle NM, Klama LN, Griffith GR, et al. A prospective study to identify the risk factors associated with acute reactions to platelet and red cell transfusions. Transfusion. 1993;**33**:794-797

[42] Izbicki G, Rudensky B, Na'amad M, et al. Transfusion-related leukocytosis in critically ill patients. Critical Care Medicine. 2004;**32**:439-442

[43] Fransen E, Maessen J, Dentener M, et al. Impact of blood transfusions on inflammatory mediator release in patients undergoing cardiac surgery. Chest. 1999;**116**:1233-1239

[44] Aguilar-Nascimento JE, Zampieri-Filho JP, Bordin JO. Implications of perioperative allogeneic red blood cell transfusion on the immune-inflammatory response. Hematol Transfus Cell Ther. 2021;**43**:58-64

[45] Bilgin YM, van de Watering LMG, Versteegh MIM, et al. Effects of allogeneic leukocytes in blood transfusions during cardiac surgery on inflammatory mediators and postoperative complications. Critical Care Medicine. 2010;**38**:546-552

[46] Ho J, Sibbald WJ, Chin-Yee IH. Effects of storage on efficacy of red cell transfusion: When is it safe? Critical Care Medicine. 2003;**31**:S687-S697

[47] Donadee C, Raat NJ, Kanias T, et al. Nitric oxide scavenging by red blood cell microparticles and cell-free haemoglobin as a mechanism for the red cell storage lesion. Circulation. 2011;**124**:465-476

[48] Baek JH, D'Aguillo F, Vallelian F, et al. Hemoglobin-driven pathophysiology is an in vivo consequence of the red blood cell storage lesion that can be attenuated in Guinea pigs by haptoglobin therapy. The Journal of Clinical Investigation. 2012;**122**:1444-1458

[49] Hod EA, Spitalnik SL. Stored red blood cell transfusions: Iron, inflammation, immunity, and infection. Transfusion Clinique et Biologique. 2012;**19**:84-89

[50] Stark MJ, Keir AK, Andersen CC. Does non-transferrin bound iron contribute to transfusion related immune-modulation in preterms? Archives of Disease in Childhood. Fetal and Neonatal Edition. 2013;**98**:F424-F429

[51] Yazdanbaksh K, Bao W, Zhong H. Immunoregulatory effects of stored red blood cells. Hematology. American Society of Hematology. Education Program. 2011;**2011**:466-469

[52] Straat M, Böing AN, Tuip-De Boer A, et al. Extracellular vesicles from red blood cell products induce a strong pro-inflammatory host response, dependent on both numbers and storage duration. Transfusion Medicine and Hemotherapy. 2016;**43**:302-305

[53] Koch GC, Li L, Sessler DI, Figueroa P, et al. Duration of red-cell storage and complications after cardiac surgery. New Engl J Med. 2008;**358**:1229-1239

[54] van de Watering L, Lorinser J, Versteegh M, et al. Effects of storage time of red blood cell transfusions on the prognosis of coronary artery bypass graft patients. Transfusion. 2006;**46**:1712-1718

[55] van Straten AH, Soliman Hamad MA, van Zundert AA, et al. Effect of duration of red blood cell storage on early and late mortality after coronary artery bypass grafting. The Journal of Thoracic and Cardiovascular Surgery. 2011;**141**:231-237

[56] van de Watering LM. Age of blood: Does older blood yield poorer outcomes? Current Opinion in Hematology. 2013;**20**:526-532

[57] Cooper DJ, McQuilten ZK, Nichol A, et al. Age of red cells for transfusion and outcomes in critically ill adults. The New England Journal of Medicine. 2017;**377**:1858-1867

[58] Lelubre C, Vincent JL. Relationship between red cell storage duration and outcomes in adults receiving red cell transfusions: A systematic review. Critical Care. 2013;**17**:R66

[59] Sadallah S, Schmeid L, Eken C, et al. Platelet-derived ectosomes reduce NK cell function. Journal of Immunology. 2016;**197**:1663-1671

[60] Keating FK, Butenas S, Fung MK, et al. Platelet-white blood cell (WBC) interaction, WBC apoptosis, and procoagulant activity in stored red blood cells. Transfusion. 2011;**51**:1086-1095

[61] Blumberg N, Gettings KF, Turner C, et al. An association of soluble CD40 ligand (CD154) with adverse reactions to platelet transfusions. Transfusion. 2006;**46**:1813-1821

[62] Silliman CC, Moore EE, Kelher MR, et al. Identification of lipids that accumulate during the routine storage of prestorage leukoreduced red blood cells and cause acute lung injury. Transfusion. 2011;**51**:2549-2554

[63] Silliman CC, Ambruso DR, Boshkov LK. Transfusion-related acute lung injury. Blood. 2005;**105**:2266-2273

[64] Goldman M, Webert KE, Arnold DM, et al. Proceedings of a consensus conference: Towards an understanding of TRALI. Transfusion Medicine Reviews. 2005;**19**:2-31

[65] Silliman CC, Paterson AJ, Dickey WO, et al. The association of biologically active lipids with the development of transfusion-related

acute lung injury: A retrospective study. Transfusion. 1997;**37**:719-726

[66] Spiess BD, Royston D, Levy JH, et al. Platelet transfusions during coronary artery bypass graft surgery are associated with serious adverse outcomes. Transfusion. 2004;**44**:1143-1148

[67] Bilgin YM, van de Watering LM, Versteegh MI, et al. Postoperative complications associated with transfusion of platelets and plasma in cardiac surgery. Transfusion. 2011;**51**:2603-2610

[68] Sreeram GM, Welsby IJ, Sharma AD, et al. Infectious complications after cardiac surgery: Lack of association with FFP or platelet transfusions. J Cardiothoracic Vasc Anesthesia. 2005;**19**:430-434

[69] Karkouti K, Wijeysundera DN, Yau TM, et al. Platelet transfusions are not associated with increased morbidity or mortality in cardiac surgery. Canadian Journal of Anesthesia. 2006;**53**:279-287

[70] McGrath T, Koch CG, Xu M, et al. Platelet transfusion in cardiac surgery does not confer increased risk for adverse morbid outcomes. The Annals of Thoracic Surgery. 2008;**86**:543-553

[71] Ranucci M, Pazzaglia A, Bianchini C, et al. Body size, gender, and transfusions as determinants of outcome after coronary operations. The Annals of Thoracic Surgery. 2008;**85**:481-486

[72] Banbury MK, Brizzio ME, Rajeswaran J, et al. Transfusion increases the risk of postoperative infection after cardiac surgery. Journal of the American College of Surgeons. 2006;**202**:131-138

[73] van Straten AH, Soliman Hamad MA, Martens EJ, et al. Effect of storage time of transfused plasma on early and late mortality after coronary artery bypass grafting. The Journal of Thoracic and Cardiovascular Surgery. 2011;**141**:238-243

[74] Khorana AA, Francis CW, Blumberg N, et al. Blood transfusions, thrombosis, and mortality in hospitalized patients with cancer. Archives of Internal Medicine. 2008;**168**:2377-2381

[75] Shohat N, Ludwick L, Goh GS, et al. Blood transfusions increase the risk for venous thromboembolism events following total joint arthroplasty. Scientific Reports. 2021;**11**:21240

[76] Marusic AP, Locatelli I, Mrhar A, et al. Influence of prescribed blood products on the incidence of deep vein thrombosis and pulmonary embolism in surgical patients. Clinical and Applied Thrombosis/Hemostasis. 2017;**23**:938-942

[77] Ghazi L, Schwann TA, Engoren MC, et al. Role of blood transfusion product type and amount in deep vein thrombosis after cardiac surgery. Thrombosis Research. 2015;**136**:1204-1210

[78] Tuinman PR, Vlaar AP, Cornet AD, et al. Blood transfusion during cardiac surgery is associated with inflammation and coagulation in the lung: A case control study. Critical Care. 2011;**15**:R59

[79] van Manen L, van Hezel ME, Boshuizen M, et al. Effect of red blood cell transfusion on inflammation, endothelial cell activation and coagulation in the critically ill. Vox Sanguinis. 2022;**117**:64-70

[80] Parolari A, Mussoni L, Frigerio M, et al. Increased prothrombotic state lasting as long as one month after on-pump and off-pump coronary surgery. The Journal of Thoracic

and Cardiovascular Surgery. 2005;**130**:303-308

[81] Levi M, Cromheecke ME, de Jonge E, et al. Pharmacological strategies to decrease excessive blood loss in cardiac surgery: A meta-analysis of clinically relevant endpoints. Lancet. 1999;**354**:1940-1947

[82] Gando S. Microvascular thrombosis and multiple organ dysfunction syndrome. Critical Care Medicine. 2010;**38**:S35-S42

[83] Levi M, Keller TT, van Gorp E, et al. Infection and inflammation and the coagulation system. Cardiovascular Research. 2003;**60**:23-29

Chapter 9

Personnel for Blood Transfusion Services in Nigeria: A Multicenter Cooperative Study

Abdulrahman Abdulbasit Opeyemi, Adesola Precious Oyeyemi and Adeyeye Kamaldeen

Abstract

The intravenous infusion of blood components into someone's circulation is known as a blood transfusion. For a variety of medical disorders, transfusions are performed to replenish lost blood components. In the past, whole blood was used for transfusions, but in modern medicine, just the blood's constituent parts—such as red blood cells, white blood cells, plasma, clotting factors, and platelets—are frequently employed. A typical blood service is a multidisciplinary system that requires a wide range of specialists. These people include medical scientists, and technical professionals as well as the nursing staff. Several elements, including the workplace environment, the availability of essentials like PPE, gloves, and water, the training of employees, and the formulation of policies, affect how effective a transfusion service is. To comprehend Personnel for Blood Transfusion Services in Nigeria: A multicentre cooperative study, the study reviews pertinent literature.

Keywords: blood, hemorrhage, transfusion, blood products, blood transfusion

1. Introduction

Richard Lower at Oxford carried out the first known animal-to-animal (a dog) blood transfusion in 1665, and Jean-Denis carried out the first known animal-to-human blood transfusion in 1667. James Blundell carried out the first human-to-human blood transfusion in 1818 [1, 2]. Ottenberg performed the first pre-transfusion cross-match in 1907 using Landsteiner's classification of the ABO blood grouping system, which was created in the year 1900. In the year 1940, Landsteiner and Wiener developed the Rh-type system. Following this, significant discoveries in the twentieth century enabled the use of component therapy, including the development of anticoagulant and preservative solutions, refrigeration, plastic blood bags, component delivery, infectious disease testing, high-risk donor screening, etc. [1, 2].

Since its beginning in the early twentieth century, transfusion medicine has advanced. Among these was the realization that blood can be separated into its parts and supplied individually [1, 2]. Nowadays, blood transfusions almost invariably involve the infusion of one or more blood products. Whole blood transfusions are now only performed in cases requiring intensive restoration (trauma). The most well-known cellular constituents are packed red blood cells (PRBC), washed PRBC, leuko-reduced PRBC, and pooled or aphaeresis platelets. Hemophilic factor (CRYO), FFP, and cryoprecipitate are examples of plasma-derived products [1, 2]. In perioperative and peripartum settings, the transfusion of red blood cells (RBCs), platelets, fresh frozen plasma (FFP), and cryoprecipitate has the potential to improve clinical outcomes.

Blood transfusions can save lives, but they can carry hazards, such as noninfectious and infectious consequences [3]. Despite significant advancements in blood safety since the 1980s, when it was revealed that HIV could be transmitted through blood transfusions, blood transfusions still carry a distinct risk of poor patient outcomes [1–4]. Blood transfusions have been linked to higher mortality rates, longer hospital stays due to infections and sepsis, and malfunction of several organ systems [4, 5]. In a recent meta-analysis of 19 prospective, randomized studies comparing restricted with liberal transfusions in more than 6000 patients, it was discovered that adherence to restrictive blood transfusion reduced hospital mortality and postoperative infections. These observed negative patient outcomes may be partially explained by erythrocyte damage related to the length of blood storage. Old blood may have a predisposition to hemolyze in vivo, producing vaso-constrictive cell-free hemoglobin, according to canine studies. Post-transfusion, patients also have lower erythrocyte membrane deformability that is correlated with blood storage time [4–6]. Finally, some people appear to limit the use of blood transfusions due to potential recognized and unknown hazards such as the spread of blood-borne viruses. Similar to the last example, transfusion is only necessary to enhance viscosity in extreme cases of hemodilution. Circulation may be hampered by high viscosity on its own. Additionally, the delivery or consumption of oxygen at the tissue level is not instantly increased by transfused blood [6, 7]. There are, therefore, few clinical circumstances in which a blood transfusion is advantageous to the patient and improves results. After assessing the advantages and disadvantages of blood transfusion, the decision to administer blood should be made [6, 7].

All medical professionals who deliver blood or blood-derived products must complete specialized training regarding safe transfusion techniques and have a comprehensive understanding of the transfusion administration procedure. Most commonly, people refer to them as Transfusion Personnel (TP). The phrase "Transfusion Personnel" or "Transfusion Practitioner" (TP) is a term used in the workplace to refer to a variety of positions, including those of transfusion nurse, transfusion instructor, transfusion health and safety committee, transfusion control officer, transfusion clinical nurse, and hemovigilance officer. The TP role has been in place for many years in some nations [7, 8], and more lately, additional nations are putting it into practice.

The majority of the TP activity is concentrated on patient blood management, transfusion governance, monitoring practice, adverse event management, and education (PBM). Very frequently, the TP serves as the informational hub, bringing together the available resources, studying the activities carried out by transfusion colleagues in other centers, gathering audit data, and assessing how these efforts might be advantageous within their healthcare facility [7, 8]. However, there is a need for all personnel involved in transfusion service to have a common goal and work together efficiently, this research will examine Personnel for Blood Transfusion Services in Nigeria: A multicentre cooperative Study.

2. Blood transfusion

The World Health Organization (WHO) recommends 10 units of blood per 1000 people, which means that in order to meet the demand for transfusions for an estimated 800 million people, 8 million units of blood are now required [7–9]. Blood transfusion is still a life-saving medication. While blood supply and blood safety are well recognized in developed countries, access to blood is extremely limited in Africa, and the availability of hazardous blood raises serious public health concerns about blood safety. A blood transfusion may be necessary in cases of obstetric hemorrhage, auto accidents, armed conflicts, sickle cell disease, anemia, particularly in youngsters, malnutrition, HIV, malaria, parasitic diseases, cases obstetric hemorrhage, auto accidents, violent conflicts, sickle cell disease, anemia, particularly in youngsters, malnutrition, HIV, malaria, and parasitic diseases, a blood transfusion may be necessary. Therefore, it is crucial to consistently draw attention to the reaction to blood transfusions, potential causes, anticipated symptoms and indicators, preventive measures, and suitable therapy [9, 10].

Intravenous infusion of blood components into a person's circulation is known as a blood transfusion [3, 11]. For a number of medical disorders, transfusions are performed to replenish lost blood products. Early transfusions used whole blood, but in contemporary medical practice, only blood components including red blood cells, white blood cells, plasma, clotting factors, and platelets are frequently employed. Hemoglobin is a component of red blood cells (RBC), which carry oxygen to the body's cells. White blood cells, which are a component of the immune system and combat infections, are not frequently employed during transfusion [10, 11].

Transfusion of blood employs either the donor's or the recipient's own (autologous transfusion) blood as a supply of blood (allogeneic or homologous transfusion). The second is significantly more typical than the first. Blood donation is the initial step in the process of using someone else's blood. Whole blood taken intravenously and combined with an anticoagulant is the most common type of blood donated. Donations are typically anonymous to the recipient in developed nations, but blood bank products are always individually traceable throughout the entire cycle of donation, testing, component separation, storage, and administration to the recipient [3, 4]. As a result, any suspected infection transfer or transfusion reaction can be managed and investigated. In less developed nations, the donor may occasionally be specifically sought out by or for the receiver, who is often a family member, and the donation takes place right before the transfusion. It is not known whether using an alcohol swab alone or in addition to the use of an antiseptic can lessen contamination of the donor's blood [10, 11].

Blood and blood products cannot be synthesized or kept in storage for an extended period of time, making blood transfusion services a vital component of healthcare services. Therefore, it is essential to control blood demand and availability properly to maintain a sufficient provision of safe blood [12]. Because sustaining a sufficient supply of safe blood is essential for many patients, the inability to manage blood inventory and the ensuing blood shortage is regarded as dangers to national and worldwide health security. If health officials do not take rapid corrective action, blood shortages cause the failure of blood transfusion services, which leads to the breakdown of the health system and health insecurity [11–15]. In addition to endangering public health, an imbalance between blood supply and demand is one of the biggest dangers to the stability of the national and global economies and security. The view of health concerns as a danger to global health security has advantages because it gets the support and attention of government and policy-makers. The management of blood supply and demand should be handled in accordance with international health rules and policies, which should be periodically updated [12, 16].

Replace the entirety of this text with the main body of your chapter. The body is where the author explains experiments and presents and interprets data of one's research. Authors are free to decide how the main body will be structured. However, you are required to have at least one heading. Please ensure that either British or American English is used consistently in your chapter.

2.1 Personnel for blood transfusion services in Nigeria: a multicentre cooperative study

A typical blood service is a multidisciplinary organization that employs a wide range of specialists. These people include laboratory scientists and technical professionals, as well as the nursing staff. The efficiency of the staff who are properly trained for the jobs they must do in the service determines the effectiveness of a blood service in addition to the availability of appropriate tools and other working materials in a supportive working environment. Different fundamental academic and professional requirements apply to each category of professionals, although blood handling and management skills are exclusive to this workforce and are necessary for all cadres. One of the elements that contribute to an effective and efficient blood service is the availability of facilities and mechanisms for pertinent training [17, 18].

Any health intervention approach needs organization and oversight to be successful, and both are essential when developing a blood safety infrastructure. In order to build a working blood transfusion service, there must be national cooperation, backing from the government, and policy that is tailored to the requirements of a specific nation. One size does not, however, suit all [18]: despite their geographic proximity, the regional nations frequently have wildly dissimilar resources and infrastructure, thus it is important to understand each environment and customize policy making to it. In contexts with limited resources, it is crucial to develop goals that take into account the nation's overall health issues as well as the logistics and cost. Although legislation can be used to enforce policy, it should not be utilized as a substitute for organized development [17, 18]. Liberal transfusion practice with poor standards is a result of prescribing physicians' lack of expertise and training. Similar to this, strict adherence to laboratory transfusion triggers rather than clinical anemia leads to needless blood supply depletion. Additionally, the transfusion service is usually fragmented, resulting in little connection between the blood center and the hospitals or prescribing physician, which makes it impossible to supervise transfusion practice [19].

The requirement for strong organizational support is reiterated in strategies addressing the policy. The ministry of health collaborated with international and nongovernmental organizations, such as WHO-African Region, who would be potential candidates to oversee this on a regional basis [19, 20]. Regional transfusion services with more advanced infrastructures can potentially take the lead and support their neighbors. For instance, the South African National Blood Service (SANBS) now conducts donation serology and Nucleic Acid Testing (NAT) laboratory testing for Namibia blood transfusion service. Utilizing transfusion committees prepared to track blood usage and audit practice in accordance with established logical principles, national frameworks must be disseminated at the hospital level. Staff members who hold dual appointments at the hospital and the blood center may also help to close the gap between the two institutions. Finally, the successful implementation of clinical recommendations depends on education and training [20, 21].

Currently, a large number of both private and public institutions in Nigeria operate hospital-based transfusion services to sustain the country's blood supply [20, 21]. In this case, each institution finds its own blood donors, checks them for TTIs, and then stores the units for use in clinical procedures. Blood units are frequently saved for intended recipients in hospital-based transfusion services [12, 16, 22], even if they might not need them until after their shelf life has passed. Due to this technique, there are more discarded blood products and few available blood products. Another significant drawback of decentralized hospital-based transfusion programs is the tendency for blood units to be "mal-distributed;" at one hospital, there may be an abundance with a propensity for waste due to expiration, while in a nearby hospital, there may be a severe shortage [20, 21, 23].

Effective blood usage is a part of rational blood use. Differential fractionation of whole blood into derived red cells, plasma, cryoprecipitate, and platelets—also known as component therapy—is a method to increase effectiveness [24]. In the developed world, when parent blood products can be varied, this is the predominant practice. In contrast, given the significant plasma portion that contains antibodies, entire blood must be transfused to a patient whose ABO type matches the donor. A group O unit of whole blood, for instance, must be given to group O receivers only until it has been determined that the recipient has a low antibody titer. Group O red cell components, however, can be safely given to any recipient. Additionally, the enormous amount of whole blood puts recipients at risk for circulatory overload brought on by transfusion. In the WHO study from 2006, only seven of the 46 nations had a national policy for the distribution of fractionated plasma products, and 24 of the 39 responding countries were still transfusing more than 75% of their blood as whole blood. The more recent assessment of 7 blood centers in Francophone, Africa [24] confirmed these findings.

Critical steps that must be taken to guarantee the safety of blood units include screening donor blood and quarantining blood and blood components. They should be released for clinical or manufacturing use, or they should be discarded, depending on the screening results. Blood samples taken at the time of donation should undergo laboratory testing for TTIs. All blood tests must be carried out and recorded using standardized protocols in laboratories that are fully equipped to do so [23–25].

TTI indicators (HIV antigen-antibody, HBsAg, anti-HCV, and syphilis) are regularly screened for in blood transfusion facilities at the same time [25, 26]. In order for the blood or blood components, particularly labile ones like platelets, to be discharged right away, screening time must be minimized. Reactive contributions are initially isolated and separated. The donor is then either disregarded or additional testing is done, depending on the technique the laboratory utilized. Sequential screening may be used in some labs by initially looking for one or two infection indicators. No additional testing is done on this donor if a reactive outcome is received. The prevalence of infections in the population of blood donors will have an impact on the screening approach for selecting the test or tests that are conducted first. In nations where the incidence of one TTI is higher than that of another, sequential screening may be used. For instance, HBsAg may be checked first when the prevalence of hepatitis B is higher than that of HIV and HCV [25–27]. Only HBsAg negative contributions would subsequently be subjected to syphilis, HIV antigen-antibody, and anti-HCV testing in this scenario. On donations that show a positive result on the HBsAg screening test, no assays for these viral markers would be run. There is hence a chance for cost reductions, particularly if donations that have already tested positive for HBsAg do not require the more expensive assays [25–27].

2.2 The need for laboratory staff in transfusion services

When performing the tests and assessing the data, laboratory staff should always follow the national screening approach, protocol, and standardized methods. The likelihood of analytical and transcribing errors, particularly false negative results, will be reduced when laboratory tests are conducted in a high-quality environment with knowledgeable employees and a functional documentation system [27]. Blood screening seeks to identify infection-related indicators in order to stop the distribution of contaminated blood and blood components for clinical use. Strategies for blood screening are intended to ensure the security of blood units; nevertheless, they should not be utilized to inform blood donors of reactive test findings. Before informing donors of their infectivity status, the proper confirmatory testing technique for blood donor management should be used. When deciding whether to release blood units for clinical use, all testing for infection indicators for TTIs and blood group serology should be considered.

In most cases, donors must consent to the procedure; as a result, minors cannot donate without the approval of a parent or legal guardian. In some nations, such as the United States, names are maintained in order to compile lists of ineligible donors, while in others, such as several European nations, only the donor's blood is associated with the responses to ensure anonymity. A potential donor is "delayed" if they do not meet these requirements. Due to the possibility of later approval for many ineligible donors, this word is utilized.

The following skills are anticipated of a competent Medical Laboratory Scientist in the field of blood transfusion services [12, 17]:

- In the blood transfusion laboratory, have a working knowledge of quality management systems (QMS), validation, and good management practices.
- Understanding the clinical significance of all blood group systems' serological features
- Mastery of all laboratory techniques for blood safety in terms of serology and microbiology
- Preparation and standardization of reagents used in blood transfusion procedures, such as antisera
- Proficiency in blood donation protocols, as well as in the handling, processing, and storage of blood and blood-related materials
- The resolution of unusual and negative situations, medical-legal concerns, and blood transfusion procedures.
- Using Electronic medical systems and being familiar with automation (BECS)
- understanding of the scientific techniques involved in hemopoietic stem cell transplantation and its immunology

With these skills in place, Nigerian medical laboratory scientists are trained to produce professionals who can work productively in the core laboratory functions of any blood service or hospital blood transfusion department.

2.3 Role of nurses in transfusion services

Nursing plays a significant part in ensuring transfusion safety since the nurse practitioner is responsible for understanding the indications for transfusions, double-checking data to prevent errors, educating patients on blood transfusion, identifying and responding appropriately to transfusion responses, and recording the procedure [27, 28]. Nursing's role is essential for the effective management of transfusion reactions to achieve the desired outcomes for two primary reasons: nurses are the final link in the chain of the transfusion process and nursing-related tasks dominate the transfusion process. As a result, nurses must possess sufficient skills and knowledge in the transfusion of blood and blood products [29].

As the nursing team is responsible for recognizing the indications for blood transfusion, examining data to prevent errors, disseminating information about blood transfusion, diagnosing transfusion responses, and documenting the processes, a nurse plays a critical role in ensuring blood transfusion safety [29, 30]. As a crucial process, blood transfusion requires knowledge and skilled specialists to preserve patient safety. The risk of blood transfusion is reduced by qualified and experienced nurses. There are four phases associated with nursing performance, including pre-transfusion preparation, pre-transfusion actions, blood bag collection, and post-transfusion activities to maintain the patient's safety. The preparation phase includes checking the written prescription of the physician [29, 30]. This gives sufficient details regarding the indications, risks, and advantages of blood transfusion. The second stage involves drawing blood from the blood bank, which is crucial for enhancing patient safety. In order to prevent blood incompatibility, the nurse must accurately match the patient's identification details on the blood bag and collection paper. Transporting blood from the blood bank to the ward should be done using a special blood carrier box. Two authorized individuals verified the blood's compatibility prior to transfusion. Checking the patient's vital signs is necessary. Since this is the final opportunity to introduce any unsuitable blood component, it is a very sensitive step in the safety of blood transfusions. Blood transfusion must begin slowly during post-transfusion activities during the first 15 min after it begins. The nurse should continue to monitor the patient to look for any reactions. While receiving a blood transfusion, it is advised to take normal saline intravenously and morphine at 1 mg/ml, but no more medication is permitted [30]. To save a patient's life, the nurse must be aware of any blood response signs and know how to treat them [31]. A handbook manual on blood transfusion services must be provided to nurses in order to continue their education in all healthcare institutions, and they must be continuously urged to attend national and worldwide blood transfusion workshops and conferences.

2.4 Establishing multicenter cooperative transfusion service

The community must get high-quality medical care through hospitals, which serve as the primary organization for the delivery of public services. In accordance with these provisions, there are four sections pertaining to hospitals' obligations in providing medical services, namely: Responsibility for employees: competent personnel must be hired through an open and transparent hiring process, professional responsibility for quality: Professional bodies are always required to set up ongoing training programs for their members in blood transfusion services in order to comply with international best practices, responsibility for facilities and equipment; appropriate financing should be available to supply the tools and supplies that medical professionals, particularly those working in blood transfusion units, need; and Last but not least, the hospital is responsible for the building's safety and upkeep [32–34]. This includes making sure that both patients and staff are safe inside the institution. Therefore, blood transfusion services must be safe for the patient, and the patient must be protected against the risk of developing an infectious disease through blood transfusion and even death.

Toward this shared objective, medical practitioners must collaborate. Every important participant in the transfusion chain must, therefore, share a shared objective. Healthcare facilities in Nigeria should make every attempt to keep everyone's values and presumptions in mind as it may affect interactions with team members who are other professionals. Regardless of the talents and limitations of various team members, effective teamwork contributes to the provision of high-caliber and safe healthcare [33, 34]. Hospitals must create a blood transfusion committee that meets regularly to examine the current transfusion strategy, and best practices, compile a transfusion manual and handbook, as well as to take training sessions to stay informed about the current state of transfusion services [34].

3. Conclusions

In Nigeria, health professionals who provide transfusion-dependent patients' care have a real and compelling responsibility to uphold their end of the bargain when it comes to being held accountable for the human, financial, clinical, and other resources involved in managing blood donations. All parties involved—from patients to laboratory scientists, physicians, blood collectors, and distributors—must collaborate if they are to use these priceless donations of human blood with judiciousness and excellence.

Acknowledgements

All glory to the Almighty for making it possible to write this paper. Likewise, I thank my mentors whose guidance and constructive criticism yielded this write-up in the person of Professor A.O Hassan, Professor Abubakar, A.A., Dr. Adeniyi T.D., and Mr. Ismail A. The contributory effort of Mr. Abdulkareem Aliyu is well appreciated and we say special thanks to all of you. We will also like to note that this review receives no funding.

Notes/thanks/other declarations

Special thanks to the publisher and editor of this journal for finding it worthy to place this review in their reputable journal.

DOI: http://dx.doi.org/10.5772/intechopen.107301

Author details

Abdulrahman Abdulbasit Opeyemi*, Adesola Precious Oyeyemi
and Adeyeye Kamaldeen
Department of Medical Laboratory Science, Achievers University, Owo, Ondo State, Nigeria

*Address all correspondence to: aabdulbasit5@gmail.com

References

[1] Karim S, Hoque E, Hoque M, Rahman SM, Islam K. Blood component therapy. Anwer Khan Modern Medical College Journals. 2018;**9**(2):142-147. DOI: 10.3329/akmmcj.v9i2.39211

[2] Poterjoy BS, Josephson CD. Platelets, frozen plasma, and cryoprecipitate: What is the clinical evidence for their use in the neonatal intensive care unit? Seminars in Perinatology. 2009;**33**(1):66-74. DOI: 10.1053/j.semperi.2008.10.004

[3] Lacroix J, Hébert PC, Hutchison JS, TRIPICU Investigators. Canadian critical care trials group; Pediatric acute lung injury and Sepsis investigators network. Transfusion strategies for patients in pediatric intensive care units. New England Journal of Medicine. 2007;**356**(16):1609-1619. DOI: 10.1056/NEJMoa066240

[4] Isbister JP, Shander A, Spah DR, Erhard J, Farmer SL, Hofmann A. Adverse blood transfusion outcomes: Establishing causation. Transfusion Medicine Reviews. 2011;**25**:89-101. DOI: 10.1016/j.tmrv.2010.11.001

[5] Musallam KM, Tamim HM, Richards T. Preoperative anaemia and postoperative outcomes in non-cardiac surgery: A retrospective cohort study. Lancet. 2011;**378**:1396-1407. DOI: 10.1016/S0140-6736(11)61381-0

[6] Frank SM, Abazyan B, Ono M. Decreased erythrocyte deformability after transfusion and the effects of erythrocyte storage duration. Anesthesia and Analgesia Journal. 2013;**116**:975-981. DOI: 10.1213/ANE.0b013e31828843e6

[7] Yaddanapudi S, Yaddanapudi L. Indications for blood and blood product transfusion. Indian Journal of Anaesthesia. 2014;**58**(5):538-542. DOI: 10.4103/0019-5049.144648

[8] WHO. Global Database on Blood Safety. Geneva: World Health Organization; 2015

[9] Olaniyi JA. Blood transfusion reactions. In: Tombak A, editor. Blood Groups. London: IntechOpen; 2019

[10] Land KJ, Townsend M, Goldman M, Whitaker BI, Perez GE, Wiersum-Osselton JC. International validation of harmonized definitions for complications of blood donations. Transfusion. 2018;**58**(11):2589-2595. DOI: 10.1111/trf.14948

[11] Adjepong KO, Otegbeye F, Adjepong YA. Perioperative management of sickle cell disease. Mediterrian Journal of Hematology and Infectious Disease. 2018;**1**(10):e20

[12] Yahia AI. Management of blood supply and demand during the COVID19 pandemic in king Abdullah Hospital, Bisha, Saudi Arabia. Transfusion and Apheresis Science. 2020;**4**:102836

[13] Siddon AJ, Kenney BC, Hendrickson JE, Tormey CA. Delayed haemolytic and serologic transfusion reactions: Pathophysiology, treatment and prevention. Current Opinion in Hematology. 2018;**25**(6):459-467. DOI: 10.1097/MOH.0000000000000462

[14] Carson JL, Stanworth SJ, Roubinian N, Fergusson DA, Triulzi D, Doree C, et al. Transfusion thresholds and other strategies for guiding allogeneic red blood cell transfusion. Cochrane Database of Systematic Reviews. 2016;**12**(10):CD002

[15] Webster J, Bell-Syer SE, Foxlee R. Skin preparation with alcohol versus alcohol followed by any antiseptic for preventing bacteraemia or contamination of blood for transfusion. Cochrane Database of Systematic Reviews. 2015;**12**(2):CD007

[16] Yahia AIO. Management of blood supply and blood demand to ensure international health security. In: Stawicki SP, Papadimos TJ, Galwankar SC, Miller AC, Firstenberg MS, editors. Contemporary Developments and Perspectives in International Health Security. London: IntechOpen; 2021

[17] Medical Laboratory Science Council of Nigeria (MLSCN). New curriculum for training programme. 2013. https://web.mlscn.gov.ng/index.php/mdocs-posts/mlscn-act/

[18] Shander A, Goodnough LT. Objectives and limitations of bloodless medical care. Current Opinion in Hematology. 2006;**13**(6):462-470. DOI: 10.1097/01.moh.0000245692.32085.bd

[19] W.H.O. Blood transfusion safety—Safe and appropriate use. 2010. https://www.who.int/health-topics/blood-transfusion-safety#tab=tab_1

[20] Allain JP, Sarkodie F, Boateng P, Asenso K, Kyeremateng E, Owusu-Ofori S. A pool of repeat blood donors can be generated with little expense to the blood center in sub-Saharan Africa. Transfusion. 2008;**48**(4):735-741

[21] Barro L, Drew VJ, Poda GG, Tagny CT, El-Ekiaby M, Owusu-Ofori S, et al. Blood transfusion in sub-Saharan Africa: Understanding the missing gap and responding to present and future challenges. Vox Sanguinis. 2018;**113**(8):726-736. DOI: 10.1111/vox.12705

[22] Chand NK, Subramanya HB, Rao GV. Management of patients who refuse blood transfusion. Indian Journal of Anaesthesia. 2014;**58**(5):658-664

[23] Bates I, Hassall O, Mapako T. Transfusion research priorities for blood services in sub-Saharan Africa. British Journal of Haematology. 2017;**177**(6):855-863. DOI: 10.1111/bjh.14577

[24] Bloch EM, Vermeulen M, Murphy E. Blood transfusion safety in Africa: A literature review of infectious disease and organizational challenges. Transfusion Medicine Reviews. 2012;**26**(2):164-180. DOI: 10.1016/j.tmrv.2011.07.006

[25] WHO. Global Database on Blood Safety, World Health Organization. Geneva; 2008

[26] Roback JD. CMV and blood transfusions. Review in Medical Virology. 2002;**12**(4):211-219. DOI: 10.1002/rmv.353

[27] Obeagu E. Safe blood transfusion through proper donor screening correspondence to. 2019;**6**:01-07

[28] Tavares JL, Barichello E, De Mattia AL, Barbosa MH. Factors associated with knowledge of the nursing staff at a teaching hospital on blood transfusion. Revista Latino America Enfermagem. 2015;**23**(4):595-602. DOI: 10.1590/0104-1169.0024.2593

[29] Bediako AA, Ofosu-Poku R, Druye AA. Safe blood transfusion practices among nurses in a major referral center in Ghana. Advances in Hematology. 2021;**2021**:13

[30] Haseena M, Kousar P, Muhammad H, Muhammad A, Sayed AG. Assessment of Nurses' practices regarding blood transfusion. Merit Research Journal

of Medicine and Medical Sciences. 2020;**8**(8):396-402

[31] Elhy AHA, Kasemy ZAAJ. Nurses' Knowledge Assessment Regarding Blood Transfusion to Ensure Patient Safety2011. pp. 104-111. DOI: 10.9790/1959-060202104111

[32] Kusumaningrum A. Hospital responsibilities in blood transfusion services as a patient protection. Advances in Economics, Business and Management Research. 2021;**14**:34-38

[33] Katib IK. Quality management in the Nigerian health system; A case study of Isalu hospital limited, Ogba Lagos. International journal of economic development Research and investment. 2011;**2**(1):161-169

[34] Muhammed SSA, Bahia GA, Magda AA, Mamdou MA. Nurses performance regarding care of patients undergoing blood transfusion. Port Said Scientific Journal of Nursing. 2015;**3**(2):1-13. DOI: 10.21608/pssjn.2016.32525